Physical Assessment Skills for Nursing Practice

Physical Assessment Skills for Nursing Practice

Second Edition

EDITED BY

Josephine M. Sana, R.N., M.A.
Professor of Nursing, The University of Michigan
School of Nursing, Ann Arbor

Richard D. Judge, M.D.
Clinical Professor of Internal Medicine
The University of Michigan Medical School, Ann Arbor

Little, Brown and Company, Boston

Preface

Reader recommendations have guided the revisions incorporated into this second edition. We appreciate the reactions to our first edition and hope that our revisions will enhance this text's usefulness.

The illustrations have been expanded greatly both in number and in detail to facilitate reader comprehension. We are indebted to Professor Gerald P. Hodge, Director, Medical and Biological Illustration Unit of The University of Michigan, Associate Professor Lou Sadler, and their staff artists for their help in planning and preparing the new illustrations.

The sectioned format has been maintained to serve the varying reference needs of clinicians and students.

The nursing framework perspective, fundamental to clinical applications of the assessment process presented in Sections II and III in the first edition, has been retained in Section I. New material related to the very crucial quality assurance component in nursing has been added to Chapter 3.

All chapters have been reviewed and modified as contributing authors and editors considered necessary in light of changing knowledge and practice needs.

References and suggested reading lists have been updated. Our central focus remains, as before, to provide a nursing context for the physical assessment process with sufficient detail for application by the nurse or student in different clinical settings. A new feature has been added to serve as a quick reference source: major considerations are briefly outlined at the end of most chapters in Sections II and III and pocket-sized cue cards carrying the same information also appear in a pocket at the back of the book. We hope that they will be useful ready reference guides.

The secretarial assistance of Ms. Bernice Gittens deserves mention, and we are especially grateful for the invaluable counsel and assistance of Ann West, Nursing Developmental Editor, Little, Brown and Company.

J.M.S.
R.D.J.

Contents

Contributing Authors

Suzanne Brunner, R.N., M.S.
Clinical Nurse Specialist, Pediatric Nursing, C.S. Mott Children's Hospital and University Hospital, The University of Michigan, Ann Arbor

Candace M. Burns, R.N., Ph.D.
Associate Professor and Assistant Dean, University of Florida College of Nursing, Tampa

Patricia Mitchell Butler, R.N., M.S.
Assistant Professor of Nursing, The University of Michigan School of Nursing, Ann Arbor

Joyce Crane, R.N., M.S.N.
Professor of Nursing, University of Oregon Health Sciences Center, Portland

Jo Waylan Denton, R.N., M.S.
Supervisor, Health Care Services, Home Health and Counseling Services, Inc., Castro Valley, California

Carol Gilbert, R.N., M.S.N., Ph.D.
Associate Professor, Hunter College, Hunter-Bellevue School of Nursing, New York

Marjorie M. Jackson, R.N., M.S.
Associate Professor of Nursing, The University of Michigan School of Nursing, Ann Arbor

Judy M. Judd, R.N., M.A.
Professor of Parent-Child Nursing, The University of Michigan School of Nursing, Ann Arbor

Phyllis M. Coindreau Patterson, R.N., M.S.
Assistant Professor of Nursing, The University of Michigan School of Nursing, and Clinical Nurse Specialist, University Hospital, Ann Arbor

Susan Mengel Pinney, R.N., M.S.
Formerly Assistant Professor of Nursing, University of Cincinnati College of Nursing and Health, Cincinnati

Barbara A. Sachs, R.N., Ph.D.
Associate Professor of Nursing, Wayne State University College of Nursing, Ann Arbor

Josephine M. Sana, R.N., M.A.
Professor of Nursing, The University of Michigan School of Nursing, Ann Arbor

Samuel Schultz II, Ph.D.
Professor of Nursing and Director, Computing Laboratory, The University of Michigan School of Nursing, Ann Arbor

Linda K. Tanner Strodtman, R.N., M.S.
Clinical Nurse Specialist, Endocrinology and Metabolism, University Hospital, The University of Michigan, Ann Arbor

Margie J. Van Meter, R.N., M.S.
Coordinator, Nursing Quality Assurance Program, University Hospital, The University of Michigan, Ann Arbor

I. Physical Assessment Perspectives

1. Expanded Nursing Practice

A popular phrase in nursing parlance today is the "expanded role of the nurse." Ever so quickly, like a burst of Chinese firecrackers, the phrase has caught the fancy of the nursing profession. In haste, it has been rejected or endorsed in its embryonic stage without being seriously studied, completely understood, and fully tested in practice. *Expanded role* is a term that means whatever the user wishes it to mean. It is used interchangeably with "extended role" or to characterize a variety of new nursing roles: nurse practitioner, nurse clinician, or clinical nurse specialist. A selective use of the term emphasizes changing role and function; a wider and richer perspective focuses on changing nursing practice. The position presented here is that true expansion of nursing practice will be achieved when nurses assume greater responsibility and accountability for patient cure and restoration in acute, chronic, and preventive health care settings.

Expanded role has had its roots in the management concept of job enlargement, which grew out of an orientation toward and concern for the development of human resources in organizations. The enlargement concept includes a triad: (1) variety of knowledge and skills in doing a job; (2) a better utilization of the worker's total skills and abilities; and (3) responsibility and freedom in the performance of the job. True job enlargement is not the addition of the same kinds of tasks, but an expansion of job content with a wider variety of tasks and an increased freedom of methods.

EXTENDED ROLE VERSUS EXPANDED ROLE

Murphy [7] provides an important conceptual distinction between the job enlargement of the nurse who is a role extender and the nurse who is a role expander. She describes role extension as a unilateral lengthening, an additive process, and role expansion as a spreading out, a process of diffusion. With expansion, by definition, there is a richer mix both in the variety of tasks and in the new relationships among the tasks. The very nature of nursing practice is dynamically changed. With extension, by definition, there is continued addition of similar tasks and techniques, so that the nature of nursing practice is essentially unchanged. Nurses have always been in an extended role for, like it or not, a substantial portion of clinical nursing practice has and continues primarily to be inherited medical practice. Many of the major clinical functions in nursing are predominantly medical orders translated into action. This is strikingly evident in hospitals, which constitute the professional center of the health care world. Historically, nurses have been the physicians' assistants, implementing medical regimens and applying medical technology. The current controversy about roles and role alignments was ignited by the advent of a new breed, the physician's assistant, and is significantly influenced by the women's liberation movement's emphasis on equity and autonomy. This controversy revolves around the scope of nursing practice as distinct from medical practice.

THE NATURE OF NURSING PRACTICE

Definitions of nursing abound, and while there is no consensus, there is consistent recognition of its nature as human service and assistance. The primary goal of nursing is to assist persons to attain and maintain optimal physical, psychologic, and social functioning. The assistance ranges along the entire health-illness continuum from birth to death and is offered in a variety of health care settings, including the home. This helping role of nursing encompasses both instrumental and expressive functions. These evolve from the needs of patients and from the needs of medical practice and of the medical practitioner. The persistent dilemma of nursing is the proper marriage of instrumental and expressive functions, and this conflict is intensified by the acceleration in the technology of therapy and the escalating demand for health care.

To care and comfort is said to be the special province of the nurse. To cure and restore is said to be the special province of the physician. Murphy has superimposed the extender-expander role concepts on this cure-care model in terms of physician-nurse responsibilities. When viewed in Murphy's juxtaposition, the nurse who takes on primarily the cure functions of medicine becomes an extender of cure, while the nurse who undertakes the care function becomes an expander of care. Yet does it not distort the reality of the bedside, of the neighborhood clinic, or of the family the public health nurse assists to distinguish care and comfort from treatment and cure? To say that cure is a secondary function of the nurse is to ignore the paradoxes that often occur at times when nurses find it impossible to secure patient comfort and preserve personal integrity because they are responsible for the very procedures that produce the discomfort or demean the patient's personal dignity.

Compounding these dilemmas is the growing complexity in the delivery of health services. Kelly [6] contends that the nurse's clinical role is shrinking and dwindling to coordinator and traffic director as more and more of the tasks central to patient care are reallocated to others: the clinical pharmacist, the inhalation therapist, the IV team. She comments that "The role is shrinking because the nurse is incapable of controlling the care situation or exerting instrumental influence over her work."

Not only is the content of nursing practice changing daily, but the emphasis and the context of practice are also rapidly shifting. Social forces and education are orienting the modern nurse to health rather than illness, to prevention rather than crises, to a holistic rather than a technical approach, to the community rather than the hospital. The National Commission for the Study of Nursing and Nursing Education [8] and the Department of Health, Education, and Welfare [3] document the urgent need for a refocusing and redefinition of roles and practice. Both these reports underline the complementary roles of physician and nurse in a new professional realignment in the vast area of primary health care and in acute and chronic health care settings. It is beyond the province of this chapter to consider the urgent issues of role and function raised by these reports, but the reports are commended as essential resources.

The development of congruent roles of the physician and the nurse can resolve many current functional and jurisdictional disputes in scope of practice. Only through mutual understanding and agreement will a synthesis occur in the two divergent perceptions about nurses' roles, i.e., the nurse as a caretaker or the nurse as an assistant to the overburdened physician.

CLINICAL DECISION-MAKING

Basic to the expansion of practice and central to the complementary roles of nurse and physician is clinical decision-making. Cleland [1] has defined the role extender and role expander in terms of decision-making and has identified the number and quality of cues each uses in clinical judgment. On the basis of the range of cues brought to bear in clinical judgments, Cleland has postulated that critical distinctions can be made between levels of practice and among roles. She states:

At the first level of nursing there are general nurses and nurse practitioners, at the second level there are nurse specialists and nurse clinicians. General nurses and nurse specialists work in structured and defined settings, and with narrow ranges of cues involved in the decision-making and with the dimension of time extending through the patient's current hospitalization, and often extending only through the current 8 hour day. Nurse practitioners and nurse clinicians utilize data gathered from many sources to plan a broad program of patient care with a space focus which also involves the family, and a time dimension which includes the entire course of the illness [1].

Within Cleland's important framework, the crucial question is no longer whether or not the best direction in which to expand the practice of nursing is toward the assumption of more of the tasks of medicine. Rather, the crucial question is how the nurse and physician may become a decision-making team in the diagnostic and therapeutic problems of clinical care. Despite the performance of the nurse as a diagnostician and therapist in the past decade of coronary care and, more recently, in respiratory care, physicians and some nurses have been reluctant to see the nurse as a diagnostician. My use of *team* and *diagnosis* here recognizes that insofar as accuracy and validity of clinical observations and scope and continuity of management are relevant to diagnosis and treatment, and insofar as the nurse accurately validates observations and adds scope and continuity in management, the nurse and physician are interdependent, responsible, and authoritative. They are both clinicians in assessing the clinical variables at the bedside, in the clinic, or in the home and in making clinical judgments about the therapeutic management of patient care. Imperative in the concept of role expansion based on clinical decision-making is the acknowledgment that the nurse in expanded practice prescribes nursing care as independently as the medical clinician prescribes medical therapy. The fundamental strategies for this expansion must be derived from direct clinical experience with patients and from enhanced competencies in the methods and techniques of precise and objective clinical assessment.

Defining expanding nursing practice as expansion in the scope and methodologies of clinical decision-making turns our attention to the complexities of clinical judgments. How does the nurse acquire the clinical evidence to support her clinical judgments? One of the reasons for the selective ignorance practiced by nurses in restricting their clinical judgments has been the failure to distinguish between the different types of observational data and to understand the rigor of the reasoning processes that characterize the total diagnostic procedure. Feinstein [4] has examined the nature of clinical judgments and has identified the kinds of clinical data and relationships among them that constitute the intellectual technology of decision-making. There are data that describe disease in impersonal terms (morphologic, clinical, microbiologic, and physiologic), data that describe the host in whom disease occurs, and data that describe the interaction between the disease and its host. Feinstein has proposed that the first be referred to as the evaluation of the disease, the second as evaluation of the patient as a person, and the last, as the evaluation of illness, i.e., the consequences of pathologic processes in the patient.

Nurses tend to make gestalt observations and inferences and also to couch their observations and judgments in guarded and tentative language. "A good day," "usual night," "seems anxious" typify the all too familiar subjective and unsubstantiated documentation of patient response. The ability to make objective and measurable observations and to process them through systematic reasoning distinguishes the nurse in expanded practice. In processing clinical information and in making clinical decisions, important distinctions must be made between pure description, designation, and diagnosis. Feinstein [4] defines description as an account of an observed sensation, substance, or phenomenon. In designation, a name or classification is given to the observed entity. In diagnosis, the anatomic or other abnormality that is responsible for the observed entity is indicated.

The Nature of Clinical Judgment

Within Feinstein's perspective, the clinician makes two types of decisions: explanatory decisions and management decisions. Explanatory decisions are the name, mechanisms, and causes of disease or disability. Management decisions are therapeutic and environmental: the choosing and evaluating of the modes and technology of therapy, and the environmental strategies that enable the patient to adapt to the burdens of ailment and treatment. Feinstein [5] says the following about managerial decisions:

Physicians have developed a splendid clinical science for explanatory decision, mechanisms of disease, etiology and pathogenetic inquiry decisions, and a magnificent technologic armamentarium of therapy, but our managerial decisions generally continue to be made as doctrinaire dogmas immersed in dissension and doubt.

As these conflicting decisions in therapeutic management inevitably merge when nurses implement medical therapy, nursing has a significant opportunity to develop and enrich the clinical decision base of expanded practice. Nursing can and does contribute to the orderly evaluation of therapy and to the management decisions about the clinical and environmental variables observed in therapy. Donabedian [2] notes that a cursory review of the nursing literature suggests that nurses are much more systematic and self-conscious than physicians in developing quality criteria of patient care. "In contrast to studies of physician care that focus on purely technical performance, there is also greater attention to social and psychological aspects of patient management."

Increasingly utilized, Lawrence Weed's [10] approach to patient record-keeping, in which medical and nursing observations and plans of care are integrated, illustrates only one methodology, but an important one, for making conjoint diagnostic and therapeutic decisions operational. For 20 years, nursing education has emphasized the problem-solving approach in nursing care, but its effectiveness has been limited by the traditional medical record and the reliance of both physicians and nurses on spoken communication. The precise skills called for in a problem-oriented system of care are specifically those required for expanded clinical judgments.

Let me amplify my definition of expanded practice. Expanded practice within a framework of patient problems and solutions demands increased skill in clinical description, in reporting observations in objective terms, in designation of observed entities, and the development of explanatory and managerial decisions that result in significant patient care outcomes. I mean, significant in that the patient and his family know they have benefited from nursing care as well as medical care. Rather than describe isolated symptoms or signs, or isolated behavior on the part of the patient, the nurse in the expanded perspective designates the patient's functional and clinical status, such as ability to walk, feed himself, maintain excretory continence, participate in activities of daily living, comply with therapeutic regimens, work at a chosen occupation, and make intellectual decisions. The severity of a symptom is indicated by an account of its concomitant effect on the patient's total function.

Even more important than developing skills in accumulating the quantitative and qualitative data base for clinical judgment is the ability to make managerial decisions, i.e., to plan and carry out care in environmental and therapeutic decisions such as how the mode and agent of therapy should be managed or modified for this particular patient in his particular situation. In addition to analyzing historical and current information about a patient's functional status, the ability to predict future clinical or environmental events becomes a necessary and new skill in expanded practice. Therefore, anticipation and forecasting based on knowledge of the natural history of health and illness, growth and development, and the aging process, as well as on understanding ethnic and cultural variations, becomes part of expanded clinical judgment.

PHYSICAL ASSESSMENT SKILLS

At nursing's present stage of development, it is difficult for nurses themselves, and for physicians, to accept the ultimate imperative of the concept of expanded nursing practice. The new focus demands a new order of interdependence and temporary dependence on physicians while the nurse learns (1) how to use diagnostic tools and reasoning and (2) the therapeutic measures to function in the decisions of cure and restoration. The dependence on the physician occurs as the nurse masters the techniques of physical examination, interview, inspection, palpation, percussion, and auscultation. The nurse moving into expanded practice needs instruction, verification, and confirmation from the physician until he or she appreciates the wide range of normal, understands the significance of negative data, and develops the ability to characterize symptoms specifically by the seven dimensions of bodily location, quality, quantity, chronology, setting, aggravating and alleviating factors, and associated manifestations. When problems of testing reliability of clinical observation and standardization of physical assessment performance are resolved, the nurse can move from dependence to interdependence in physical assessment skills.

THE NURSING PROCESS

Two challenges confront the nurse in gaining competence and mastery in expanded practice. The first challenge, the development of sound clinical judgment based on objective clinical evidence, has been discussed; the second resides in the ability to optimize the nursing process as a vehicle for expanded practice. The challenge is to transcend definitions that confine the nursing process to interpersonal or communication models. The nursing process is all these, but more. The nursing process is diagnostic and therapeutic clinical decision-making, resulting in clinical judgments that explain clinical evidence and delineate the plan and management of treatment and care.

The current debate over issues of role and function, that is, the distinction between medical and nursing practice, power, and authority, is not addressed here. The thesis here is that true expansion in nursing practice occurs within the legal definition of nursing through validated clinical judgment and in the management of therapy. The nurse as clinician does not trespass into the licensed precincts of medicine. Rather, the heretofore supporting role becomes a complementary relationship consistent with the concept of the nurse "carrying out treatment and medications prescribed by the licensed physicians" and "rendering care consistent with clinical orientation, training, and experience [9]."

Meaningful expansion of nursing practice in any health-care setting is rooted in a common focus: decision-making in patient cure and care. Expanded practice demands a critical concern with clinical judgment—the ways in which decisions are made, alternative decisions are proposed, and the consequences of decisions are examined and weighed in the balance of therapeutic accomplishment and human benefit.

REFERENCES

1. Cleland, V. *Nurse Clinicians and Nurse Specialists: An Overview*, In *Three Challenges to the Nursing Profession—Selected Papers from the 1972 ANA Convention*. New York: American Nurses Association, 1972.
2. Donabedian, A. Part II. Some issues in evaluating the quality of nursing care. *Am. J. Public Health* 59:1834, 1969.
3. Extending the Scope of Nursing Practice, a Report of the Secretary's Committee to Study Extended Roles for Nurses. Washington, D.C.: Department of Health, Education, and Welfare. November 1972, p. 22.
4. Feinstein, A. R. *Clinical Judgment*. Baltimore: Williams & Wilkins, 1967.
5. Feinstein, A. R. What kind of basic science for clinical medicine? *N. Engl. J. Med.* 283:849, 1970.
6. Kelly, N. S. The nurse's role: Is it expanding or shrinking? *Nurs. Outlook* 21:236, 1973.
7. Murphy, J. Role expansion and role extension: Some conceptual differences. *Nurs. Forum* 9:380, 1970.
8. National Commission for the Study of Nursing and Nursing Education. *An Abstract for Action*. New York: McGraw-Hill, 1970.
9. *Regan Report on Nursing Law* (vol. 14, No. 1) Providence, R.I.: Medical Press, 1973.
10. Weed, L. L. Medical records that guide and teach. *N. Engl. J. Med.* 278:593, 1968.

SUGGESTED READINGS

Barnoon, S. *Measuring the Effectiveness of Medical Decisions*. Springfield, Ill.: Thomas, 1972.

Elstein, A. S., Shulman, L. S., and Sprafka, S. A. *Medical Problem Solving: An Analysis of Clinical Reasoning*. Cambridge: Harvard University Press, 1978.

Janis, I. L., and Mann, L. *Decision Making*. New York: Free Press Publishing Co., Macmillan, 1977.

2. Physical Assessment: An Aspect of the Nursing Assessment

MORE than a decade has passed since the concept of nursing by assessment was introduced by McCain [9]. While considered innovative in 1965, systematic nursing assessment is widely recognized and implemented today as a vital, integral part of the nursing process. Few would deny that systematic assessment is essential to the practice of professional nursing; that nursing is, in fact, a problem-solving process that incorporates assessment in its modus operandi. This is certainly a basic tenent in the development of new nursing roles. Yet, as nursing practice continues to expand, there is considerable discussion and debate about the depth and scope of the assessment process appropriate to nursing practice. Does expanding nursing practice dictate the need for expanded assessment skills? To what extent should physical assessment be incorporated into the nursing role? What are the skills needed by the nurse who is engaged in physical assessment activities? How do these skills relate to others required for systematic nursing assessment? Such questions must be contemplated and answered by those teaching and learning assessment skills, as well as by those who employ and collaborate with this "new breed" of nurse.

WHY PHYSICAL ASSESSMENT SKILLS FOR NURSES?

Increasing numbers of nurses are learning physical assessment skills today—not only those who are preparing for nurse practitioner roles, but also students enrolled in undergraduate and graduate nursing programs, the faculties in these programs, and nurses already practicing in a variety of roles and settings. With increasing regularity, nursing literature is emphasizing physical assessment. In its broadest context, the literature suggests that physical assessment skills serve to enrich the data base from which nursing judgments are made and therefore belong in the repertoire of practicing nurses. Some authors, however, caution against placing disproportionate value on physical assessment skills themselves [8].

Physical assessment skills are not new to nursing. Certainly, nurses working in intensive care areas have relied on physical assessment methods to monitor alterations in patients' conditions and determine the need for nurse or physician intervention. Similarly, these skills have been utilized by nurses in a variety of other settings and, to a limited extent, have been a component of the nursing assessment from its inception. There is little question, however, that the trend toward expanding nursing practice has accentuated the need for expanded nursing skills for nurses in general, and particularly for those already engaged in physical assessment. Lynaugh and Bates [8] highlight several uses of these skills in nursing practice:

To confirm hypotheses growing out of the assessment interview;

To enhance the investigation of nursing problems;

To increase the nurse's capacity for decision-making;

To enable nursing management of a greater range of patient care problems.

Physical assessment skills are requisite to functions inherent in the nurse's expanded role, such as entering people into the health care system on the basis of an assessment of health status; referral to other health care professionals; monitoring the patient's condition to detect changes or trends in his health-illness status; assessing functional abilities and assisting the patient in making necessary adaptations in his life-style; and making independent and interdependent judgments about patient care management.

To the extent that nurses use these skills to make more reasoned nursing judgments, there is justification for their inclusion within expanding nursing practice. Physical assessment skills have rational uses for nurses if they are incorporated within the context of nursing and are not used primarily to substitute for the physician's role in physical diagnosis.

PHYSICAL ASSESSMENT: AN INTEGRAL PART OF SYSTEMATIC NURSING ASSESSMENT

Systematic nursing assessment is a deliberate, problem-solving process comprising the diagnostic component of the nursing process and serving as the essential first step to its other three components: planning, implementing, and evaluating patient care. McCain [9] has defined nursing assessment as an orderly and precise collection of data about the physiologic, psychologic, and social behavior (or functional abilities) of a patient. Activities inherent in this process are those of analysis and synthesis. Analysis involves the classification of and distinction between differences in data, whereas synthesis includes establishing relationships among data, deriving trends, and performing deductive and inductive analysis [3, 11]. The assessment process, with its subprocesses of data collection, analysis, and synthesis, culminates in the identification of functional disabilities that require nursing therapy as well as recognition of the patient's most significant functional abilities. This assessment process begins as soon as possible after the patient is admitted to the agency or on an initial home visit and continues as the nurse assesses and evaluates on an ongoing basis, modifying the plan of care as the patient's behavior or functional abilities change.

The process of systematic assessment places all of nursing practice on a consciously planned, problem-solving basis. In addition, it:

1. Provides a format that ensures consistency in data collection.
2. Individualizes nursing care.
3. Maximizes the amount and quality of information that one can obtain from the patient in a short period of time.

4. Provides baseline information about the patient's functional abilities, which can be utilized later to identify changes over time in functional status, as well as to evaluate the effectiveness of care.
5. Facilitates the establishment of an early relationship with the patient.
6. Provides a basis for decision-making regarding management of nursing care.

The primary resource for collecting data for the nursing assessment is the patient. When the patient is unable to respond or communicate, or when he is an unreliable historian, the data may be supplemented through the use of secondary resources. Secondary resources for data collection are the family or others significant to the patient, health team members, and the patient's records. The particular use of secondary resources is to validate the data collected from the primary resource [10].

The skills required by the nurse in collecting data for the nursing assessment include interviewing, observation, and the physical assessment skills, namely, inspection, auscultation, palpation, and percussion. In early references to the process of systematic nursing assessment, data collection by the nurse was largely dependent on the use of such techniques as interviewing, direct observation, and inspection. Physical assessment per se was primarily the physician's responsibility and generally outside the realm of nursing practice. Today, physical assessment skills are increasingly found in the nurse's repertoire and are looked on as providing a mechanism for enriching the data base from which clinical judgments are made [6]. Physical assessment, when incorporated as an integral part of the nursing assessment, gives credence to the nurse's hypotheses about the patient's functional abilities and disabilities; it enables the nurse to validate observations and to make reasoned judgments about patient care problems and their management. In addition, physical assessment skills provide a dimension that enhances the evaluation of the effectiveness of nursing care through the monitoring of physiologic outcomes of care.

The prominent place that systematic assessment, including physical assessment, holds in the practice of nursing is exemplified in the flow chart in Figure 2-1, which illustrates the nurse practitioner's role in the patient-care process. Bates and Lynaugh [2] describe the patient care process as:

. . . familiar to nursing as well as medicine. Given her basic professional knowledge, the nurse gathers data, makes hypotheses, identifies problems, implements management, and evaluates the results. In the expanded role of the medical nurse practitioner, the basic process is the same, but the scope of practice and decision-making is greater.

The process depicted in Figure 2-1 is one of continual interplay between systematic assessment and analysis and nursing action. Note the significant role of physical assessment in the overall process. These authors add that their reasons for the nurse's extensive involvement in new patient assessments are as follows:

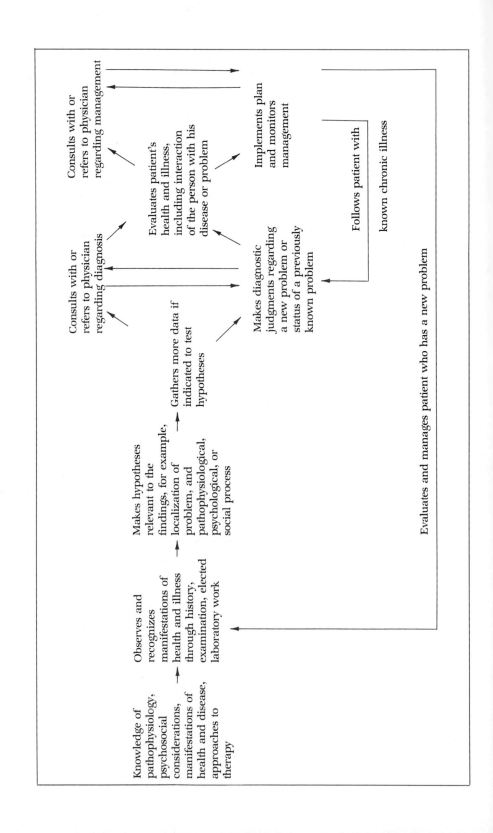

Knowledge of pathophysiology, psychosocial considerations, manifestations of health and disease, approaches to therapy

Observes and recognizes manifestations of health and illness through history, examination, elected laboratory work

Makes hypotheses relevant to the findings, for example, localization of problem, and pathophysiological, psychological, or social process

Gathers more data if indicated to test hypotheses

Consults with or refers to physician regarding diagnosis

Makes diagnostic judgments regarding a new problem or status of a previously known problem

Evaluates patient's health and illness, including interaction of the person with his disease or problem

Consults with or refers to physician regarding management

Implements plan and monitors management

Follows patient with known chronic illness

Evaluates and manages patient who has a new problem

First, the process of interview and physical examination helps the nurse to establish an early relationship with the patient. The team is thus able to avoid the "separation anxiety" and dissatisfactions that both patient and physician may feel when the patient is transferred to the nurse.

Second, significant initial involvement by both professionals helps to broaden the data base and the perception of patient problems.

Third, where medical services are scarce, the physician is the bottleneck at the entry point into the system. Nursing involvement enhances access to health care [2].

SKILLS REQUISITE FOR PHYSICAL ASSESSMENT

The physical assessment examination usually follows the assessment interview and history-taking activities and consists of systematically examining the patient for physical evidence of functional abilities, or disabilities, or both. It enables the assessor to explore hypotheses derived from the data collected during the interview, as well as to uncover new physical data.

The assessor must be systematically thorough and deliberate in conducting the examination to ensure complete and accurate data collection. Each nurse performing physical assessment develops her own systematic approach and should attempt to follow this procedure as closely as possible with each examination, while allowing flexibility in order to meet the patient's particular needs. In many situations it is a new experience for the patient to have a nurse perform a physical examination. If this is the case, the patient might well find it confusing without an explanation (particularly if the physician also performs an examination). Generally speaking the assessor should be prepared to tell the patient that the physical assessment will be used by the nurse as the basis for planning nursing care and will be shared with the physician as it relates to the patient's need for health care within a broader context.

To become successful at physical assessments, the nurse must not only be well versed in distinguishing normal from abnormal findings, but she must also be able to discriminate variations in normal among patients as well as ranges of normal in a given patient. In addition, Judge and Zuidema [4] refer to two irrevocably independent elements required for accurate and complete data collecting: the sensory or perceptual act and the conceptual process. The first step involves perceiving the sensory stimuli; the second relates the sensory stimuli to some relevant knowledge or past experience. Performing the mechanics of physical assessment is a relatively simple task, but relating the finding to the decision-making process that follows demands knowledge as well as rigorous training and experience.

Figure 2-1.
The nurse practitioner's role in the patient care process. (Copyright 1973, The American Journal of Nursing Company. Reproduced with permission from the *American Journal of Nursing*, August, Vol. 73, No. 8, and Bates and Lynaugh [2].)

Skills pertinent to problem-solving in general are already within the repertoire of nurses who base their practice on the process of systematic nursing assessment. Skills requisite for physical assessment that are new to many nurses include inspection, palpation, percussion, and auscultation. Their general characteristics are described here. Their specific applications to physical assessment are discussed in subsequent chapters.

Inspection   Inspection may be defined most simply as the visual examination of the patient for detection of significant physical features. It involves detailed and focused observations coupled with comparison of the findings with established standards or norms. Critical examination should note both the general appearance of the area being inspected and its specific characteristics: the presence or absence of usual or unusual landmarks and color, texture, location, position, temperature, size, vital signs, type and degree of movement, symmetry, and comparison with the opposite side of the body. Inspection requires the nurse to discern what is normal, what is unusual but within normal range, and what is abnormal and needing attention.

While seemingly the least complex physical assessment skill, inspection demands of the assessor an adequate knowledge base and skill in observing. It may well be the most important technique used in the physical assessment of a patient. Alexander and Brown [1] suggest that one should never underestimate the value of the naked eye coupled with the perceiving mind as a physical assessment tool.

Preliminary inspection begins during history-taking. However, inspection is most profitable in yielding pertinent assessment data when the assessor gives full concentration and careful scrutiny to what is being observed. Like other techniques used in examination, inspection should be conducted in a routine, systematic fashion. Although used alone initially, it is often combined with other physical assessment skills throughout the examination. Inspection and palpation are often best conducted together.

Palpation   Palpation is the process of examining the body through the use of tactile senses for the purpose of determining the characteristics of tissues or organs. More simply stated, palpation uses the sense of touch to detect physical signs (Fig. 2-2). This physical assessment technique involves not only the senses of touch and temperature, but also the perception of movement (e.g., vibration), position, consistency, and form. Palpation is used to examine all accessible parts of the body, including organs, glands, blood vessels, skin, muscles, and bones. By palpation one can assess the presence or absence of masses, pulsatility, organ enlargement, tenderness or pain, swelling, muscular spasm or rigidity, elasticity, vibration of voice sounds, crepitus, moisture, and differences in texture. Frequently, this assessment is used in conjunction with inspection.

In assessment by palpation, it is essential that the patient be relaxed and positioned comfortably; muscular tension during the examination may interfere with the assessor's ability to use this technique effectively or may even distort findings. Deep breathing through the mouth may enhance the patient's ability to relax during deep palpation. Tender areas should be palpated last. To maximize data collection, the assessor should progress in a systematic manner, using a bilateral and symmetric pattern, so that similar areas on opposing sides of the body can be compared with each other.

Figure 2-2.
The successful use of palpation requires not only the sense of touch, but also the ability to interpret the significance of what is being sensed. (Reproduced with permission from R. D. Judge, G. D. Zuidema, and F. Fitzgerald (Eds.). *Methods of Clinical Examination* (4th ed.). Boston: Little, Brown, 1982.)

Tactile pressure should be applied with warm hands, in a slow, gentle, deliberate manner, first using light palpation and then progressing to deeper palpation. Different parts of the examiner's hands are used during palpation, depending on what is being evaluated. For fine tactile discriminations, such as texture of the skin and size of lymph nodes, the tips of the fingers are used because they are the most sensitive area of the hand. For temperature, the dorsa of the hands and fingers are used because on the dorsa the skin is thinner and therefore more sensitive to temperature differences. The palmar aspects of the metacarpophalangeal joints are most sensitive to vibration. For position and consistency, the grasping action of the fingers is used. To determine rebound tenderness, ballottement is used, in which pressure is exerted on the organ and then rapidly released to assess the impact on rebound. When palpating the abdomen, particularly when using deep palpation, a bimanual technique is used. In this case, both hands are used, with a passive or "sensing" hand placed against the abdomen and the other serving as an active hand, applying pressure to the sensing hand. In this case, palpation is accomplished with the cushions and palmar surface of the sensing hand.

The successful use of palpation as a physical assessment technique depends not only on palpatory skills, but also on the examiner's ability to discriminate and interpret the significance of what is being sensed.

Percussion   Percussion is the striking or tapping of the body surface, lightly but sharply, to produce sounds that reflect the position, size, and density of an underlying structure. The effect of percussion is both heard and felt by the examiner. The quality of the sounds obtained vary according to the density of the underlying tissue. Percussion is particularly valuable in determining the relative amount of air or solid material in the underlying lung and the boundaries of organs or parts of the body that differ in structural density. Borders of certain organs, such as the heart, can be mapped out by gradually comparing densities in the organ with surrounding tissues. Percussion can also be used to ascertain if there is a change from normal density; for example, when a solid mass exists within a hollow organ.

Methods of Percussion

There are two methods of percussing: direct and indirect. *Direct or immediate percussion* is performed by striking the body surface directly with the fingers, either with one finger, usually the middle or ring finger, or with several partly bent fingers held close together. This technique is particularly valuable in percussing over the clavicle or for defining the cardiac border. *Indirect or mediate percussion* is performed by placing the index or middle finger (which becomes the *pleximeter,* i.e., the object receiving the blow) against the body surface and with the palm and fingers remaining off the skin, using the tip of the middle finger of the other hand (which becomes the *plexor,* i.e., the object striking the blow) to strike the base of the distal phalanx of the pleximeter finger. To execute this movement properly, strike a quick, sharp stroke with the middle finger, holding the forearm stationary and making the striking motion, using the wrist. If the blow is not sharp, the sound is damped. The plexor is withdrawn immediately to prevent attenuation of vibrations. The lightest blow that produces the desired sound is preferred. Both the sound elicited and the sense of resistance and vibration underneath the finger are evaluated. Percuss gently though firmly, making a special effort to apply equal force at all points (Fig. 2-3). It is necessary to percuss more firmly in heavy individuals.

Percussing the thorax is much like playing staccato notes on the piano, and as in playing the piano, practice makes perfect. Practice on another person is essential in learning percussion skills, but you can begin practice with a few simple exercises done by yourself. Practice flexing the wrist while keeping the forearm stationary by placing your hand and forearm on a table and striking the surface of the table with the tip of your middle finger. Use individual blows so that you are sure you are quickly rebounding to the flexed wrist position. You might want to also practice percussing your thigh and other parts of the body, such as the thorax and abdomen, to become familiar with percussion of a less firm surface and to compare differences in sounds elicited.

Several common errors of percussion should be avoided:

1. Make sure that only the distal phalanx of the pleximeter is resting on the body surface.
2. The pleximeter must be firmly placed on the skin; if not, vibrations are poorly transmitted.
3. Use a very short blow and rebound immediately. If the blow is not sharp, muffling of vibration may occur due to sustained pressure on the plexor.

Figure 2-3.
Basic method for mediate
percussion of the chest.
(Reproduced with
permission from R. D.
Judge, G. D. Zuidema, and
F. Fitzgerald (Eds.).
*Methods of Clinical
Examination* (4th ed.).
Boston: Little, Brown,
1982.)

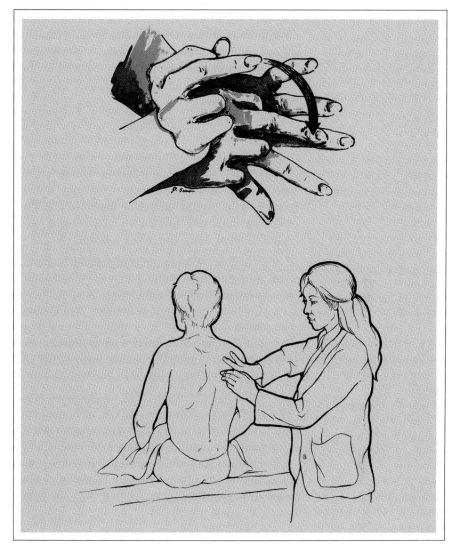

4. Do not use too forceful a blow. Your pleximeter finger will soon become sore. More important, you should concentrate on characteristics of the sound other than loudness—pitch, duration, and quality—for which lighter percussion is often superior.

5. Keep the forearm stationary and try to deliver strokes with equal force. If the motion comes only from the wrist, the momentum of the hand generally produces strokes of equal force.

6. Do not thump repeatedly in one area. Two or three staccato blows should be all that are needed before moving the pleximeter on to another area to compare sounds.

Percussion Tones

The tones of percussion have intensity, pitch, quality, and duration. *Intensity* of tone is determined by the amplitude of the vibration; loud tones such as those produced over the lung have a greater amplitude than soft tones heard over the heart. The *pitch,* or frequency, refers to the number of vibrations per second. The greater the number of vibrations, the higher the pitch (for example, over a consolidated lung); the fewer the number of vibrations, the lower the pitch (for example, over the normal lung). *Duration* is determined by the time period of the vibrations and is the length of time the sound lasts. *Quality* is a purely subjective characteristic, but serves to distinguish the source of the sound; it varies in relation to the density of the underlying tissue. *Sonorous percussion* is used to determine the density of a specific tissue; over low-density tissue as lung, one hears a resonant sound, whereas over moderately dense tissue, such as the heart, a dull sound occurs. A flat sound, without resonance, is heard over such high-density tissues as the thigh. *Definitive percussion* is used to distinguish between two structures with markedly differing densities, for example, the heart and lungs.

Percussion Notes

Percussion notes are most difficult to describe with words and can actually be comprehended only after hearing them. They are classified into the following qualities that reveal certain acoustic characteristics of tone:

Resonance. *Resonance* is the clear hollow note that is the normal sound in lung percussion. It is low-pitched, well sustained, and, although not loud, is heard with ease. The resonant note is always longer than the flat note and has a more definite and lower pitch.

Tympany. The word *tympany* comes from tympanum, or kettle drum, and the sound is truly like the sound resulting from the soft beating of this instrument. It is somewhat high-pitched, musical with rich overtones, clear, hollow, and well sustained. A like sound can be produced by filling the cheek with air and tapping it lightly with a finger. Tympany is higher-pitched than resonance. This seems to defy the rule that the less dense the underlying area, the lower the percussion note. However, in the stomach, the tympanic note is formed when the air in that closed chamber vibrates in unison with its elastic wall. Adding more air to the stomach is analogous to tightening the drum head—it causes greater tension and a higher pitch.

Hyperresonance. Like resonance, hyperresonance is a well-sustained, intense sound and can be described as a cross between resonance and tympany. Hyperresonance has a lower pitch than normal resonance, since it is due to an area with greater air/solid ratio, or less density. It therefore indicates an increased amount of air, or decreased amount of tissue, or both. Hyperresonance is accompanied by a distinct feeling of vibration sensed by the pleximeter finger. It is usually pathologic in origin.

Dullness. Dullness occurs with increased density and solidity. The sound is high-pitched, short, soft, and thudding. The pleximeter finger does not receive a vibrating sensation as with resonance or hyperresonance. Variations between resonance and dullness are often termed "impaired resonance" or "slight dullness."

Flatness. Flatness is absolute dullness, a very short, high-pitched sound that is nonmusical in quality. It has no resonance or vibration and is normally obtained when percussing over solid tissue such as the thigh.

You can demonstrate most of the percussion sounds for yourself on any normal person. First, listen to resonance by percussing the lung at the right anterior third interspace. Then have your subject exhale as completely as possible and percuss again—the note you hear should be impaired resonance. Next, have him inhale as deeply as possible, and the note should become more resonant, perhaps slightly hyperresonant. Now move down to the fourth right interspace. Here, the resonant note should be slightly impaired, due to the underlying liver. The note becomes duller as the fifth and sixth interspaces are percussed. Percussing the seventh interspace should elicit a flat note, because only the liver is present underneath.

Auscultation   Auscultation is the process of listening to sounds produced by various organs of the body for the purpose of detecting variations and deviations from their usual characteristics. This physical assessment skill is particularly demanding for the learner, since abnormal sounds are distinguishable only if one has developed a clear appreciation of the normal variations in sounds arising from body structures. In addition, the listener must understand the basic facts of sound production within the body, including the distinguishing characteristics of sounds arising in each body structure and the location in which they can be heard most clearly. Auscultation is a useful tool in appraising sounds arising from the heart, lungs, and abdomen and from bruits or murmurs in the neck and abdomen. The techniques of auscultation and the nature of the sounds specific to each of these are discussed in detail in subsequent chapters (see Fig. 2-4).

Characteristics of Sounds

Regardless of location, there are four characteristics of sound to consider in auscultation: frequency (pitch), intensity (loudness), quality (timbre), and duration. These characteristics, as defined by Lehmann [5], follow.

Frequency. The frequency of a vibration is the number of wave cycles generated per second by the vibrating body. Frequency determines the pitch of the sound; the higher the frequency, the higher is the pitch of a particular sound. Low-frequency vibrations produce low-pitched sounds.

Intensity. The intensity of sound is related to the height or amplitude of the sound wave produced by the vibrating object. Vibrations of high energy pro-

Figure 2-4.
Indirect auscultation.
(Reproduced with
permission from R. D.
Judge, G. D. Zuidema, and
F. Fitzgerald (Eds.).
*Methods of Clinical
Examination* (4th ed.).
Boston: Little, Brown,
1982.)

duce waves of high amplitude and are heard as loud sounds, for example, the clanging of cymbals. A low-energy system produces waves of low amplitude which are heard as soft sounds, such as the light tapping of one's fingertips on a table.

Quality. Two sounds with the same degree of loudness and the same pitch, but coming from different sources, are distinguished by their quality [timbre]. Sounds of equal loudness and pitch from different organs, such as the heart and the lungs, can be differentiated.

Duration. Duration refers to the number of continuous vibrations. As the energy given to the vibrating system is diminished by frictional resistance, the duration of the vibration is reduced. When this occurs, it is known as damping. Vibrations coming from the internal organs of the body are damped by the soft tissue that cover these organs.

Types of Stethoscopes

As with percussion, auscultation can be achieved by the direct or indirect method. In the *direct, or immediate, method,* the ear is applied directly to the body surface. Although this technique may be used if necessary, it is not the procedure of choice. *Indirect, or mediate, auscultation* is accomplished with the use of a stethoscope as in Figure 2-4. The selection of a stethoscope is crucial to effective auscultation; many nurses prefer to purchase their own to ensure adequacy of the instrument to meet their particular purposes. Stetho-

Figure 2-5.
The stethoscope. (Modified
from Judge and Zuidema
[4].)

scopes are equipped with one or both of two general types of pickups or chest-pieces: the open bell and the closed diaphragm (Fig. 2-5).

Littman [7] has described in detail the characteristics of each type of stetho-scope, highlighting their inherent advantages and disadvantages. He compares the open-bell chestpiece to the old-fashioned trumpet-type hearing aid. It consists of a short, cone- or funnel-shaped bell joined to a binaural headset and eartips by flexible tubing, and conducts sounds with practically no distortion. The diameter of the bell does not usually exceed one inch, therefore limiting the volume of sound it can accumulate. A wider bell would be unlikely to conform to the surface of the body, and the resulting leaks would minimize the air pressure vibrations within the stethoscope; these are pressure variations that are essential for the perception of sound. With the bell-shaped stethoscope, it is necessary to obtain a perfect seal with the skin, which acts as the stethoscope's diaphragm.

The closed diaphragm chestpiece is usually the preferred instrument. It is larger than the open-bell type and is sealed by its own diaphragm to form a closed system; a perfect seal with the skin is not necessary. Its large diameter permits it to accumulate a greater quantity of sound. For this reason, it is more sensitive to faint noises. The diaphragm filters out low-frequency vibrations, so that sounds appear of higher pitch.

Combination stethoscopes with at least two chestpieces are commonly used by those who need them for precise discrimination among various abnormal sounds. The open bell is more effective for the perception of certain low-pitched sounds, such as diastolic murmurs and some gallop rhythms. The closed diaphragm type is used for most screening and general purposes and, especially, for the detection of high-pitched sounds, including the first and second heart sounds. It can be used to pick up most heart and lung sounds and is convenient for placement under blood pressure cuffs [7].

Use of the Stethoscope

Each assessor develops his own procedure and sequence of steps as he learns to perform auscultation. All areas should be covered systematically and symmetrically. The room and the stethoscope should be warm, and the patient relaxed, so that involuntary muscle contractions do not occur and mask findings. Before beginning to auscultate the chest, make sure that you are in a quiet room. The level of background noise may not seem high, but very little noise is necessary to interfere with the low-intensity sounds which are important to detect on auscultation. It is important to eliminate as many extraneous sounds as possible. If the entire rim of the chestpiece does not touch the skin and a leak occurs, extraneous noise in the form of a roaring sound is heard by the examiner. Also, if the chestpiece is not held firmly, sounds of respiratory excursion (such as movement of intercostal muscles, joints, or skin) are heard and may mimic a friction rub. Movement of the chestpiece over hair can produce a factitious sound that resembles rales. This can be eliminated by wetting the hair. Breathing on the tubing or sliding one's fingers over the chestpiece may also cause confusing sounds. The learner should purposely produce all these sounds and become familiar with them, in order to recognize and eliminate them during the examination.

The key to successful auscultation lies in listening to one thing at a time and concentrating on what one is hearing. Auscultation is the most complex of the physical assessment skills. To be successful in utilizing this assessment technique, the learner needs to concentrate first on normal sounds and must achieve the first level of discrimination in auscultation—detecting abnormal from normal sounds—before progressing to the level of discerning the nature and significance of abnormal auscultatory findings.

Recording of Data   Competency in performing the technical skills inherent in inspection, palpation, percussion, and auscultation is only made manifest as it is reflected in the problem-solving process that follows. Just as the nurse must be systematically thorough and deliberate in collecting complete and accurate data, similar rigor must be employed in data analysis and synthesis. The data collected through physical assessment must be classified and distinctions made as to what is functional versus dysfunctional as well as significant and nonsignificant. In some instances data are incomplete and the appraiser must return to collect more information.

The system for recording these data should be logical and orderly, one that condenses and concentrates the relevant findings into a usable, problem-solving form. The problem-oriented recording system, described in Chapter 3, provides one such logical approach to record-keeping. Regardless of the recording format, however, the synthesis of data is facilitated if it is kept in logical sequence and suitably condensed so as to eliminate nonessential and lengthy detail.

Analysis and synthesis of assessment data culminate in the identification of functional disabilities that require nursing action as well as those that merit referral to the physician. In addition, particular attention should be given to the person's most significant functional abilities, those that should be maintained and fostered throughout implementation of prescribed health care regimen.

Physical assessment findings, when incorporated within the context of a complete nursing assessment, enable the nurse to make more enlightened decisions about the individual's health care needs.

REFERENCES

1. Alexander, M. M., and Brown, M. S. Physical examination: The why and how of examination. *Nursing '73* 3:25, 1973.
2. Bates, B., and Lynaugh, J. E. Laying the foundations for medical nursing practice. *Am. J. Nurs.* 73:1375, 1973.
3. Carrieri, V. K., and Sitzman, J. Components of the nursing process. *Nurs. Clin. North Am.* 6:115, 1971.
4. Judge, R. D., and Zuidema, G. D. (Eds.) *Methods of Clinical Examination: A Physiologic Approach* (3rd ed.). Boston: Little, Brown, 1974.
5. Lehmann, J. Auscultation of heart sounds. *Am. J. Nurs.* 72:1242, 1972.
6. Lewis, E. (Ed.) A rolè by any name. *Nurs. Outlook* 22:89, 1974.
7. Littmann, D. Stethoscopes and auscultation. *Am. J. Nurs.* 65:82, 1965.
8. Lynaugh, J. E., and Bates, B. Physical diagnosis: A skill for all nurses? *Am. J. Nurs.* 74:58, 1974.
9. McCain, R. F. Nursing by assessment—not intuition. *Am. J. Nurs.* 65:82, 1965.
10. McCain, R. F., et al. Systematic Nursing Assessment. Unpublished materials developed at The University of Michigan School of Nursing, Ann Arbor, Michigan.
11. Parker, J. C., and Rubin, L. J. *Process as Content: Curriculum Design and the Application of Knowledge.* Chicago: Rand McNally, 1966.

SUGGESTED READINGS

Alexander, M. M., and Brown, M. S. Physical Examination: History-Taking. *Nursing '73* 3:35, 1973.

Alexander, M. M., and Brown, M. S. *Pediatric History Taking and Physical Diagnosis for Nurses* (2nd ed.). New York: McGraw-Hill, 1979.

Bates, B. *A Guide to Physical Examination* (2nd ed.). Philadelphia: Lippincott, 1979.

Beaumont, E. For the Latest Word on Stethoscopes—Listen Here! *Nursing '78* 8:32, 1978.

DeGowin, E. L., and DeGowin, R. L. *Bedside Diagnostic Examination* (3rd ed.). New York: Macmillan, 1976.

Fowkes, W. C., and Hunn, V. K. *Clinical Assessment for the Nurse Practitioner.* St. Louis: Mosby, 1973.

Judge, R. D., Zuidema, G. D., and Fitzgerald, F. (Eds.). *Methods of Clinical Examination* (4th ed.). Boston: Little, Brown, 1982.

Malasanos, L., et al. *Health Assessment.* St. Louis: Mosby, 1977.

Traver, G. A. "Assessment of Thorax and Lungs." *Am. J. Nurs.* 73:466, 1973.

Margie J. Van Meter

3. Problem-Oriented Documentation and Measurement of Nursing Care

THE processes and tools for diagnosing, planning, documenting, and measuring successful nursing care have common and interrelated components. Problem-oriented records, nursing diagnoses, standard nursing care plans, and quality assurance criteria will be defined, the components and processes will be discussed, and then the interrelationships of the components will be diagrammed.

THE PROBLEM-ORIENTED RECORD (POR)

Historically, the nursing records of patient care have been a chronologic narrative of somewhat random observations about the patient and the effects of medications and treatments, activities of the nurse, monitoring data for medical decisions, and legally pertinent facts. The nursing plan of care, the independent actions of the nurse, and the results of nursing intervention have not been consistently in evidence on the patient's permanent records. The identification of patient care problems, the degree to which they can be resolved, and the activities needed to achieve this resolution have been recorded in pencil on the Kardex and erased when no longer current. Data, then, are not available for measuring the quality of the nurse's contribution to patient welfare, comparing outcomes of various nursing interventions, or developing research programs.

The concept and role of the professional nurse is changing. The psychologic and intellectual dependency of nurses is beginning to be replaced by the building of interdependent relations among health team members. This change is being reflected in the nursing records of professional nurse practitioners who want to facilitate patient care, publicly document evidence of their contributions, and leave sufficient permanency for accountability, peer review, and clinical nursing research. Interdisciplinary patient care documentation systems have been developed. The nurse's records are showing evidence of the whole of the nursing process: data collection, formulation of problems (nursing diagnoses), formulation of solutions, intervention, and evaluation. Nurses recognize that only as trends and patterns in patient outcomes are identified will it be possible to have objective delineation of nursing care approaches that have high probability for success [18].

A health care record system that is being widely adapted by a variety of care settings is Weed's problem-oriented record system [19]. Nurses reading current nursing and medical journals are familiar with this documented problem-solving process. It guides the practitioner in his/her approach to the patient and the patient's discrete problems. The process teaches others in the health care disciplines who read the record, because clinical judgments, rationale, and results are readily discernible. This process and record system consists of four main components:

The initial data base is as significant and complete as is realistic. It includes a profile of the patient's way of life, subjective symptoms, and objective findings. The compiling of the data is begun on the initial contact with the patient. The data base is standardized so that the type and quantity of data are the same for all patients, regardless of the extent of their presenting complaints.

The data provide the identification of the patient's problems. Each problem must be supported by data and stated at the level that it is understood at the time. An abnormal weight gain or frequent crying episodes may be the level at which problems are initially identified. There are no leaps to probable diagnoses, "rule-outs," or question marks. All the known problems are listed and given a title and number. The problem list is updated as more information is obtained: problem titles are changed as the diagnosis evolves; new problems are identified and added; and problems are terminated when they are resolved.

A separate sheet on the front of the record lists all the problems and the number assigned each problem. This problem list serves as a dynamic table of contents to the patient's record and a summary of all the identified past and current problems. The date of identification and resolution of problems is indicated on this list.

The plan for each problem states specifically how the care planner is going to approach the problem in regard to (1) diagnostic plan, (2) therapeutic measures, and (3) patient education.

All plans, orders, subsequent data, and progress notes are recorded under the numbered and titled problem in the record. This makes it possible to determine from the record the reason for the test, the treatment, and so on.

The periodic progress notes are a record of the follow-up of the problems and the patient's responses to the planned program. This is the evaluation phase. The progress notes consist of narrative notes, flow sheets, and final summaries of problems. Narrative data about a problem are recorded in a structured format. SOAP is the acronym for the format.

S — subjective observations (the patient's or significant other's point of view and data).

O — objective observations of the care provider.

A — analysis of the observations. For example: Has the status of the problem changed? On what criteria?

P — plan for continued treatment (Rx), diagnosis (Dx), and patient education (Ed).

Flexibility in using the POR format permits concise and chronologic sequencing of data, such as providing *Objective* data before *Subjective* data in progress notes (see Fig. 3-4, Problem 1—Pacemaker; Fig. 3-2, Skin) or grouping Dx-Rx-Ed (see the plans in Fig. 3-4, Problem 6—Communication with Sons; Fig. 3-4, Problem 2—Shoulder, and Problem 4—Brain Tumor).

Problems with multiple and interrelated variables may be more easily followed by the creation and use of flow sheets on which values are recorded in time sequence and in relationship to therapy. Not only does this facilitate the use of the data, but it may avoid voluminous progress notes (see Fig. 3-5).

In Weed's concept, all disciplines of a health care delivery system contribute to one record and problem list. The departments of medicine, nursing, social work, and dietetics may all be assisting the patients with aspects of the same problem. With a single record and problem list, the contributions of each is seen, and redundancy of recording and effort is prevented.

A combined record is dependent on all disciplines' being in agreement with the adoption of the system, the creation of appropriate record forms, and the reorganizing of such processes as patient admission. Because of these requirements, the initiating of this effective approach is delayed considerably in some health care settings. Nurses can facilitate patient care and upgrade the quality of their documentation of care by using the process individually until the entire health team accepts the idea of a common record and problem list. This is actually desirable for nursing because in this way nurses can learn much about their independent functions and become accustomed to public documentation of their nursing judgments, plans, and outcomes. Nurses can become as aware of and effective in their independent role as in their dependent role and make uniquely nursing contributions to the patient care process and record, beyond obtaining and recording data needed for medical decisions. Using the problem-oriented method, nurses also learn the nature of the data base needed to make nursing decisions and gain skills in obtaining and describing these data objectively. These skills further enable nurses to contribute data of substance and significance to the common record and problem list.

The examples in the literature provide evidence of the nature of the data the nurse collects, how he/she identifies problems, and what his/her nursing contributions are [6]. Elaboration of the nurse's contribution is illustrated by an approach used by a nursing staff. The nursing record of a patient in one hospital setting from admission through the first few days of hospitalization is shown in Figures 3-1 to 3-6. It is presented and discussed as one useful model and as a

Figure 3-1.
Problem list. Problems
identified on admission
assessment (see Fig. 3-2)
and problems indicated on
progress notes (see Fig.
3-4) are entered here.

PROBLEM LIST

Name

1 058 771
Gannon, Mary Louise
6132 Riverview
Palmroy, MI 48176

NO.	PROBLEM TITLE	DATE IDENTIFIED	DATE RESOLVED
1	Pacemaker Function: No self-monitoring	3-14-79	
	Tenderness over battery pack	3-14-79	
	Lt. chest muscle twitching	3-14-79	3-17-79
2	Rt Shoulder Rom guarded	3-14-79	
3	Laxative regularly uses	3-14-79	
4	Brain tumor possible - experiencing diagnostic process	3-14-79	
5	Self Breast Exam - Vague about	3-14-79	
6	No communication with sons	3-17-79	
7			
8			
9			
10			

Figure 3-2.
Admission nursing
assessment form.

DATA BASE

1 058 771

Gannon, Mary Louise

DATE ___3-14-79___ ADDRESS ___6132 Riverview___

BIRTHDATE ___8-3-1920___ ___Palmroy, Mich. 48176___

PHONE ___313-820-4176___ COUNTY ___Peninsula___

OCCUPATION ___Homemaker___ MARITAL STATUS S (M) W D

EDUCATION ___9th grade___ RELIGION ___Baptist___ TYPE HOUSING ___2 story   Own___

INSURANCE _____ ALLERGIES: ___Adhesive tape, Ampicillin___

PERSON(S) TO CONTACT: ___Husband - Homer___ _____

PATIENT ASSESSMENT

Include reason for admission and initial observations about status of functional areas: Respiratory, Circulatory, Motor, Temperature, Nutrition, Elimination, Skin, Special Senses, Reproductive, Rest and Comfort, Mental Emotional, Social

FUNCTIONAL AREA:	OBSERVATIONS: Subjective and Objective
Social	Retired laundromat attendant. Retirement forced by MI 2 yrs. ago. Does housework, embroidery, active member of church. Husband continues to do odd jobs for local people. He had rt. arm amputated at age 10. Has always had difficulty getting jobs even though described by wife as very capable. Both receive Soc. Sec. Medicare and Blue Cross. MI and pacemaker inserted 2 yrs. ago. Battery changed 2 months ago. Admitted for first time to University Hospital for work up for possible brain tumor.
Respiratory	S- Uses stairs. No DOE. Sleeps flat c̄ one pillow. No cough. Nonsmoker. Bedroom and bath on 1st floor. O- Rate 20 during interview
Circulatory	S- Pacemaker changed 1/79. Does not know type of pacemaker or how to monitor functioning of it. Appt. in 1 month c̄ cardiologist. Has fleeting, sharp, midchest pain occasionally (i.e. Several days may pass between episodes.) Pauses in activity and breathes deeply. Several brief, dizzy spells accompanied by sights and smells and rt. arm twitching "until batteries

31

Figure 3-2.
Continued.

Functional Area	Observations: Subjective and Objective
	changed." Taking Dilantin now. O-BP sitting Rt. 110/76 Lt. 112/80. Apical, Rt. and Lt. Radial pulses full volume, regular rhythm. 72/min. Hands and feet warm and pink.
Motor	No pedal edema. S - Arthritic pain on rt. side in 1972 for which took "orange pill." Rt. shoulder painful today; attributes to position when sleeping and arthritis.
	O - Guarded complete active ROM rt. shoulder. Slight ulvar deviation both hands R > L. Good strength all extremities. Ambulates c̄ smooth gait s̄ ataxia.
Nutrition	S - Reg. diet s̄ food allergies. Eating pattern 8^{30}a 12n 5^{30}p 9^{00}p.
	O - Wt. 140 Ht. 5'4½". Most excess wt. around abdomen. Upper denture plate. Lower teeth good repair.
Elimination	S - Voids approx. 4 x day. No nocturia. Has used Exlax twice a week for 5 yrs. Constipated s̄ Exlax O - Abd. soft.
Skin	O - 3 inch incision over rt. chest. Same incision for battery change as for original insertion. Well healed.
	S - Tender since prone on table for brain scan.
Reproductive	S - no vaginal discharge. Last pap 2 months ago. Checks breasts for lumps. Not specific about method or frequency.
Special Senses	O - Hears conversation s̄ requesting repetition. Reads newsprint c̄ ease. Pupils equal, reactive directly and consensually to light.
Rest and Comfort	S - Up at 7^{30}a to bed at 9^{00}p. Sleeps on rt. side. Supine and lt. lateral positions cause "jumping" of lt. chest muscle. Can give no possible cause; expressed concern.
	O - Pulsations or muscle twitching palpated over lt. chest when in lt. lateral position.
Mental Emotional	S - Aware reason for admission is possible brain tumor. Does not think she has a tumor because brain scan was negative. "Was pretty worried." Views self as calm, hard-working person - asks no questions - independent.
	O - Alert; Oriented x 3; Expressive interested affect. Visiting with other patients.
	A. Augustine, R.N.

Figure 3-3.
Form for problems
identified on assessment
plans for resolving
problems.

No.	Problem Title	Initial Plans 3-14-79
1	Pacemaker - not checking function	Expected outcomes: 1) Demonstrates monitoring of pacemaker 2) Battery site tenderness cleared. 3) Informed of cause of twitching
		Dx - Apical P. q.s.
		Observe battery site q.d.
		Discuss twitching c̄ cardiology nurse specialist
		Rx - Note on chart front when going for dx studies about positioning
		Ed - Pt. Ed. booklet on Pacemakers
2	Rt Shoulder ROM guarded	Expected Outcome: Comfortable - complete use rt. arm.
		Rx - Active ROM bid. Ask MD for analgesic if remains painful this p.m.
		Ed - Encouraged to persist in using.
3	Laxative used regularly	Expected Outcome and Rx: BM minimum q 3 days. Has MOM ordered PRN
		Dx - Assess bowel pattern etc.
		Ed - Informed and instructed to request MOM
4	Brain Tumor diagnostic phase	Expected Outcome: Discussing fears and diagnostic results
		Rx - Daily contact c̄ A. Augustine
		Dx - Neuro check q. shift
		Ed - Each eve inform and teach about next day's dx studies.
5	Self Breast Exam	Expected Outcome: Demonstrates self-breast exam c̄ appropriate technique. Identifies frequency to perform.
		Dx/Ed - Assess further for details and teach after current brain tumor problem resolved.
		A. Augustine, R.N.

Figure 3-4.
Progress notes form.

DATE/TIME	PROBLEM NO. & TITLE	PROGRESS NOTES
		PROGRESS NOTES **S**ubjective — Patient's Perceptions **O**bjective — Observable **A**nalysis — Interpretation of Data **Pl**an — Plan of Care: Diagnostic, Therapeutic, Pt. Education 1 058 771 Gannon, Mary Louise
8/15/79 8-4p	3 Laxative usage	S - Does not like MOM. Causes gagging. Desires pill form.
		O - MOM taken last PM and had BM today. Pharmacy has nothing comparable to Exlax nor MOM pills.
		A - Prefers pill form lax. even though MOM effective.
		P - Rx - Discuss c̄ MD possibility of using own Exlax.
		Dx - Assess measures used to promote regular BM.
		Ed - Explore other measures that will promote BM s̄ dependency on laxative.
		Goal - Dependency on laxative limited.
		L. Moore, R.N.
4-12p	4 Experiencing Brain Tumor Work Up	S - No episodes of hallucinatory smells or sights. No rt. arm twitching. Focused on negative brain scan in discussion of possible tumor.
		O - Strength 5+ all 4 extremeties. Pupils equal & reactive. BP and P continue in same range. Calling nurses by name.
		A - Hopeful. Neuro status stable.
		P - Dx/Rx continue neuro monitoring and talking.
		C. Farner, R.N.
8/16/79	2 Rt. Shoulder	S - No pain O - Moving freely. No ASA used.
		A - Improved. **Pain etiology** she suggested probably correct.
		P - Rx/Dx Continue Active ROM and monitoring .
		Ed - Re-enforced using is key to maintaining function of any joint.
		A. Augustine, R.N.

Figure 3-4
Continued.

DATE/TIME	PROBLEM NO. & TITLE	
8/17/79 9A	1 Pacemaker	O - Consult c̄ cardiology nurse --- muscle twitch that occurs only in *these* particular positions is probably the conduction of the pacemaker impulse through the heart apex to the chest wall. Pt. informed. Reg. Apical - 72
		S - Expressed relief and gratitude for information.
		A - Muscle twitch from pacemaker conduction.
		P - Dx - Continue pacemaker q d
		Rx - Place on rt. side when on stretcher
		Ed - Pacemaker Booklet given to read and will discuss this afternoon. See Pt. Ed. Record.
		Cardiology nurse to visit 8/19.
		S - Only children are two married sons in this state. Rarely visit parents. Once a yr is shortest interval between visits of 1-2 hrs. No letters or phone calls. Youngest son visited during hospitalization for M.I. Oldest son had no contact then. Gives no reason for sons' alienation.
		O - Only visitors have been husband and 2 sisters.
	6 No communi-	A - New problem
	cation with	P - Dx/Rx Pt. outcome: Discussing meaning of no contact c̄ sons to her.
	sons	A. Augustine to provide time q d for her to talk about this and functional limitations from MI, pacemaker, plus possible B.T.
		A. Augustine, R.N.

Figure 3-5.
ADL treatment activities and clinical parameters.

ADL, TREATMENTS and CLINICAL PARAMETERS

1 058 771

Gannon, Mary Louise

		3-14-79 N	D	E	3-15 N	D	E	3-16 N	D	E
DATE / SHIFT		N	D	E	N	D	E	N	D	E
Hygiene:	BODY					Independent			Self	
	ORAL					Independent			Self	
Activity:	AMBULATORY			Independ.		Up frequently			Independent	
	BED REST									
	CHAIR			X			X		X	X
	VISITOR(S)		0	0		Husband			2 sisters	
	DIVERSIONAL						Embroidery			
Diet:	TYPE			Reg	Reg →				Reg	↑fiber
	APPETITE			ate all		good	good		ate well	good
Stool:										
Safety:										
Problem Number	TREATMENTS and CLINICAL PARAMETERS									
1	Apical Pulse			Reg	Regular	Reg	Reg	Extra beats		Reg
				72	73	72	72	75	73	72
	Elastic Stockings			applied	✓	x2	✓	✓	x2	✓
	off 1/2 hr					slight redness small toe - lt			Redness cleared	
	q. shift								Skin intact	
2	Rt. Shoulder					Guarded	Slow full range		Uses more freely	
	Active ROM					x2	x2	Ṫ	x2	x2
	Procedures Taught		Brain Scan			EEG				
	Procedures Done		Brain Scan	EKG						EEG
	Specimens Sent			Urine						
	Signature of Nurse		A. Augustine, R.N.	F. Worder, R.N.	G. Demmer, R.N.	L. Moore, R.N.	C. Farmer, R.N.	G. Demmer, R.N.	A. Augustine, R.N.	K. Parker, R.N.

Figure 3-6.
Patient education record.

| PATIENT EDUCATION RECORD | | | | LOCATION | DATE | SERVICE |

PATIENT EDUCATION RECORD

Problem(s) No. and Title

Recipient(s) of Teaching _____

#1-Having a pacemaker is a unique experience and will require ongoing adherence to a health care regimen as well as a personal commitment to monitor the pacemaker rate and other pacemaker parameters.

LOCATION   DATE   SERVICE

Reg. No.   Class

                                                            Name

                                                            Address

Areas to consider are: Disease Process, Medications, Activity, Skill, Signs of Complications, Growth and Development, and Discharge Planning for Home Management

Expected Outcomes or Content of Teaching	Teaching 1 Initial 2 Reinforcement	Outcomes Achieved by Recipient		Comments/Evaluation
	Date and Sign	Date		
		Yes	No	
A. Verbalizes need for pacemaker, especially related to symptoms.				
B. Understands operative procedures and postoperative routine.				
C. Has the booklet "You and Your Pacemaker" as a reference tool.				
D. States the immediate activity restrictions and also verbalizes that there are no restrictions for most activities after the first two weeks.				
E. Pacemaker Rate:				
1. Knows how to check pulse (or has alternate method, i.e., family, telephone monitoring).				
2. Knows importance of assessing pulse *daily*.				
3. Knows rate of pacemaker.				
4. Knows 4 beat pacemaker rate drop indicates generator failure.				

Figure 3-6.
Continued.

Areas to consider are: Disease Process, Medications, Activity, Skill, Signs of Complications, Growth and Development, and Discharge Planning for Home Management				
Expected Outcomes or Content of Teaching	Teaching 1 Initial 2 Reinforcement	Outcomes Achieved by Recipient		Comments/Evaluation
	Date and Sign	Date		
		Yes	No	
F. Knows the complecations that might occur and where to get help if one occurs (see booklet).				
G. Understands replacement procedures.				
H. States which electrical devices might interfere with pacemaker (see booklet).				
I. Identification:				
1. Has appropriate pacemaker identification cards.				
2. Has Medic alert form.				
J. Knows appropriate information regarding suture removal: (7-10 days)				
1. Date 2. Place				
K. Has a followup pacemaker clinic appt. in Heart Station. (Followup Interval) New pacemaker = 1 mo. Generator only = 3 mo.				
l. Knows name, dose, purpose, side effects for discharge meds.				

stimulus and generator of ideas for nurses who wish to adapt the process to their practice and setting. Adaptations were made by the nurses for their particular unit and patient population. Potential users of the record need to develop the format and process for their particular setting in harmony with their philosophy and needs. Format, use, and revisions were decided on by the staff.

The example of POR presented is detailed and complete. It is based on an actual patient's record. All the data and problems are factual. Beyond that it was revised to provide a comprehensive example for the reader. It is not expected, given the realities of health care delivery systems, that all the problems of a patient can typically be so thoroughly planned and documented. The example provided here is intended to illustrate several concepts, but not to defeat the reader and inhibit usage. My initial use of POR concepts was simply a label (problem title) on the left-hand side of progress notes.

The patient assessment presented incorporates few data from physical examination, thus demonstrating that the nurse does not have to have highly developed physical assessment skills or be in an expanded role to facilitate patient care through the use of the problem-oriented record. The interventions under "plan" (Figs. 3-3, 3-4, and 3-6) are independent functions of nurses, not physician-directed activities.

When the patient is admitted to the nursing unit, nursing assessment is done. "Systematic Assessment of the Functional Abilities of a Patient," developed by McCain [15], is used as the approach for data collection. The initial data are recorded in the data base (Fig 3-2).

The patient's problems identified from the initial assessment, together with the expected outcomes and nursing actions for treating and resolving the problems, are listed in Figure 3-3. The problems are listed next to the plan, so that relationships can be readily seen. The problems also appear on the problem list form (see Fig. 3-1), which is the index to the patient's nursing care record.

The problems identified for nursing intervention are stated in terms of functional status or specific patient behaviors. Nursing interventions are directed toward assisting patients and families in attaining and maintaining a state of optimal functional ability; the physician's goal is to prevent, cure, and alleviate disease. By focusing on functional abilities, the effect of nursing on the patient's status can be determined.

Follow-up of problems is recorded on the progress notes. Observations are noted in S–0 division, decisions under A. This makes nurses aware of when they are recording only one component of the observations. The interventions are detailed as diagnosis (Dx), treatment (Rx), and education (Ed) under P (see Fig. 3-4). These interventions include present activities, future actions, and nursing orders. The progress notes are used for ongoing data collection and evaluation of identified problems, patient data not related to identified problems, and newly identified problems. New problems are identified by recording the data and the problem and plan in the progress notes; each problem is also recorded on the problem list (for example, see Figs. 3-1 and 3-4). Analysis of previously identified problems is indicated by revised plans, retitled problems on the problem list, or indication on the problem list that the problem is resolved (see Problem 1, Fig. 3-1).

The dependent functions of the nurse can readily be recorded on check sheets and flow sheets; the documentation system illustrated here also included a medications record form, a fluid balance sheet and a vital signs sheet. The goal is to avoid repetition in recording, so that available forms that are satisfactory may be retained. The ADL treatments and clinical parameters form was created for more efficient recording of the services the nurse continually provides for patients during their hospitalization. Generally, such information tends to be the major content of the nursing record. Using a system such as the one illustrated here makes readily apparent to a nurse whether he/she is recording only what he/she has done for the patient or is actually observing and recording the patient's responses and status.

The ADL treatments and clinical parameters nursing form (Fig. 3-5) can be used to quantify the distance the patient has walked and the patient's appetite, independence level, treatment schedule, and response. If, instead of a checkmark, descriptive words are used to record in the blocks, much can be learned about the patient's status, and measurements for quality assurance are more readily available.

In the hospital setting, where it is required that the responsible nurse be identified on the record for each 8-hour shift, this can be achieved by providing a convenient place for signatures on the treatment activities sheet like the sections shown in Figure 3-5. Placing flow sheets at the bedside facilitates charting and keeping the patient informed of his or her progress.

The area of most difficulty in records of this kind is problem identification. Nurses vary in their ability to see the interrelationships of multiple behaviors of a patient. A problem may have been identified at one level by one nurse, while another nurse with more limited knowledge and experience may identify components of that problem as separate problems. This difficulty is not unique to the setting or to nursing. Goldfinger [9] discusses this in a critique of the problem-oriented record. Redundancy in the problem list is less likely to occur in a primary care setting in which the nurse practitioner works with a caseload of patients for whom she alone identified the nursing problems.

Placing the key word at the beginning of the problem statement facilitates use of the problem, for example, Pacemaker, Shoulder, Laxative, Brain tumor, Breast examination (see Fig. 3-1).

It is helpful to develop a list (taxonomy) of the most common problems or nursing diagnoses for a particular care setting [14]. Redundancy and wordiness in the Problem List can sometimes be diminished by this. A taxonomy for a neuro inpatient unit might include:

Level of consciousness altered

Skin integrity impaired

Bowel elimination

Depression

Mobility deficits

Self-image altered

Communication deficit

These are broad categories to which a descriptive word or etiology may be added to communicate the specific nature of the problem.

A problem list might contain the following:

Problem		Onset	Resolved
Bowel elimination	diarrhea	3/18/79	3/25/79
	constipation	4/1	4/5
	tarry stools	4/15/79	
Depression related to dependency		4/10/79	
Skin integrity impaired			
left heel		4/1	4/5

The problem list for the patient example presented here (see also Fig. 3-1) was originally organized as follows:

No.	Problem	Onset	Resolved
1.	Not checking pacemaker function	8-14-79	
2.	Guarded ROM right shoulder	8-14	
3.	Regularly uses laxative	8-14	
4.	Tenderness over battery pack	8-14	
5.	Left chest muscle twitching	8-14	8-17
6.	Experiencing diagnostic work up for brain tumor	8-14	
7.	Vague about self-breast examination	8-14	
8.	Not communicating with sons	8-17-79	

The problems are the same as those identified in Figure 3-1. In Figure 3-1, the nurse recognized that several symptoms were components of the basic problem—the pacemaker. Either problem list is workable and is reflective of the nurse's skill in problem statements or knowledge about cardiac pacemakers. Brief problem lists are desirable. Extensive problem lists, like those that occur in the acute care setting, become dysfunctional for the busy staff nurse.

A clear statement of the problem or diagnosis provides the basis for a relevant and effective solution. The patient problem is stated, not the care needed. A statement of the problem may point to a need for multiple solutions. The generation and classification of nursing diagnoses are discussed in the following section.

POR documentation provides for comprehensive health-oriented care even in an acute care setting. Mental Health (Problems 4 and 6), Patient Education (Problem 1), and Health Maintenance (Problems 2, 3, and 5) are readily incorporated into the care process for nursing intervention at appropriate times. Problems that are unrelated to the current hospitalization, but may hamper health, can be addressed. The plan of care can evolve over time, as in Problem 3. By initial planning (see Fig. 3-3) and continued planning in the progress notes (see Fig. 3-4), plans for discharge can be made before the day of discharge. Discharge outcomes can be identified early on the basis of admission data (see Fig. 3-3, Initial Plan—Expected Outcomes).

This record system does not automatically ensure superb nursing care or make everyone an excellent practitioner. It is a tool with which comprehensiveness, continuity, and quality can be promoted and more easily evaluated. Staff development is needed to help groups of nurses with a variety of abilities to use the record system more effectively for patients' benefit and their own professional and clinical development.

Articulation of problem lists and summaries of acute and long-term problems and hospital and primary care settings are goals that are essential for patient care continuity. For effective implementation of the nursing care plans written in the problem-oriented record, nurses also must write on the Kardex the plans that others are to follow. Traditionally, this information was written on the temporary record, the Kardex. With the problem-oriented system the reverse may be seen—the plan is entered only in the permanent record and not placed on the Kardex daily working records.

The major benefit of instituting the problem-oriented nursing record forms is that the system will require all nurses to collect and interpret data, develop nursing care plans, evaluate the outcome of the plans, and document their use of the nursing process. It is a dynamic process with ongoing assessment and planning.

In some hospital settings, a decision might be made to set some minimal expectations for all nurses and request the nurse or nurses with the most effective assessment skills and the best clinical judgment to begin the process by doing the initial assessment, problem identification, and planning. All nurses would contribute from that point in implementing the plan and documenting patient response in the progress notes. Most decisions are then being made by the most clinically expert nurses.

The nurses who developed the nursing care documentation system described here are experiencing the rewards of writing the data in the "Resolved" column on the problem list, knowing by documented evidence that patients have progressed because of planned nursing intervention and because follow-up was possible without dependence on an olympian memory (see Problem 5 in Figs. 3-1 and 3-3). Another benefit that is occurring is the potential for examining patient outcomes in relation to the interventions. The ability to audit nursing records is an important step in making possible the establishment and evaluation of standards of nursing care in terms of patient outcomes and in facilitating clinical nursing research.

NURSING DIAGNOSES   The benefits of consistency in terminology in problem lists for the problem-oriented record have been discussed. The need and potential benefits of consistent terminology for nursing diagnosis are multiple for the nursing profession. The development of standard nomenclature and the classification of nursing diagnoses are the goals of the National Group for the Classification of Nursing Diagnoses [16].

The step involved in the generation and classification of nursing diagnoses are: (1) identify all those conditions that nurses locate or diagnose in clients/patients; (2) reach some agreement about consistent nomenclature for the findings identified in step one; (3) group the identified diagnoses (the labels) into classes and subclasses so that patterns and relationships among them can emerge [8].

The definition of nursing diagnosis utilized by the First National Conference on Classification of Nursing Diagnoses was: "the judgement or conclusion which occurs as a result of nursing assessment" [8]. This was viewed as the end point of nursing assessment and a starting point for nursing intervention.

The Third National Conference on Classification of Nursing Diagnoses identified the components of a nursing diagnosis to be (1) the label, (2) defining characteristics, and (3) etiologic factors. An example of a nursing diagnosis follows [16].

ALTERATION IN COMFORT: PAIN

A. ETIOLOGY
  1. Injuring agents
     a. Biologic
     b. Chemical
     c. Physical
     d. Psychologic
B. DEFINING CHARACTERISTICS
  1. Subjective
     a. Communication (verbal or coded) of pain descriptors
  2. Objective
     a. Guarding behavior—protective
     b. Self-focusing
     c. Narrowed focus
        (1) Altered time perception
        (2) Withdrawal from social contact
        (3) Impaired thought process
     d. Distraction behavior
        (1) Moaning
        (2) Crying

(3) Pacing

(4) Seeks out other people and/or activities

(5) Restless

e. Facial mask of pain

(1) Eyes—lackluster, "beaten look," fixed or scattered movement

(2) Grimace

f. Alteration in muscle tone

(1) May span from listless to rigid

g. Autonomic responses (these signs are not seen in chronic stable pain)

(1) Diaphoresis

(2) Bp and P increases or decreases

(3) Pupillary dilation

(4) Increased or decreased respiratory rate

The generation of nursing diagnoses is the domain of all professional nurses. The activity is inherent in the role of the professional nurse. The most recent compilation of agreed upon nursing diagnoses and nomenclature is the work of the Third National Conference for the Classification of Nursing Diagnoses, April 1978. This can be obtained and/or diagnoses submitted for discussion through the Clearinghouse for Nursing Diagnoses [16].

The lack of a taxonomy of nursing diagnoses is a restraint for nursing research and nursing quality assurance activities. There have been no universally accepted labels and defining characteristics of a particular diagnosis for data collection across time, care provider, and care settings. Neither has there been a coding system for patient record retrieval by nursing diagnoses. Record retrieval for a particular patient population is by medical diagnoses and code numbers.

The medical profession has been approximately 300 years in developing the medical diagnoses and classification system. It is anticipated that the nursing profession will proceed with remarkable speed in comparison, given the technologic advances for information processing.

The Standards for Nursing Practice of the ANA state that nursing diagnoses are derived from health status data [1]. Problems identification is an integral component of POR systems. These two movements require daily application of and experience with nursing diagnoses. Drawing from this experience will strengthen the labeling and classifying process.

STANDARD NURSING CARE PLANS
The standard nursing care plan (SNCP) is a protocol for nursing care of large numbers of patients with the same diagnosis or condition. It defines the problems common to the population, the expected patient outcomes of the nursing care, the frequency for evaluating and documenting, and the nursing activities to achieve the expected outcomes. Thus, the SNCP is: the framework in which individualized nursing care is planned; a mechanism for orienting new nursing

personnel to expected standards of nursing care; and an effective tool for the provision and evolution of quality nursing care.

SNCP are developed by nurses knowledgeable in the care of specific patient populations. The plans are based on clinical expertise and nursing research. Key nursing activities and patient outcomes are extracted from the SNCP and utilized in developing quality assurance criteria. The SNCP nursing orders for respiratory congestion problem #3 (Fig. 3-7) are the same as the Critical Preventive Management factors on the Criteria Set (see Fig. 3-9). The three discharge criteria on both the SNCP and the criteria set are exactly the same. The SNCP example for a hospitalized patient (Fig. 3-7) utilizes Mayers' format [12].

Quality Assurance   Quality assurance is the establishment of standards of good or excellent care and the taking of steps to ensure that this level of care is consistently reached [10]. There are two parts to the definition, establishment of good care and taking steps for consistent achievement of good care. Quality assurance is the assurance of quality to the consumer.

The American Nurses Association quality assurance model (Fig. 3-8) consists of seven segments. The first two (Identify Values and Identify Standards & Criteria) segments relate to the first part of the definition, and the remaining five steps relate to the taking of steps for consistent delivery of good care.

Once values, criteria, and standards are identified for a specific population, data must be collected to compare actual performance with expected standards. Strengths and weaknesses are analyzed from the data secured. Corrective action is planned to increase strengths and overcome deficiencies. Once the deficiencies have been corrected, nursing care for that patient population is reaudited, using essentially the same criteria. The results of the reaudit should show improvement. Correction of deficiencies and periodic reaudits are essential for *assuring* quality care.

Health can be evaluated from three perspectives, that is, the focus of the criteria used to measure performance can be: (1) the structure of the health care delivery system (the institution is the subject); (2) the process of the health care delivery itself (the provider is the subject); (3) the outcome of the health care delivery for the client/patient, as demonstrated by a measurable change in the state of the client's health (the client/patient is the subject) [7]. An example of each criterion follows:

Structure—The nursing department shall be directed by a qualified nurse administrator.
Process—The patient is taught steps of ostomy care.
Outcome—The patient demonstrates steps of ostomy care.

Several criteria, judged to be reflective of successful nursing care, are identified for the selected patient population. Nurses directly involved in the provision

Figure 3-7.
Standard nursing care plan
for patient having lumbar
laminectomy.

| STANDARD NURSING CARE PLAN FOR* Lumbar laminectomy for disc, tumor, trauma |
| Postoperative period |

DISCHARGE CRITERIA: 1. Patient performs ADL (activities of daily living) independently.
2. Verbalizes alterations in life style related to status of back.
3. States at least 2 principles of correct body mechanics.

Date	Usual Problems	Expected Outcomes	Deadlines	Nursing Orders
Post-op	1. Impaired mobility related to pain, stiffness and muscle spasms from surgery	Initiates moving about in bed Ambulate to bathroom with increasing ambulation to a minimum 3 × day without assistance Increasing independence in ADL and independent by 5th postop day Verbalizes reasonable comfort	(√ qd) Postop day 2 Postop day 5 (√ qs)	1A. Instruct, assist (prn), remind pt. to: a. Log roll q 2 hrs. b. Exercise: active ROM isometrics q 1-2 hrs. c. OOB qid with increasing time span each day (unless 1B occurs) d. Request and use analgesics freely first few days to decrease pain and increase mobility 1B. Flat in bed for 4 days if dura entered so dura can seal and heal (if occurs, add 4 days to deadline for outcome 2 and 3)
	2. Potential wound complications A. Wound infection	Dressing dry and intact Afebrile	(√ q8°) Sutures removed (√ qd) Dischg.	2A. If any drainage, reinforce dressing with sterile ABD and report immediately a. Temp q 4 hrs. × 48 hrs. then q shift b. Keep dressing dry and intact until sutures removed c. No tub bath or shower until sutures removed
	B. Spinal fluid leak with possible meningitis	Early detection and prompt treatment for leakage received Clear sensorium	(√ qd) Ongoing and dischg.	2B. Observe for halo sign on dressing or linens a. double ring effect from blood and spinal fluid b. report signs of meningitis STAT: fever spike, headache, lethargy, nuchal rigidity
	3. Potential respiratory congestion related to post-anesthesia and decreased mobility	Breath sounds clear if no underlying respiratory disease Afebrile	(√ qs) Postop day 3	3A. Temp q 4 hrs. × 48 hrs. then q shift 3B. C & DB q 2° for 24 hrs. then while awake if temp 99.6 (o). If temp 100.6° awaken q 2° to C & DB.

*This care plan to be adapted for the individual patient and to be compatible with the physician's orders.
Developed: Date: May 1975   Unit: Neuro
　　　　　Persons: Van Meter, Peters
Revised: 2/77 J. Cantor, A. DeLane, A. Louks, K. Swenson
　　　　　Nursing Services
　　　　　University Hospital
　　　　　Ann Arbor, Michigan

of care identify the criteria for measurement of care. Outcome criteria that is intended to measure quality of nursing care should be measurable by nurses, influenced at least in part by nursing care, and be realistic based on the available resources.

Quality assurance criteria specify the patient population, the measurable criteria, the point at which measurement of achievement is to occur, how and when the measurement is to be done. The point in time for achievement may be:

Figure 3-8.
Quality assurance model.
(Copyrighted by the
American Nurses'
Association and used with
permission.)

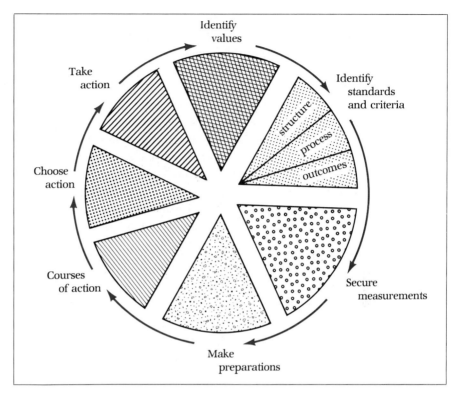

Admission—defined time during period of admission.
Interim—defined time during period of care.
Discharge—at the time of discharge from care.

The data may be obtained by direct observation, patient opinion (interview or questionnaire), or auditing of patients' records. The data retrieval may be done concurrently (while care is being given), or retrospectively (review after care is completed and the patient is discharged).

Currently the trend is to use process and outcome discharge criteria evaluated by the retrospective chart audit method.

The aggregate data from repeated measurements of quality assurance criteria in a variety of locations is needed to establish standards. A standard is the range of acceptable variation from achievement of a criterion. It is a percentage; what percentage must be achieved and in what percentage of situations is it acceptable to fall short of the criterion. The ANA Standards of Nursing Practice use the word standard to mean a declarative statement, not a range of achievement [1-3].

Professional accountability and the desire for self-regulation on the part of individual nurses and the professional nursing organizations; consumer demand for cost effective care; government requirement especially for Professional

Services Review Organizations to assure quality health care for recipients of Medicare, Medicaid, and Maternal Child Health Programs; corporate liability; insurance companies; and the Joint Commission for Accreditation of Hospitals have all had a major role in highlighting the necessity of quality assurance programs.

An individual nurse can apply quality assurance concepts in his/her own practice and accountability behaviors [13]. The ANA Standards, particularly the specialty standards, can be used for measuring one's own practice. Quality Assurance materials available from the ANA are listed in the references [1-5]. The expected outcomes and nursing orders of SNCP or some individually developed criteria would also be appropriate. Sharing the activity of evaluating one's practice with just one colleague is the beginning of peer review. These activities would evolve an experience base from which wider ranging quality assurance efforts could grow.

Three major aspects of the person, the recipient of care, are to be considered when identifying criteria. The three areas are the person's health status, adaptive behaviors, and knowledge and skill for self-care [10]. Audit a few patients' charts and determine if these three major areas were considered when assessing, intervening, and documenting.

Several criteria for a specific patient population form what is commonly called a criteria set. The criteria set defines the audit topic or patient population, the elements to be measured, any exceptions to achievement, complications, critical management of complications, and instructions for data retrieval. An example of a patient outcome at hospital discharge retrospective chart audit is shown in Figure 3-9.

RELATIONSHIP OF NURSING DIAGNOSIS, SNCP, QA CRITERIA, AND POR COMPONENTS

There are corresponding relationships in the components of the four nursing practice tools discussed. Sometimes there is exact duplication of components, such as process criteria and nursing orders or expected outcomes and outcome criteria. This duplication causes nurses who are learning POR documentation, SNCP development, and QA criteria identification to view them as redundant activities. Each has a distinct purpose (Fig. 3-10). A clear concept of the purpose of each and what components correspond (Fig. 3-11) help the nurse with abilities in utilizing one tool to apply those abilities in the development of the other tools. Nurses have quickly identified QA from SNCP criteria and, conversely, have used a criteria set as the basis for developing a SNCP.

An area that is commonly neglected, as demonstrated by chart audit results, is the adaptive behavior (psychosocial-spiritual status) of the patient. The *Subjective* component and patient *Education* component of POR progress notes provide nurses with the potential (if disciplined in using POR) for planning, delivering, and documenting objective and subjective results of care and for having continuous validation from the recipient of the care. Improved care that is documented yields improved audit results.

Figure 3-9.
Nursing care quality assurance discharge criteria set for patient having lumbar laminectomy.

Criteria Set for: Nursing   Lumbar Laminectomy

Elements	Standard 100%	0%	Exceptions	Instructions and Definitions for Data Retrieval
Discharge Status				
1. Patient performs ADL independently	√		1. Any presurgical limitation in ADL or ambulation not related to surgery	1. ADL: Personal hygiene: Eating, feeding self, dressing, and ambulating independently Discharge summary (DS) Nurses' notes (NN) Clinical parameter sheet (CPS)
2. Patient and/or s.o. verbalizes alterations in life-style related to status of back	√		2. Transferred to extended care facility	2. Patient education sheet DS NN CPS Restrictions in life-style (any two) a. Occupational limitation b. Sexual c. No lifting or pulling d. No driving e. Climbing stairs Other adjustments a. Verbalization of fears and anxiety b. Planning for future c. Complying with restrictions in hospital d. Utilization of resource people (social workers; nurses; family; friends)
3. Patient and/or s.o. states at least two principles of correct body mechanics	√			3. Patient education sheet—Note: "Care of the Back" given to patient for reference, and patient can state any 2 principles in book. DS, NN

Elements	Standard 100%	0%	Critical Preventive and Responsive Management	Instructions and Definitions for Data Retrieval
Complications				
1. Wound infection		√	1. (P) a. Keep wound clean and dry b. √ dressing q shift c. Observe for signs of infections d. Temp q 4 hrs. for first 48 then q shift (R) a. Report to MD signs of infection b. Wound care per MD order (either soaks or irrigation) c. Temp. q 4 hrs. for temp < 100.5° (o) Temp q 2 hrs. for temp > 100.5° (o) d. Administer antibiotics per MD order	1. Signs of infection a. Redness, tenderness, warmth, drainage b. CPS c. NN d. Graphic sheets e. Med. sheets
2. Resp. congestion		√	2. (P) a. C & DB or incentive spirometer q 2 hrs. for 1st 24 then to q 4 hrs. when awake	2. a. NN or CPS b. NN–Status of BS

Figure 3-9.
Continued.

Complications	Standard 100% 0%	Critical Preventive and Responsive Management	Instructions and Definitions for Data Retrieval
		b. Auscultate breath sounds at least q. s. × 48 hrs.	
		c. Turn q 2 hrs. in bed	c. NN–CPS
		d. Dangle or OOB at bedside 1st postop night, then q shift at least in chair	d. NN–CPS
		e. Monitor TPR q 4 hrs. × 48, then q shift	e. NN–CPS graphic sheet
		(R) a. C & DB or incentive spirometer q 2 hrs, awaken during night	a. NN–CPS
		b. Blow bottles or incentive spirometer per MD order	b. NN–CPS
		c. IT sx per MD order	c. NN–CPS and graphic sheet
		d. Temp q 2 hrs if increase > 100.6°	
		e. Antibiotics per MD order	
		f. Auscultate BS q 2 hrs.	
3. Urinary retention	√	3. (P) a. Initiate measures to promote voiding within 4 hrs after return from PARU	3. a. Measures to promote voiding 1. Stand to void (if dura was not opened) 2. Running water 3. Provide privacy NN
		b. Maintain adequate hydration	b. At least 2000 cc/24 hrs. I & O sheet
		c. Monitor I & O for 48 hrs. postop	c. I & O sheet
		(R) a. If no void by 8 hrs postPARU, contact MD	a. NN & MD orders
		b. Catheterize per MD order	b. NN & MD orders
		c. Continue to monitor I & O until problem resolved	c. I & O sheet and problem list

Figure 3-10.
Purpose of nursing diagnoses, standard nursing care plans (SNCP), problem-oriented records (POR), and quality assurance (QA) criteria.

Nursing Diagnosis	*SNCP*	*POR*	*QA Criteria*
Label for organized planning, documentation, and evaluation of care	Care planning and delivery for recipients with common problems	Documentation of care planned, delivered and response for the individual recipient	Evaluation of care delivered and results achieved for a group of recipients

Figure 3-11.
The relationship of
components of SNCP, QA
criteria, and POR.

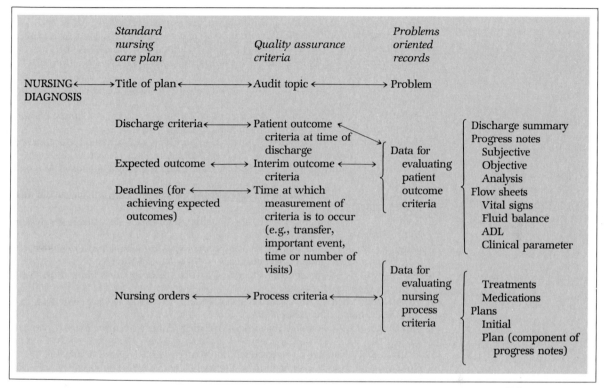

CONCLUSION AND CHALLENGE

The professionalization of nursing requires the continuous utilization of a scientific process. The nursing process is a problem-solving process, a scientific process. All of the tools and processes discussed aid in one or more of the following: collecting data, formulating decisions, planning interventions, taking action, or evaluating results—some phase of the nursing process. Nurses are enhancing their use of the nursing process by utilization of the tools and processes discussed here. Readers are challenged to identify process and outcome criteria with and for the recipients of their care and then to take steps to see that the criteria are consistently reached. The nursing practice tools described in this chapter will facilitate achievement of this level of accountability.

REFERENCES

1. *ANA Standards Nursing Practice.* Kansas City, Mo.: ANA, 1973.
2. *ANA Standards Gerontological Nursing Practice.* Kansas City, Mo.: ANA, 1976.
   ANA Standards Maternal Child Health Nursing Practice. Kansas City, Mo.: ANA, 1973.
   ANA Standard Medical Surgical Nursing Practice. Kansas City, Mo.: ANA, 1974.

ANA Standard Psychiatric Mental Health Nursing Practice. Kansas City, Mo.: ANA, 1973.

3. *ANA Standards of Cardiovascular Nursing Practice.* Kansas City, Mo.: ANA, 1975.
   ANA Standards of Neurological and Neurosurgical Nursing Practice. Kansas City, Mo.: ANA, 1977.
   ANA Standards of Orthopedic Nursing Practice. Kansas City, Mo.: ANA, 1975.
   ANA Standards of Rehabilitation Nursing Practice. Kansas City, Mo.: ANA, 1977.
   ANA Standards of Urologic Nursing Practice. Kansas City, Mo.: ANA, 1977.

4. *ANA A Plan for Implementation of the Standards of Nursing Practice.* Kansas City, Mo.: ANA, 1975.

5. *ANA Congress on Nursing Practice. Quality Assurance Update.* ANA 2420 Pershing Road, Kansas City, Mo. 64108.

6. Becknell, E. P., and Smith, D. M. *System of Nursing Practice: A Clinical Nursing Assessment Tool.* Philadelphia: Davis Co., 1975.

7. Donabedian, A. *Medical Care Appraisal—Quality and Utilization.* In *Guide to Medical Care Administration.* Vol. II. New York: Am. Pub. Health Assoc., 1969.

8. Gebbie, K. M., and Lavin, M. A. (Eds.). *Classifying Nursing Diagnosis.* St. Louis: Mosby, 1975.

9. Goldfinger, S. E. The problem-oriented record: A critique from a believer. *N. Engl. J. Med.* 288:606, 1973.

10. Hoover, J. and Zimmer, M. Nursing Quality Assurance—the Wisconsin System. *Nurs. Outlook,* Apr.: 242, 1978.

11. Lang, N. *Are Professional Nurses Ready for a Quality Assurance Program?* N.Y. State Nurses Association Convention Papers, 5:24–32, 1974 (a).

12. Mayers, M. G. *A Systematic Approach to the Nursing Care Plan.* New York: Appleton-Century-Crofts, 1972.

13. *MNA Standards for Professional Nursing Practice For Field Testing Only.* East Lansing, Mi.: Mich. Nurs. Assoc., 1976.

14. Mundinger, M. O. Nursing Diagnoses for Cancer Patients. *Cancer Nurs.* June: 221, 1978.

15. McCain, R. F. Nursing by assessment, not intuition. *Am. J. Nurs.* 65:82, 1965.

16. *National Group for Classification of Nursing Diagnosis.* St. Louis: Saint Louis University School of Nursing, 3525 Caroline Street, Rm 439, St. Louis, Missouri 63104.

17. Phaneuf, M. C. *The Nursing Audit Self Regulation in Nursing Practice* (2nd Ed.). New York: Appleton-Century-Crofts, 1976.

18. Stevens, B. J. Why won't nurses write nursing care plans? *J. Nurs. Adm.* 2:66, 1972.

19. Weed, L. Medical records that guide and teach. *N. Engl. J. Med.* 278:593, 1968.

4. The Use of Computers and Decision Theory to Enhance and Measure the Effectiveness of Nursing Assessment

AS the nursing profession moves more and more into the practice of clinical assessment methods such as physical assessment, it also becomes responsible for both *assessing the accuracy* and *improving the effectiveness* of those methods. The critical nature of these requirements for the profession of nursing is clear when we consider present shortages in health care manpower and ever-increasing health care costs. With the nurse performing physical assessment, she will be initiating a great many health services, and thus the costs of health care incurred by consumers will depend on the effectiveness of her decisions. If nurses as physical assessment practitioners are not trained to weigh the costs against the benefits or potential effectiveness of treatments, their assessments will operate in an economic vacuum and help only to further accelerate the rising costs of health care. In addition, if nursing is to assess the effectiveness of its assessment role accurately, it must do so within the full context of the whole health care system. That is, the effectiveness of nursing assessment is dependent on what happens to the patient and on the decisions made by the nurse about the patient after the assessment is made. If the patient does not properly follow the decisions made by the nurse, or if the next health care professional in the patient's path through the health care system does not maximally utilize the decisions made and information gathered by the nurse, the effectiveness of those nursing decisions will certainly be reduced. All these requirements for assessing and improving the effectiveness of nurse decision-making then require some technology and some expertise in applying it.

Because of the relative youth of the physical assessment role as a major role for nursing, one would expect that a whole new area of research need be established to do these things. This is only true to the extent that for nursing per se, research in the area of physical assessment effectiveness (PAE) is underdeveloped. On the other hand, medicine has been in the business of diagnosis for many years, and humanity has been engaged in decision-making for a much longer period. From these endeavors has developed a vast resource of technology and research in the general area of measuring and improving the effectiveness of decision-making and diagnosis. Drawing on these resources, an attempt will be made here to provide for nursing a review of these tools and how they apply to physical assessment. These tools include *decision theory, operations research, bayesian models of decision-making, sequential decision-*

making, multiphasic screening, cost/benefit and *cost/effectiveness analysis, the psychology of decision-making and information processing in general,* and the most important development of technology, *the computer.* In this chapter, a brief tutorial on the areas of technology will be provided, and their application to nursing assessment will be interpreted. Finally, relevant research into health care decision-making using these tools will be briefly cited.

COMPUTERS AND THEIR LANGUAGES

In the main, human physical characteristics are virtually universal in their similarity, regardless of geographic location. Thus the material in this book relating to these characteristics should be usable anywhere in the English-speaking world. Unfortunately, computers and their languages (programs or software) are not so universally similar. Though the machines (hardware) are becoming ubiquitous, several of their characteristics, especially their software, prevent any large degree of universality. Just as all Fords are not alike, and all Ford Pintos are not the same, all IBMs and all IBM 370s are not the same. However, the problem with the computer is still worse. While anyone who can drive a Ford Pinto can probably drive *any* Ford Pinto regardless of options, anyone who can use an IBM 370 cannot necessarily use *any* IBM 370. There are many models of the 370, none of which are alike (as, for example, are two Pintos that differ only in trim), since their options (peripherals) often are a mix of models, and manufacturers make them so different that each behaves like a totally unique machine.

The even greater diversity in software complicates the problem further. An IBM 370 model 145 in Detroit may "speak" a language different from that of the same model in Ann Arbor, only 40 miles away, because it has been programmed differently. (This is greatly oversimplified, since general-purpose computers often use several languages and often do so simultaneously, or in a very short period [microseconds] of time). However, the computer systems used in health care settings usually are not what one would call general purpose systems. The problem is further exacerbated by the fact that computer languages with the same name often have several versions, depending on when they were created, what type of machine they were written for, and the specific local variations in use when they were first written. Even the most universal languages (e.g., FORTRAN) have local variations that can be crucial in some computer applications. All these variations put us in a position analogous to our not being able to drive any other car than our own, even if it looks just like our own, without substantial training. This chapter will not and could not teach you how to use "the computer" (which should now clearly be seen as an imprecise term) for physical assessment or any other problems. As Judge and Zuidema [13] state: "You cannot learn it in the library. You must do it at the bedside." Just as this book cannot adequately transmit the behavioral skills in physical assessment neither can it transmit computer usage skills at the practice level. Rather, the purpose of this chapter is to inform, raise problems, and suggest solutions to the overlap of roles for computers, physical assessment, and clinical information processing in general and specifically for nursing.

Rather than leave the impression that this chapter will discuss several tools that you cannot use because of the lack of a universal language for computers, one can take comfort in the knowledge that computers are now speaking English or at least a rigid dialect of English. Further, one need not be a highly trained programmer to use a computer. Increasing numbers of applications involve "conversational" programs, ones that allow neophyte users to conduct a dialogue with the computer in English. Once you learn how to turn on the machine or "sign on" the computer (identify yourself to the computer as a valid user), usually taking a minute or so, many computer systems will teach you how to use the program you want to use.

COMPUTER ROLES IN NURSING ASSESSMENT

The computer currently has several primary roles in evaluating and enhancing nurse assessment: computer-assisted instruction in diagnosis and basic processes and functions; computer-aided decision-making (especially diagnosis); computer-aided analysis of research data (e.g., the assessment process); and finally, computer-aided management of clinical information. The computer also plays a plethora of auxiliary roles that affect the nursing assessment role, and these will be mentioned in passing. It will be noted as well that the functions of the computer in nursing closely follow the research, practice, learning (teaching), and administrative roles of nursing.

Jacquez [12] is the preeminent resource for all readers interested in pursuing in depth the state of the art of research into computer-aided diagnosis. Another book, particularly useful for hospital applications, is that of Lindberg [17]. Finally, the *Journal of Clinical Computing* is a continuous resource of information in this area.

Computer-Aided Data Analysis

Of all the "computer applications" in nursing assessment, computer-aided data analysis is probably the least often applied, since the clinical nursing role has typically involved little research, formal or otherwise. In the main, only nurse researchers, especially in the academic setting, are likely to use the computer-aided data analysis function. This is unfortunate, since it is precisely this ability of the computer to converse with the nurse (as a neophyte computer user) that makes it a useful tool in applied nursing settings. Figure 4-1 shows an example of an interaction between a nurse and a computer produced by a nurse researcher using a computer terminal in the University of Michigan School of Nursing Computer Laboratory. This figure demonstrates the application of conversational computing to the area of statistical analysis. It is clear that a dialog is occurring (all of the nurse's entries are underlined for purposes of illustra-

Figure 4-1. Conversational computer print-out from the University of Michigan Statistical Research Laboratory Midas Program. User's entries are underlined for purposes of illustration.

```
GO
MTS (LA01-0036)
WHO ARE YOU?

#          $COPY  *CCHOURS
#$SIGNON K1U3
#ENTER USER PASSWORD.
?███████████
#JOB-TYPE=TERMINAL, PRIO=NORMAL, CLASS=UNIV/GOVT
#**LAST SIGNON WAS: 14:03.18
# USER "K1U3" SIGNED ON AT  14:10.12 ON FRI AUG 23/74
#$RUN STAT:MIDAS
#EXECUTION BEGINS


  M I D A S
  STATISTICAL RESEARCH LABORATORY
  UNIVERSITY OF MICHIGAN
  14:11.56
  AUG 23, 1974




  COMMAND
?READ INTERNAL FILE=ALL30
  VARIABLES TO READ (E.G., 1-10)
?ALL


  READ OBSERVATIONS
  FROM INTERNAL FILE

     33 CASES READ FOR   96 VARIABLES


  COMMAND
?HISTOGRAM OPTION=HIST%
  VARIABLE(S) FOR HISTOGRAM/FREQUENCY
?8
  INTERVAL EXPRESSION -- #INT:(MIN,MAX)  (MIN,MAX)/WIDTH  #PER/(MIN,MAX)
?/500


  HISTOGRAM/FREQUENCIES

  MIDPOINT   HIST%  COUNT FOR ME9MATP$     (EACH X =1)

    9450.0    8.0    2 +XX
    9950.0    0.     0 +
   10450.     8.0    2 +XX
   10950.    16.0    4 +XXXX
   11450.    12.0    3 +XXX
   11950.    16.0    4 +XXXX
   12450.    20.0    5 +XXXXX
   12950.     8.0    2 +XX
   13450.     4.0    1 +X
   13950.     0.     0 +
   14450.     0.     0 +
   14950.     0.     0 +
   15450.     4.0    1 +X
   15950.     4.0    1 +X

  MISSING           8
  TOTAL            33  ( 500.00   = INTERVAL WIDTH)
```

Figure 4-2.
Example of a computer-
produced histogram.

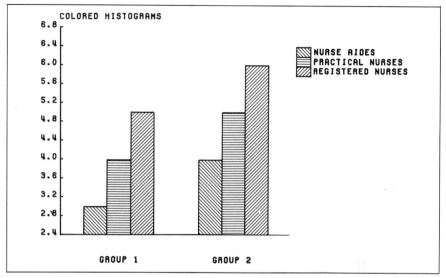

tion) because of the obvious two-way interactive nature of the "conversation." Figure 4-2 shows an example of a figure produced by a nurse in the nursing computer laboratory in order to illustrate a particular clinical phenomenon. This figure was produced in less than two minutes of the nurse's time for a cost of less than five dollars and is in a form that is camera ready for publication in any medium. It is clear, then, that a substantial amount of computer technology is now available to nurses (at least those in an academic setting) for the purpose of analyzing and displaying clinical data. That is, since more data will be generated and available as the computer becomes ubiquitous in various nursing settings, with the expansion of nursing roles such as assessment, it will then become imperative, as well as easier, for nurses to analyze those data in order to monitor and enhance the effectiveness of nursing procedures.

The convenience of the computer as a tool further amplifies its utility. A computer terminal* is likely to become *the* essential tool of nursing, more used than charts, Kardex, or stethoscopes, and it will be used multifunctionally, not in just one, but in all of the roles mentioned. Through one terminal, nurses should be able, for example, to retrieve and analyze data, or engage in self-instruction in any area of nursing. More precisely, the nurse should be able to converse with several computer systems, depending on which function or combinations of functions are needed at a particular moment.

---

*A computer terminal is essentially just a typewriter-like keyboard and some display device, such as a printer or a video screen, that allows two-way communication between a user and a computer by telephone or other communications line (see Fig. 4-4).

**Computer-Assisted
Instruction**

As nursing moves into the assessment role, a substantial educational effort will have evolved out of the need to develop these skills on a profession-wide basis. This book is obviously one part of that effort. Because most of this training will be in-service, because a great deal of instructional technology is available to help develop assessment skills, and finally because of the likely availability of the computer at nursing stations and in other nursing environments, the "computer-as-teacher" role can be useful to nursing.

A computer network for instruction in the health professions, one that is readily accessible and usable by telephone from anywhere in the United States and elsewhere, is the Health Education Network Users Groups (HENUG) of the Association for the Development of Computer-Based Instruction Systems (AD-CIS). It links the vast resources of Massachusetts General Hospital (MGH) Computer Science Laboratory and Ohio State University Medical Center to users of the network. Figure 4-3 shows an MGH program for instruction in cardiopulmonary resuscitation, a simulated encounter with a patient who has had cardiopulmonary failure of some sort, a patient who could "die" before you on the computer terminal unless proper action were taken. It is this kind of patient-encounter simulation which typifies the reality orientation of the MGH programs and which makes them so effective instructionally. This technique could certainly be applied to nursing assessment. Most of the programs give either a running account of the effectiveness of an action or a diagnosis or a recapitulation in full detail after the encounter is over. Currently, some nursing assessment programs are being developed by the nursing staff at the MGH Computer Science Laboratory.

The programs at Ohio State University are more numerous and more traditional in subject matter and approach, comprising somewhat less than 100 programs in such basic sciences as pathology and histology, as well as in applied clinical instruction. Some of these programs are more than 10 hours long, allowing users to leave and return days or hours later and begin where they left off. One could easily obtain an extensive education in the health sciences with this resource. Another program on the Ohio State system is CASE, developed at the University of Illinois Medical Center at Chicago, a computer-aided simulation of a patient encounter which allows the user to type in free-format English as though she were speaking normally with the patient. This is currently a useful approach, but the free-format English gives an illusion of reality at the expense of the richness of a real patient encounter. Nevertheless, this is another instructional technique from which nursing appraisal could easily gain.

Few of these programs are designed specifically for nurses, although their content and style certainly make most of them useful for nursing. Also, many other institutions have computer-assisted instruction in the health sciences. PLATO system, developed at the University of Illinois in conjunction with the Control Data Corporation, also has a wide distribution and many applications

Figure 4-3.
Three different segments of
a student's interaction with
the Massachusetts General
Hospital Computer
Laboratory
cardiopulmonary
resuscitation program.
User's entries are
underlined for purposes of
illustration.

THE PATIENT IS AN 81-YEAR OLD MAN WHO IS 2 DAYS POST CATARACT EXTRACTION.
YOU ARE A STAT CONSULT BECAUSE THE PATIENT DOES NOT LOOK RIGHT.
   WHAT DO YOU DO FIRST?

1. TAKE AN EKG
2. START AN IV
3. CHECK MAJOR VESSELS FOR PULSES, SEE IF PATIENT IS RESPONSIVE
4. GIVE A SHOT OF INTRACARDIAC EPINEPHRINE

>1

   THAT WILL TAKE SEVERAL MINUTES ASSUMING YOU HAVE AN EKG MACHINE IN THE ROOM AND LONGER IF YOU HAVE TO GET ONE. . . . . .
THE PATIENT, IF TRULY ARRESTED, WILL BE BEYOND RESUSCITATION BY THE TIME YOU DOCUMENT THE FACT.

....

   THE BICARB IS RUNNING. NOW IT IS TIME TO TRY SOME SPECIFICS. LET'S TAKE A LOOK AT THE PATIENT'S RHYTHM.

THE RHYTHM STRIP IS SHOWN ON PAGE 6; IS THIS

1. VENTRICULAR FIBRILLATION
2. VENTRICULAR TACHYCARDIA
3. SLOW IDIOVENTRICULAR RHYTHM
4. ELECTROMECHANICAL DISSOCIATION

>2

   CORRECT. NOTE THAT IT COULD ALSO BE THE SINE WAVE OF HYPERKALEMIA, A CHOICE YOU WERE NOT OFFERED.

....

   THE FIRST SHOCK TOOK YOU FROM V TACH TO VF SO AN IMMEDIATE RESHOCK IS REASONABLE, IN FACT. . .

   A FEW SECONDS OF ASYSTOLE. . .
THEN GOES TO THE RHYTHM SHOWN ON PAGE 3.
WHAT WOULD YOU LIKE TO DO. . .

1. DEFIBRILLATE AGAIN
2. GIVE 1 MG EPINEPHRINE IV, MASSAGE, THEN SHOCK
3. START A LIDOCAINE DRIP THEN SHOCK

>3

   THAT MAY WORK, THOUGH IN THE SETTING OF FINE FIBRILLATION MY FIRST CHOICE WOULD HAVE BEEN EPI. THE XYLOCAINE IS RUNNING AT 4 MG/MIN, SHOCK, AND. . .

in nursing education [3]. Brigham et al. [4] have published a complete compendium of available programs, and those interested should read the volume and contact the relevant institution or Robert Votaw, HENUG coordinator at the University of Connecticut Health Center, Farmington, Conn. 06032 (telephone 203-674-2403).

Computer-Guided Assessment

The computer can also serve to its maximum potential in nursing assessment as an active aid in the assessment process, structuring and guiding the assessment process; helping nurses make decisions about the relative weights (costs, benefits) which should be applied to signs and symptoms; and helping to combine in the most effective way all the information the nurse obtains. There is strong research evidence to show that although humans may be effective in gathering information, their ability to combine that information efficiently is usually biased and conservative—conservative in the sense that they collect more information than is necessary to establish confident estimates about the likelihood of the events, processes, or functions in question. This evidence has tremendous implications for nursing assessment and for the usefulness of the computer in such assessment. Nursing can avail itself of the computer in structuring the assessment process from beginning to end: guiding the collecting of the data; helping to combine the data; and producing statistically likely diagnoses with estimates of confidence about those decisions. These programs can be based on the combined opinions of the experts in the different areas of assessment, or on existing data on the signs and symptoms usually associated with particular diagnoses, or on both. Whichever method is used, it must be made clear to nurses that the computer is a tool, not an obtrusive mechanical monster that will separate the nurse from the patient, patient care, and "true nursing"—a tool that allows the nurse to do a better, less expensive job in assessment and to spend *more time in direct patient care activities and less in paperwork.*

The current rapid development of computer technology in the areas of computer graphics and micro computing hold much promise for the development of computer-assisted physical assessment. The current rapid development of inexpensive micro computer equipment available for less than $1000 for a self contained computer terminal with a micro computer in it can be expected to lead to the development of a great deal of computer assistance for health care delivery in even the most remote and least equipped sites. Because micro computers do not depend on a large centralized computer and since they are available for less than $1000 (sometimes less than $500), a great deal of independence and autonomy is afforded the micro computer user. Thus, today a nurse could go to a local retail computer store, purchase a micro computer with a terminal for about $500, and easily implement some of the existing computer programs written by nurses for assessment [10,16]. The technology of computer graphics also holds much promise for computer-assisted nursing assessment. There currently exists several graphics programs which display all or part of the human body in color on a graphics terminal with a light pen such that a nurse could utilize this hardware with the proper nursing assessment software to assist in the proper sequence and data collection during a physical assessment or after the occurrence of the assessment [20]. One could imagine a pair of nurse clinicians working as a team, one performing the physical assessment, the other sitting in front of a graphics terminal with a light pen indicating the direction and outcome of the physical as it occurs. Clearly the likelihood of occurrence of this image depends greatly upon the development of proper hardware and software by nursing for its activities as well as a thorough continuing program of research to determine whether the technology is indeed cost effective and cost beneficial to the patient, to nursing, and to the health care system.

Computer-Aided Nursing Diagnosis

Computer-aided diagnosis is now probably one of the least frequent yet most promising applications of computer technology in the health professions. Some reasons for its infrequent use are (1) resistance by health professionals, often because of a perceived threat to their professional territory; (2) the failure of many programs to utilize expert opinion based on past experience, in lieu of requiring years of patient data, which usually do not exist; (3) the failure of health professionals to develop a common computer language so that all parties, including the computer, can communicate; and finally, (4) the enormous stresses on the health care delivery system to *deliver* services in times of shortages rather than discovering ways to improve the delivery of those services. Again, the volume by Jacquez [12] is excellent in covering this problem area.

Two programs, written by nurses, are good examples of computer-aided nursing assessment. Lagina [16] has written a program that allows nurses to assess the anxiety level of preoperative surgical patients quickly. Goodwin and Edwards [10] have devised an extensive computer-aided nursing assessment program for appraisal of the skin, which conducts a conversational dialogue concerning all aspects of skin pathology and then displays a complete assessment for the patient. Unfortunately, these programs have yet to be fully adopted in any ongoing health care system. The problem seems to be that these programs are developed by nurses in academic settings, and implementing them in any existing health information system (HIS) is difficult. What is needed is a channel of communication between the nurses who write these programs and the people who design and implement HISs. Before readily available computer systems for appraisal, instruction, and so on, are found in most nursing settings, there will probably have to be economic justification for purchasing the expensive equipment needed. As nurses take a more active role in deciding the types, quality, and quantity of care, they will also become responsible for these decisions and thus be required to support them empirically.

Health Information Systems   Most of the applications discussed have been somewhat peripheral in terms of their immediate justifiability in reducing the costs of health care. There is, however, one application that stands an excellent chance for such justification, namely, the health information system as implemented in some large setting (e.g., community, hospital) and referred to earlier as "computer-assisted management of clinical information." Barker et al. [1] have prepared an excellent survey of the extent of the role of these systems in many nursing settings, which identifies the positive and negative attitudes of nurses toward these systems. This group defined a nursing application as [1]:

. . . a procedure which assists the nurse in decision-making via a systematic collection of data, and summarization of data utilizing electronic data processing as an interface. Development of [sic], is the responsibility of nursing with the assistance of EDP personnel. Nursing applications may fall into any one of five categories; i.e., patient centered, personnel centered, educational, research, and miscellaneous.

Notable is the distinction between personnel- and patient-centered systems— this is surely a sign of the influence of nursing. The earliest systems, often misnamed "health care" systems, were simply accounting systems primarily for bookkeeping (revealing the background of the system designers). Now that nursing is beginning to exert its influence on how these systems are built, we are beginning to see patient-oriented systems, designed to monitor and enhance health rather than fiscal integrity.

Also notable in this report are the new expanded nurse roles mentioned, e.g., "systems analyst nurse," "coordinator, computer nurse." Perhaps the designers of these systems are beginning to realize that the nurse is really at the center of the action and the major source of information about the patient and that, because of this, these systems should be oriented more toward nursing. Some of the advantages of such systems for nursing listed in the survey were [1]:

. . . "more complete and accessible information," "improved nursing assessment," "more time for patient care," "more time at bedside," "reduce non-nursing function," and "improved educational programs."

Some criticisms were [1]:

. . . "extensive training requirements," "adaptation to change," "computer oriented rather than patient oriented," "could limit creativity," "cost of system," "getting nurse away from patient care," and "implementation problems."

Obviously, computers appear to be a mixed blessing, but we can also see some contradictions that might imply that it depends on the specific nurse and the specific computer and how much each can change to work together. This will probably occur by necessity, since these systems appear to be an economic inevitability; therefore, nursing must see that computers perform the way nurses want them to. Wesseling [23] describes the automation of the nursing history and care plan, and Farlee and Goldstein [9] describe a role for nurses in implementing these systems. Both papers are suggested reading for those who may have to, or want to, perform such a role.

An ongoing system at the El Camino Hospital (453 beds), Mountain View, California, illustrates how one HIS works. Beginning in March, 1971, the directors of the hospital and the Technicon Medical Information Systems Corporation, also of Mountain View, signed a contract to design and implement probably the most extensive HIS of any hospital anywhere in the United States. The Technicon system, called MIS-I for *Medical Information System*, consists of eight basic subsystems:

1. *Admissions system* for immediate processing of admission data, including emergencies and outpatients, and patient and bed census data for location and utilization.
2. *Pharmacy system* for automated medications due list, review of past and current medication orders, with the options for unit dose, label generation, prescription records, and billing.
3. *Nursing system* which eliminates manual processing of requisitions, Kardex, charge slips, and most paperwork. It also allows patient care planning and nursing notes, with instant production of patient status, location, history, and so on.
4. *Business office system* for the standard patient billing, accounts receivable, payroll, and other fiscal functions.
5. *Physician system* which allows instant retrieval of current orders and their completion status, test results, prestored personal order sets, and immediate access to patient data in convenient format.
6. *Radiology system* for automatic prep orders, radiologic summary, and provision for reviewing the chart.
7. *Laboratory system* for capturing physician orders, placing results in the record, specimen pickup, recording tests, cumulative test summaries, and so on, and connection to automated laboratory systems.
8. *Ancillary systems* such as diet ordering and hospital diet lists, requisitions, and reporting for ECGs, EEGs, EMGs, pulmonary function tests, and inhalation and physical therapy.

Thus this system attempts to handle most of the information that is processed in this health care system. In doing so it has eliminated the many time-consuming and error-prone manual procedures too well known to health professionals.

The system is especially easy to use (the author has seen and used it) because of Technicon's Video Matrix Terminals. These computer terminals consist of a video display monitor (which resembles a small television set), a standard keyboard, and an attached light pen (Fig. 4-4). The nurse need simply touch the

Figure 4-4.
Technicon Medical
Information System MIS in
use. (Courtesy of the
Technicon Medical
Information Systems Corp.)

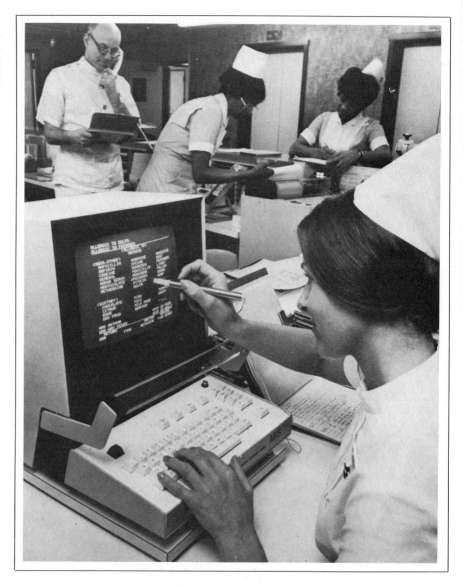

Figure 4-4.
Technicon Medical
Information System MIS in
use. (Courtesy of the
Technicon Medical
Information Systems Corp.)

word that appears on the screen in order to retrieve the information. For example, if the nurse wants the medical record of a particular person, she simply touches the words *patient list* and her particular floor, e.g., *9W*, and a patient list is displayed; she then touches the patient's *name* and *medical record* with the light pen, and the medical record for that person is displayed. If she wants a permanent printed version of that record, she simply again touches the print function word and a nearby printer prints a copy or two at the rate of 250 print characters per second. Figure 4-5 is an example of such a print-out for a patient care plan. Each nursing station has at least one video terminal and one

Figure 4-5.
Print-out of patient care
plan. (Courtesy of
Technicon Medical
Information Systems Corp.)

```
1WEST-8690              TECHNICON HOSPITAL
 4/19/78  9:01 AM                  PAGE 001           NURSING CARE PLAN
TOPEZ DANIEL                 M 37 211B  SERV:
 359807      ADM: 04/12/78   MATSON,RALPH J.,MD       7:00 AM 4/19/78
=====================================================================
RESP. NURSE:NORMA                      ALT. NURSE:
DX: PRIMARY DX: CHRONIC CHOLECYSTITIS....       **:      PAS:
    127 575.1 ...SECONDARY DX:
    CHOLELITHIASIS....127 574.0 ...
    PROCEDURE: CHOLECYSTECTOMY WITH
    CHOLANGIOGRAPHY ...47605 51.1; 98.3...
    *INCIDENTAL APPENDECTOMY, NEEDLE BIOPSY
    OF LIVER....04-13-78:CHOLECYSTECTOMY
    APPENDECTOMY LIVER BIOPSY...


REAL & POTENTIAL PROBLEMS:

   4/13  ALTERED BOWEL ELIM, POT, D/T--SURGERY               DE
   EXPECTED OUTCOMES                              C/P:  D/L:
      4/18  SOFT ABD,PASSING FLATUS, NORM BOWEL
            PATTERN FOR PT                        QDS   4 /21  CMD
   NURSING ORDERS
      4/13  CK FOR BOWEL SOUNDS,ABD SIZE & TONE                 DE
      4/13  OOB OR AMB IF POSS                                  DE

   4/13  PNEUMONIA &/OR ATELECTASIS, POT, D/T--SURGERY, SMOKING  DE
   EXPECTED OUTCOMES                              C/P:  D/L:
      4/18  NO OBVIOUS CONGESTION,NORM RESP PATTERN,
            TEMP UNDER 100 DEG                    QSH   4 /21  CMD
   NURSING ORDERS
      4/13  CK VS/ROUT                                          DE
      4/13  PLACE PT IN EFFECTIVE POSIT TO C&DB Q2H-
            SPLINT AFFECTED AREA IF NEC                         DE
      4/13  CK COL,CONSIS & AMT OF SPUTUM                       DE
      4/13  ENC PROGRESSIVE ACTIV AS ORD                        DE
      4/13  USE ANALGESICS TO FACILITATE C&DB                   DE
      4/13  INST PT RE:IMPORT & METHOD FOR C&DB,&
            ACTIV                                               DE

   4/13  HEMORRHAGE/SHOCK, POT, D/T--SURGERY                 DE
   EXPECTED OUTCOMES                              C/P:  D/L:
      4/18  STABLE BP/P/R:SKIN WARM & DRY:NO PALLOR:
            NO SUDDEN RESTLESSNESS                QSH   4 /21  CMD
   NURSING ORDERS
      4/13  CK SKIN WARMTH,DRYNESS,COL, & SENSORIUM W
            VS                                                  DE
      4/13  CK WND & DSG,COL & AMT OF ANY TUBE
            DRAINAGE W VS                                       DE

MISC PT DATA & POSS. PROBLEMS:
   4/12  PRESENT ILLNESS--CHOLECYSTITIS, ADDITIONAL DESCRIPTION--
         INTERMITTENT UPSET STOMACH WITH VOMITING (BILE) SINCE
         FEB. 78.                                              DBD
   4/12  HOME SITUATION WHICH MAY AFFECT DISCH PLAN--LIVES WITH
         WIFE.                                                 DBD
   4/12  OCCUPATION--MACHINIST HELPER.                         DBD
   4/12  GENERAL ABILITY TO CARE FOR SELF:INDEPENDENT          DBD
```

printer, and some have more than one terminal. Terminals are used by both physicians and nurses and are also available at the other health subcenters, such as admissions and pharmacy. The important point is that both the machines (hardware) and the programs (software) have been designed expressly for and by health professionals such as nurses. In El Camino Hospital, a nurse is designated to act as a liaison between the hospital and Technicon to see that the system operates in the way nurses and others desire.

Just to dispel the idea that this could not work in a remote setting outside a large hospital, the El Camino Hospital *does not* house *any* computer to perform these functions. The computer is located miles away and is used via telephone line connections. Similarly, Technicon's installation at the National Institute of Health Clinical Center in Bethesda, Maryland actually utilizes a computer in New Jersey. Thus it is possible for nurses in any setting (now, with the advent of communications satellites, including the most remote settings) to bring computing power to the patient (with a light portable terminal). Thus, computer-aided nursing assessment can operate in any setting. The advent of micro computing, as mentioned, makes this a reality today.

Another feature is that several facilities could use one central computer, thus lowering the cost. Technicon has utilized a backup system, which can take over if the main one fails.

Currently, Technicon has installed their system in at least 11 major medical centers, including the El Camino Hospital in Mountain View, California; the Maine Medical Center in Portland, Maine; the Nebraska Methodist Hospital in Omaha; the National Institutes of Health Clinical Center in Bethesda, Maryland; the Medical College of Virginia in Richmond; and University of Colorado Hospital in Denver. These implementations represent a wide variety of combinations of hospital/vendor arrangements; such arrangements include utilizing existing hardware and purchasing the software from Technicon, utilizing a complete hardware-software package as purchased from Technicon, and other combinations. The point here is that the MIS system is now being fully field-tested in a variety of situations under a variety of circumstances, and as experience builds up in these various settings with the common system, a set of share interests will develop as a user community begins to form. This user community, as it manifests itself with the nursing staff, can be expected to provide a major source of computer software development for nursing practice. If the quantum leaps required by nursing practice are to be produced, a major link must be formed between the academic nursing science community and the clinical nursing care delivery community. It is hoped that the major contributors to the development of nursing will facilitate such a link. Clearly, the ANA, the NLN, all of the major nursing periodicals and publishing houses, as well as the major funding agents, both public and private (i.e., nursing division of NIH and Technicon), must take a major role in the development of computer technology applied to the delivery of nursing care.

The El Camino system is not the only HIS, although it appears to be unique in attempting to computerize the entire hospital system at one time. In other hospital systems, like that of Massachusetts General, the designers have chosen to proceed in steps, computerizing one function at a time (starting with a laboratory data system). Other HIS include the Spectra Medical Information System currently being developed and utilized in Illinois, the HELP System in Utah, and the IBM system now being tested in North Carolina. As these and other systems begin to develop and are offered by various vendors, some method of sharing software and problem-solving methods in the application of this technology must be developed. It is suggested that a major organization similar to IBM's SHARE should be organized as a primary forum for the exchange of information.

The El Camino system is not perfect. As with all new things, it has many flaws (most of them human, by the way), but these are gradually being corrected through the efforts of many competent health and computer professionals.

The National Center for Health Services Research in conjunction with Battelle-Columbus Laboratories has just finished a four-year evaluation of the Technicon Medical Information Systems Corporation, MIS at El Camino Hospital. In addition, El Camino Hospital itself has been conducting a continuing extensive cost-impact study of the system. An earlier report, HRA76-3144, Evaluation of a Medical Information System in a Community Hospital, and this report, HRA77-3188, Demonstration and Evaluation of a Total Hospital Information System, document the continuing evaluation effort. Without going into great detail, a few significant outcomes of this evaluation will be noted here. A nursing unit was selected as the first site for testing an on-line station for the system. Implementation took nearly 10 months, almost twice as much time as was originally anticipated. A quantum leap in the development of computer-based nursing assessment occurred with the development of a systematic approach to the nursing care plan by Mayers, 1972, as a response to the insufficiency of preexisting manual systems for nursing notes. This generalized approach to standard care plans clearly has utility for systems beyond the Technicon System [18]. Major concerns to nursing in the implementation (along with approximately a month of anxiety caused by the switch to a totally new system) were: system reliability, methods and procedure changes to maximize the benefits derived through the use of MIS, and training. Substantial effort has been put into the training of personnel in the use of the MIS system, familiarizing them with seldom-used features as well as changes and improvements in the system. Clearly a need for a standard vocabulary has emerged as a major concern from the project. Numerous major benefits for nursing have resulted from the project, including a significant decrease in required clerical tasks, an ability to shift more clerical tasks to the unit clerk, a greater availability of data both within shifts and from one shift to the next (nurses are no longer dependent on Kardex), and a substantially increased legibility of nursing notes. In addition, because of the enormous data management problems in nurse care planning, the staff has embarked upon a long-term project to develop a care planning system compatible with the computer system. Interestingly enough, the enhancement of nurses' roles as care-givers rather than as transcriptionists, although it led to an early conflict between them and the physicians who are non-users of MIS at the beginning, has led to a major benefit perceived by nursing and led to support of the system by nursing staff. Because of the shift in clerical activities, nurses recognize that they can enhance the level of care delivered and do so with a lower ratio of nursing staff to patients. The complete analysis of economic impact of the system, as it affects both the hospital and nursing, is even at this date not yet complete. The issue is an extremely complex one and certainly beyond the scope of this chapter. It is suggested that interested readers secure the referenced materials and examine the extensive economic analysis. Again, only through nursing's substantial involvement in this economic analysis can a complete and accurate picture of the impact of the system upon nursing be fully assured.

Technicon's system is not necessarily devoted to any one diagnostic or assessment method, since MIS-I allows health professionals to tailor their own idiosyncratic systems. Another system, Weed's PROMIS (Problem-Oriented Medical Information System) [22], is based on the problem-oriented method (see Chapter 3). Weed's system is a patient-oriented system, independent of a particular health care configuration or type of computer. I see no particular reason why the Weed system could not be implemented within the Technicon system because of the latter's independence of philosophy. This is, in fact, its main advantage: that as patients, professionals, and health care delivery systems change, so can the computer system.

This author visited psychiatric nursing units at NIH Hospital in Bethesda and saw the implementation of a Maslow-based hierarchical model within the highly modular Technicon system. Although this implementation is not more than two years old, it is a clear demonstration that the system is sufficiently flexible to encompass a number of widely varying nursing theories and philosophically different delivery structures. Future research with MIS has been toward a Patient Care Quality Assurance System (PACQAS) which can be overlaid on the existing total hospital medical information system. This system would be composed of four subsystems including: (1) a computer-assisted, diagnosis particular, outcome-oriented nursing care planning subsystem, (2) a computer-assisted patient care audit subsystem, which integrates both the concurrent and retrospective aspects of the nursing audit, medical audit, and utilization review into a coordinated patient care audit, (3) a computerized patient care plan base staffing requirement subsystem, and (4) a computerized services coordination subsystem for patient scheduling/services coordination from preadmission through discharge. This program will unify the multiple quality assurance programs going on in any hospital setting into a single hospital-wide patient care quality assurance system. It is suggested that nursing seriously consider a review of the major quality of care instruments (e.g., the Horn-Swain, Qualpac, Slater, Rush-Medicus) in terms of how they can be implemented into an ongoing nursing information system. It is only in this way that the quality of nursing care will be measured in a normal nonthreatening manner that is comfortable for the staff instead of by the heroic and periodic massive research efforts traditionally mounted to secure such data. It is clear that if nursing considers its quality measurement tools part of a research process and too difficult to utilize in a continuing manner, these tools eventually will become only historical curiosities. Computer-based nursing care is here and nursing's measurement tools must address it.

Automated Multiphasic Health Testing

Before turning to the methodology for evaluating the effectiveness of nursing assessment, one final application of computers to the health care system, namely, automated multiphasic health testing (AMHT), should be mentioned. AMHT systems have been in operation for several years and appear to be useful and successful tools. Cononi and Siler [5] discuss the role of nursing with respect to AMHT and conclude that nurses are especially well suited to staff AMHT centers in a supervisory role.

Simply defined, AMHT is the automated (computer-aided) administration of more than one health test to a person or persons. AMHT allows the full range of health data collection—from self-entry of history data by the patient to nurse-assisted entry of vital capacity data, with the computer recording total and one-second expired volume. The experience of the Kaiser group in California has demonstrated the cost/effectiveness of AMHT, and it has become a major component of the group's health maintenance system. Thus, again, AMHT should not be seen as a professional threat, but as a useful tool to aid the nurse in physical assessment and assessment in general. If nursing now takes an aggressive role in implementing AMHT and other systems, it will serve the profession and its goals well.

Need for a Systematic Approach

In presenting the rationale for his problem-oriented approach, Weed [22] emphasized the need for systematic data collection and processing in medical diagnosis and assessment. In his critique of the traditional system, which led to the development of the problem-oriented philosophy, he made the following eight points:

1. Physicians, seeing only a random presentation of patients for symptomatic treatment, never felt responsible for, or saw the need for, following up those patients and thus never engaged in preventive medicine.
2. This randomness of patient presentation led to a randomness in the information recorded by physicians that never clearly defined problems and associated patterns.
3. The randomness of the information recorded prevented a full examination of the effectiveness of patient treatment.
4. The foregoing (1–3) produced an educational and licensure system dependent on a pedagogy of memory, leading to a system in which the physician's entire future performance was predicted by his knowledge at licensure time—a performance-oriented system dependent on memory.

5. It was assumed that the future physician could effectively combine isolated, specialized pockets of knowledge into a comprehensive system for patient treatment.
6. There was an imbalance between the plethora of molecular biologic studies designed to serve future patients and the paucity of useful techniques applicable to existing patients.
7. Future physicians were trained without instruction in the economic realities of the cost/benefit of treatment, which led to enormous expenditures on the wrong problems at the wrong time, both at the clinical and basic scientific research levels.
8. All the foregoing led to the present nonsystem of medical education and practice which defies uniform application of sound decision-making necessary in a world of limited resources for health care.

Weed's assessment of the history of physician education may be more or less accurate, but the importance of his message for all health professionals, including nurses, is that health information processing and decision-making problems have been contained by a complex set of educational, research, and clinical heuristics which have evolved and demand the application of some sound principles and technology. The systematizing effect of Weed's problem-oriented method is one solution that incorporates some of these principles. The computer offers further advantages, including organization, efficiency, and rapid analysis.

Measuring the Effectiveness of Nursing Assessment

One can consider nursing assessment as being composed of several parts: (1) data collection, (2) data screening, (3) data aggregation, (4) data analysis, and (5) decision-making.

Data collection consists of a methodical accumulation of information about the patient. Techniques such as interviewing, observation, auscultation, percussion, palpation, inspection, and measurement are used. The kind of data collected depends heavily on the orientation of the collection process (e.g., problem-oriented, adaptation-oriented, health- or illness-oriented). *Data screening* is the act of eliminating irrelevant signs, symptoms, and cues and increasing the detectability of relevant ones. This, too, depends on one's theoretic bent. *Data aggregation* is the concatenation of all the isolated data into a meaningful, cohesive set. Again, how this is done depends heavily on one's theoretic orientation—"the medium is the message" presents this component's bias well. *Data analysis* is the process by which the ordered collection of data is tested for meaningfulness and significance and is concentrated into a relatively more efficient small set of indicators. Obviously, theory is crucial to this process. Finally, *decision-making* is the act of translating the processed and analyzed data into proposed alternatives for action. Theory's obvious importance cannot be overemphasized. These steps rarely occur in such a neat sequential order, but rather appear as both a somewhat random and somewhat orderly chain of steps, occurring as a function of the demands of the particular problem and the sequence in which critical data appear. Nevertheless, this structuring of nursing assessment can allow us to analyze the process to determine the effectiveness of each part of the process and of the process as a whole.

What we have then is a complex of people and models (theories), some who are giving off signs and symptoms, some who are receiving, screening, and processing them, and attempts to relate patterns of them to preexisting matrices or models based on experience and theory. This process then clearly involves the biases of human information processing and judgment to a large extent.

Methods of Reducing Bias

Much research has been done to demonstrate bias in human information processing and decision-making. The Oregon Research Institute is devoted primarily to the study of that topic, especially as applied to clinical decision-making. Early in the 1960s, researchers at the University of Michigan, Ohio State University, and other academic centers who were studying human behavior in gambling situations began to notice that people underused the information available to them and thus did not risk bets which the odds said they should have. In other words, people are conservative decision-makers (wait for more information than they really need). Further work showed that it is the way in which people aggregate data (put it all together) that is conservative rather than the way in which they perceive the data. That is, people devalue the data not when they collect it but when they aggregate it. However, if they wait too long to make a decision based upon some continuing aggregation of the data, they clearly waste data. What this says for nursing assessment is that, like all human information processors, nurses will be likely to be wasteful (conservative) in their collection of data (assessment), which costs money.

Edwards [7, 8] has summarized this line of research and delineated these issues and possible solutions to the conservatism problem. He mentions that training has worked to reduce conservatism, but only when the data came from the same source and were of the same nature in both the training and the test situation [8]. Another apparently more reliable solution is one of a series of methods or models proposed by Edwards, namely, probabilistic information processing (PIP). Simply described, PIP is a system in which humans in concert can protect themselves against their own conservatism. Basically, in PIP, several independent information collectors do the data collection and another independent set of human information processors estimate likelihood ratios (LRs); LRs are defined as the ratio of the probability of a symptom S given one disease D_1 to the probability of the same symptom S given another disease D_2; thus

$$LR = \left[\frac{\text{Prob } (S_1 \text{ given } D_1)}{\text{Prob } (S_1 \text{ given } D_2)} \right]$$

The LRs import is that it directly related the appraiser's evaluation of the diagnostic potential of a symptom—its ability to discriminate between two diseases. The PIP model passes on the LRs for each symptom for each pair of diseases to a bayesian processor (e.g., a computer calculating via Bayes theorem). Bayes theorem is a uniquely important statistical rule for combining evidence, especially useful in clinical situations. One of its unique features is the ability to combine "subjective" estimates by expert opinion *and* objective estimates by statistical tallies, and so on, into a numeric (probability) estimate. In one form, Bayes theorem states that the revised estimate (R) of the odds (probability) favoring one hypothesis (diagnosis) over another (the estimate of the odds after considering the latest item of evidence) is equal to the prior estimate (P) of the odds made before considering the new item of evidence, multiplied by the LR of that new item of evidence; that is, $R = (P) \times LR$. Thus, by using Bayes theorem, probabilities can be revised on the basis of new evidence.

One more fact about the assessment process which will clarify the relationship between the PIP model, the likelihood ratio, Bayes theorem, and nursing assessment is that the assessment process is a sequential process of hypothesis formation, testing, and rejection, associated with some subjective estimate on the part of the assessor of the odds or probability of each of the various hypotheses. What occurs can be described as a tree of decision-making. An example given by Kleinmuntz [15] (Fig. 4-6) illustrates a health decision tree, in which we can see this sequential process clearly. The picture looks like an inverted tree branch (often many branches of one tree are depicted). In this example, all parts of the tree are binary, with yes or no answers. Often we must attach probabilities to each node of the tree, which reflect the odds of any of the alternatives being true.

Thus, in a PIP method of assessment, a set of independent health professionals—nurses, physicians, laboratory and radiologic technicians—all collect their independent data. Then another set of health care experts assess the likelihood ratios for each pair of diseases for each symptom. This can often be stored on the computer as a pool of expert opinion or population statistics. Then these data are fed to the computer as they become available for calculation of the bayesian probabilities of each of the diseases. An action-taker (therapeutic agent) then makes a decision on the basis of the probabilities. This process, too, can be put into a PIP formulation to ensure that the proper therapeutic action will be taken, given the set of probabilities for the various diseases, again ensuring nonconservatism in the entire assessment–therapeutic measure chain. In fact, the larger picture of the health care chain says that we feed the outcomes of each of the treatments back into our treatment model to test the effectiveness of treatment continuously.

The technicalities of the assessment process and some of the accompanying jargon may, at first glance, appear to place yet another barrier between nursing

Figure 4-6.
Health decision tree.

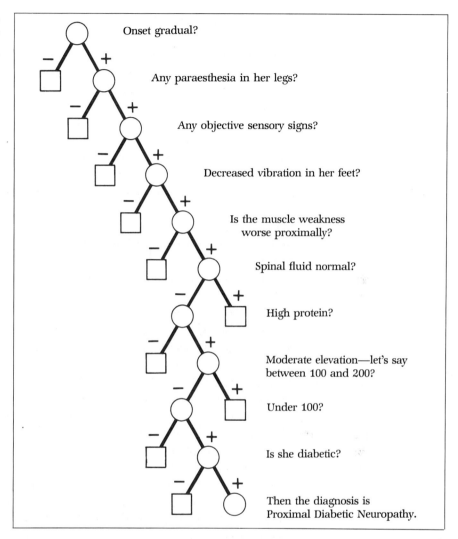

Onset gradual?

Any paraesthesia in her legs?

Any objective sensory signs?

Decreased vibration in her feet?

Is the muscle weakness
worse proximally?

Spinal fluid normal?

High protein?

Moderate elevation—let's say
between 100 and 200?

Under 100?

Is she diabetic?

Then the diagnosis is
Proximal Diabetic Neuropathy.

and the patient in the name of research. However, they are actually concerned
not with the nurse-patient relationship, but with cost/benefit and cost/effective-
ness. Their purpose is to determine the following: For the cost of the nursing
assessment and of each further component of the health care system to which
the nursing assessment sends the patient, how much health benefit does the
patient receive (e.g., increased nonhospital days, days without pain, increased
number of productive days) and how effective is the process within the health
care system (e.g., reducing the access [in time and distance] of the patient from
entrance into the system to the beginning of treatment; reducing the total system
cost for that health problem)? Nurse-patient distance and cost/benefit are definitely related, but one cannot be dismissed at the expense of the other. Com-

petent nursing professionals must contend both with the patients' social and psychologic needs and the quality of health care patients are provided. Increasing patient contact or reducing barriers between the nurse and the patient does not alone sufficiently improve the health of the patient. TLC alone does not significantly increase the effectiveness of ineffective or inefficient health care.

Obviously, the PIP model is not the only model of health information processing; nor is it a perfect model. It is, however, one attempt to maximize the effectiveness of health information processing and decision-making. A great deal of other research is under way to increase the effectiveness of human decision-making [6, 14, 19, 21].

The University of Wisconsin is engaged in a project to develop and evaluate a computer-aided medical diagnostic system which combines judgments by physicians with information from past cases, using Bayes theorem. Gustafson et al. [11] have presented preliminary results of the project, which contrast four methods of arriving at a diagnosis: (1) subjective bayesian, using expert opinion to estimate LRs; (2) actuarial bayesian, using medical record data to form LRs; (3) hybrid bayesian, using (1) and (2); and (4) contemporary standard diagnostic techniques. In diagnosing thyroid conditions, early results show the subjective bayesian method to be superior to the contemporary standard method in percentage of disease entities identified. As more actuarial data become available, the hybrid method is expected to prove superior. In this project many kinds of evidence are being gathered, and much of what is being found has to do with how health professionals are trained to assess LRs. So far this project has found several differences, which depend on data clarity and availability and whether a group or individual setting is used. These results should be heeded as training programs for nursing assessment develop.

The previous discussion encompasses much of decision theory, operations research, cost/benefit theory, and bayesian decision-making. One more important topic is that of utility and value theory in decision-making. This corpus of theories states that one should do or one does (depending on whether you think this theory is prescriptive or descriptive) things that maximize expected utility or value, where value is usually an objective, easily measured quantity, and utility is the subjective valuation of value (value can be measured in dollars, reduced bed days, and so on). There seem to be four theories here, depending on whether the probability associated with an alternative outcome is subjective or objective and whether the outcome is measured by value or utility. The theories state that if we multiply the probability of each alternative outcome by its associated value or utility if it occurs, the alternative with the largest value is the one that should be or is chosen. Figure 4-7 depicts the four theories as a function of their inputs. At this point, we shall not compare the theories, merely give an example of one, namely, the EV theory.

Figure 4-8 shows an example of a decision tree for a case in which the disease is unknown, an example given in Barnoon and Wolfe [2]. The conse-

Figure 4-7.
Four decision theories.

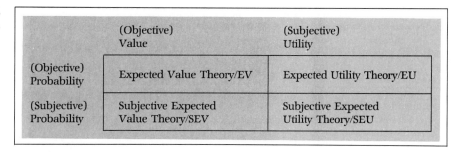

	(Objective) Value	(Subjective) Utility
(Objective) Probability	Expected Value Theory/EV	Expected Utility Theory/EU
(Subjective) Probability	Subjective Expected Value Theory/SEV	Subjective Expected Utility Theory/SEU

quences (values) are a loss of lifetime and disability, and a decision must be made to select the best treatment from five. We can see that the calculated probability of one disease, D_1, is .7 and of the other, D_2, is .3. This may have been calculated with bayesian estimates using PIP or by some other method, but we shall assume these values. The six alternative courses of action are treatments 1 through 5 and no treatment. We shall not go through the calculation here, but the alternative with the greatest expected gain (value) in life expectancy and decrease in disability, is treatment 4, since it has the highest value. (This is not obvious from Fig. 4-8, but can be calculated from the tree in the figure as in [2]. Thus, not knowing which disease was present, knowing only the likelihood of the presence of each, we are able to establish that treatment which has the greatest payoff or expected gain.

Unfortunately, some of the most difficult decisions in health care decision-making involve ethical issues that are personal and difficult to quantify at best. Edwards [8] has also treated this issue but, as yet, utility theory is of little help in these cases. However, a great many health care problems are quantifiable and are amenable to such analysis. Quality audits should be contrasted with such analyses to see if present decision-making follows any rational pattern such as utility theory. In any case, by putting assessment and other health care issues into such a framework, they are open to analysis and quality control rather than protected and masked from an effectiveness audit.

ISSUES FOR NURSING ASSESSMENT

One of the classic problems of nursing and part of its identity problem is the "What is nursing?" issue. Some of the greatest and most informed leaders of nursing have debated this issue, and I shall not attempt to answer it here. In nursing assessment, this problem is translated into "What is nursing assessment?" What is disputed is the just territory of nursing, especially in relation to medicine. The difficulty comes when the profession faces a new role such as nursing assessment, unsure of itself, and worries about whether some point in the assessment process is really nursing. For example, it is often thought that nursing can do much assessment, but is limited in its therapeutic alternatives. My suggestion for a solution is that nursing be patient-oriented rather than health-professional oriented and that people—nurses, physicians, laboratory

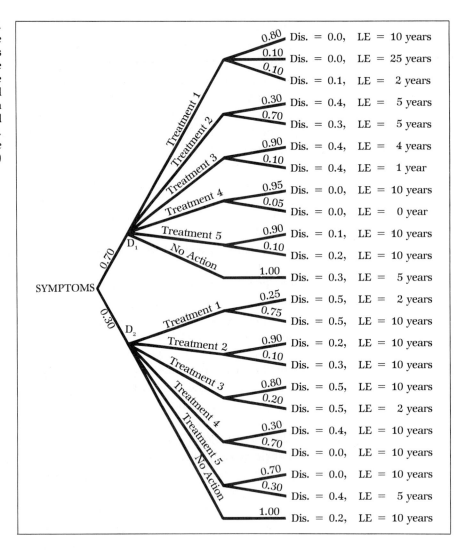

Figure 4-8.
A decision tree for the case
in which disease is
unknown, consequences are
loss of lifetime (lifetime
expectancy = LE) and
disability (Dis.), and a
treatment must be selected
from several alternatives.
(From Barnoon and Wolfe
[2].)

SYMPTOMS

0.70   D₁

Treatment 1
0.80   Dis. = 0.0,   LE = 10 years
0.10   Dis. = 0.0,   LE = 25 years
0.10   Dis. = 0.1,   LE = 2 years

Treatment 2
0.30   Dis. = 0.4,   LE = 5 years
0.70   Dis. = 0.3,   LE = 5 years

Treatment 3
0.90   Dis. = 0.4,   LE = 4 years
0.10   Dis. = 0.4,   LE = 1 year

Treatment 4
0.95   Dis. = 0.0,   LE = 10 years
0.05   Dis. = 0.0,   LE = 0 year

Treatment 5
0.90   Dis. = 0.1,   LE = 10 years
0.10   Dis. = 0.2,   LE = 10 years

No Action
1.00   Dis. = 0.3,   LE = 5 years

0.30   D₂

Treatment 1
0.25   Dis. = 0.5,   LE = 2 years
0.75   Dis. = 0.5,   LE = 10 years

Treatment 2
0.90   Dis. = 0.2,   LE = 10 years
0.10   Dis. = 0.3,   LE = 10 years

Treatment 3
0.80   Dis. = 0.5,   LE = 10 years
0.20   Dis. = 0.5,   LE = 2 years

Treatment 4
0.30   Dis. = 0.4,   LE = 10 years
0.70   Dis. = 0.0,   LE = 10 years

Treatment 5
0.70   Dis. = 0.0,   LE = 10 years
0.30   Dis. = 0.4,   LE = 5 years

No Action
1.00   Dis. = 0.2,   LE = 10 years

technicians—perform in ways in which they are capable and not according to
historical role prescriptions. What this says for evaluating the effectiveness and
efficiency of the assessment process is that it should be multidisciplinary and
patient-centered. It must analyze the nursing assessment role as part of the
health care system. This must and can be so, even though dozens of role relationships may be available to nurses as a function of the type and setting of
various health services as they evolve with the whole health care system. The
evolution of nursing assessment should not become entangled with the socio-
emotional role development nursing goes through as new independent nursing
roles emerge.

Another issue is the reticence of nursing to examine its own effectiveness.

This is changing as the nurse research role develops and as more nurse researchers are educated. Some of the problems are the overburdened state of the whole health care system in addition to the nursing role itself and a lack of perceived competence and perceived sufficient education to conduct evaluative research. *A Ph.D. is not necessary to do research*—only a willingness to solve problems and seek expert advice when it is needed. One major problem, cited by the 1973 Carnegie Commission Report on Women in Higher Education, is that the traditional societal norms have made mathematical analysis, computers, and the like nonfeminine and thus nonfemale roles. This is also changing, albeit slowly. Nursing should use evaluative research not only as a way to assess its own competency, but also as a way to enhance the stature of the profession as perceived by other health care professionals. Respect is gained by those who are self-critical and engage in evaluative research.

One final issue is the current philosophic discussion over the difference between nursing as health-oriented and medicine as disease-oriented. The problem seems to be one of efficiency in the assessment process. In trying to adapt, human beings rarely concern themselves with things that work well and proceed as expected, but pay attention to and work on things that do not work well. That is, things are noticed if humans perceive that something is not as expected or not performing properly. This is called *exception orientation*. Most TV repair technicians and plumbers, for example, work this way and have done so for a long time, probably because it is more efficient to find out what is wrong with a system than to find out what is right with it. In the health care system, physicians have been exception-oriented for good reason—it seemed to be the most efficient way. With the advent of "health" concepts, we are left with the task of seeing what is right with the patient and keeping it that way, besides correcting what is wrong. This assumes enormous amounts of assessment and data collection and thus chances for human information processing errors, such as conservatism. If health orientation of nursing is to be successful, it seems that only with the help of the computer and modern methods of machine-oriented information processing and decision-making can it become so at minimal cost and error to the patient. What is clearly needed is a self-examination by the nursing profession of its theories of health, health maintenance, and assessment in light of this recent technology. Perhaps both technology and the nursing profession could gain from the experience.

REFERENCES

1. Barker, M., Monroe, J. Mershimer, R., and McNamara, K. Hospital information Systems Sharing Group Nursing Application Study Report, 1971–1972. Ohio State University Hospitals, 410 W. 10th Ave., Columbus, Ohio 43210.
2. Barnoon, S., and Wolfe, H. *Measuring the Effectiveness of Medical Decisions.* Springfield, Ill.: Thomas, 1972.
3. Bitzer, M. A., Boudreau, M., and Arner, R. A. *Computer Based Instruction of Basic Nursing Utilizing Inquiry Approach.* Cerl Report X-40, Feb. 1973, University of Illinois, Urbana.

 4. Brigham, C., Kamp, M., and Cross, K. *A Guide to Computer Assisted Instruction in the Health Sciences (LHNCBC 73–01)*. Bethesda, Md.: Lister Hill National Center for Biomedical Communications, December 1972.

 5. Cononi, A., and Siler, M. Automated multiphasic health testing in the hospital situation. *J. Nurs. Adm.* 2:80, 1972.

 6. Dawes, R. M. Slitting the decision·makers' throat with Occam's razor: The superiority of random linear models to real judges. *Ore Res. Inst. Bull.* 12 (13): December 1972.

 7. Edwards, W. Conservatism in Human Information Processing. In B. Kleinmutz (Ed.), *Formal Presentation of Human Judgment*. New York: Wiley, 1968. Pp. 17–52.

 8. Edwards, W. N-1: Diagnosis in Unique Cases. In J. Jacquez (Ed.), *Computer Diagnostic Methods*. New York: Wiley, 1972. Pp. 139–151.

 9. Farlee, C., and Goldstein, B. A role for nurses in implementing computerized hospital information system. *Nurs. Forum* 10(4):339, 1971.

10. Goodwin, J. O., and Edwards, B. S. A computer program to assist nursing decision-making. *Nurs. Res.* 24(4):299, 1975.

11. Gustafson, D. H., Ludke, R. L., Glackman, P. J., Larson, F. C., and Greest, J. H. Wisconsin Computer Aided Medical Diagnosis Project—Progress Report. In J. Jacquez (Ed.), *Computer Diagnosis and Diagnostic Methods*. Springfield, Ill.: Thomas, 1972.

12. Jacquez, J. (Ed.). *Computer Diagnosis and Diagnostic Methods*. Springfield, Ill.: Thomas, 1972.

13. Judge, R. D., Zuidema, G. D., and Fitzgerald, F. (Eds.). *Methods of Clinical Examination* (4th ed.). Boston: Little, Brown, 1982.

14. Kahneman, D., and Tversky, A. On the psychology of prediction. *Psychol. Rev.* 80:237, 1973.

15. Kleinmuntz, B. Medical Information Processing by Computer. In J. Jacquez (Ed.), *Computer Diagnosis and Diagnostic Methods*. Springfield, Ill.: Thomas, 1972.

16. Lagina, S. A computer program to diagnose anxiety levels. *Nurs. Res.* 20:484, 1971.

17. Lindberg, D. A. B. *The Computer and Medical Care*. Springfield, Ill.: Thomas, 1968.

18. Mayers, M. *A Systematic Approach to the Nursing Care Plan, 1972*. Vols. I, II, III, KP Medical Systems, Palo Alto, California.

19. Slovic, P., and Lichtenstein, S. Comparison of Bayesian and Regression Approaches to the Study of Information Processing in Judgment. *Organ. Behav. Human Perform.* 6:649–744, 1971.

20. Sunguroff, A., and Greenberg, D. Cornell University, *Pub. in Computer Graphics*, 12:3 (August), 1978.

21. Tversky, A., and Kahneman, D. Availability: A heuristic for judging frequency and probability. *Ore. Res. Inst. Bull.* 11(6), June 1972.

22. Weed, L. Medical Records. In *Medical Education and Patient Care* (The Press of Case Western Reserve University). Chicago: Year Book, 1971.

23. Wesseling, E. Automating the nursing history and care plan. *J. Nurs. Adm.* 2:34, 1972.

II. Physical Assessment of Adults

5. Nurse-Patient Communication and Relationship in the Physical Assessment Process

THE conduct of the interview is a basic determinant of the effectiveness of the physical assessment data-gathering process and is greatly influenced by the nurse examiner's interactional behavior with the patient. The *communication skill* used to elicit data relevant to immediate assessment purposes and planning appropriate follow-up health care is but one of three concerns discussed in this chapter.

The nurse's primary objective is to initiate and maintain an open, mutually comfortable exchange of meaningful communication with the patient. This goal will be either notably facilitated or seriously compromised by the nature and tone of the nurse-patient relationship that the nurse establishes. The interaction of the nurse examiner and the individual (whether designated as patient, client, or consumer) initiated for the specific purpose of interview and physical assessment provides the foundation for what will be either a *helping* or a *nonhelping relationship*. Furthermore, the type of relationship established not only affects the quality of data obtained in the interview itself, but also—and more important—has major impact on the process and outcomes of the physical assessment. Ultimately, the individual's welfare is influenced. The first two major concerns consequently focus on the development of a helping relationship and the communication process as essential aspects of physical assessment.

When the patient views the nurse examiner as interested and caring, a helping relationship is more likely to occur. In this situation, the patient can experience less tension and is more apt to share his thoughts and feelings and be more informative generally. Mutual goals are then more easily identified and more readily established, and cooperative efforts are consequently more quickly realized. *Anxiety* is an additional concept that explains much behavior that the nurse examiner may experience herself, or observe in the patient, or both. It is generally recognized that a high degree of anxiety affects a person's thought processes, perceptual abilities, and physiologic functioning. These alterations can interfere with the nurse examiner's performance, or the nature of patient responses, or both. Because of the implications of an anxious state for both the patient and the nurse examiner, as well as for the establishment of effective communication and a helping relationship, anxiety is the third major topic considered in this chapter.

The environment in which the nurse and patient interact deserves early consideration by the nurse to ascertain its potential effects. Initial attention is therefore directed to the interview setting.

INTERVIEW SETTING   The nature of the place or setting in which the nurse examiner conducts the physical assessment examination and interview varies considerably. Although various agency settings such as hospitals, clinics, and nursing homes come immediately to mind, the importance of the home setting cannot be overemphasized. Increasingly, nurses find their practice in this environment and, of necessity, must adapt their assessment practices to the unique characteristics of each of a highly diversified range of homes. Each setting provides special opportunities or problematic considerations for the nurse and the patient.

Data-gathering in the patient's home may involve both the patient and family members as data resources. The familiar setting of the home may serve to minimize the patient's apprehensions and fears, ease the establishment of the relationship, and generally facilitate the assessment process. Adaptation in this setting rests primarily with the nurse, challenging her skills and ingenuity often, and in new and different ways. In the hospital or clinic setting the nurse usually has the advantage. She must recognize that the patient's preassessment experiences and the unfamiliar surroundings and people, as well as a whole range of environmental sensory inputs (often new, uncontrollable, and anxiety-provoking), affects his responses.

Several guidelines useful to the nurse in selecting a place conducive to the interview and examination are listed below.

1. The room should provide privacy for the patient and nurse examiner.
2. The room must not be noisy or its furnishings and equipment distracting.
3. Room temperature should be comfortable for both patient and nurse.
4. Interruptions are distracting and disruptive to interaction and communication and should be discouraged by adequate planning.
5. Both the patient and nurse examiner should be comfortably seated facing each other and sufficiently close to interact in a relaxed manner.

THE NURSE-PATIENT RELATIONSHIP   A *helping relationship* is any relationship in which one person facilitates the personal development or growth of another; in which he helps the other to become more mature, adaptive, integrated, or open to his own experience (italics added) [1]. Implicit in this definition is the need for the "helper" to collect data about the "helpee" in order to identify need for, and facilitate change in, the "helpee." For our discussion, the nurse is considered a professional helper. This signifies that she utilizes a body of knowledge and has abilities that assist her in collecting pertinent data and developing a helping relationship at one and the same time.

In recent years, there has been considerable interest in identifying the belief systems that effective helpers have in common. Coombs et al. [5] states that "What we believe to be important inevitably determines the methods we use in dealing with people"; and in their Florida studies of the helping professions, several categories of belief systems that effective helpers have in common were suggested. It was found that effective helpers were person-oriented, holding positive views of people, e.g., considering them worthy, dependable, capable, motivated, and friendly. They tended to view themselves as self-disciplined and trustworthy and felt valued and wanted, as well as adequate. Helpers had a specialized kind of knowledge in which they were well versed; manifested commitment, involvement, and altruism; and were open and revealing about themselves [5].

The nurse committed to establishing a helping relationship needs to examine her own complex of values, beliefs, and biases for their implications for, and effect on, all aspects of her practice.

Stages of the Nurse-Patient Relationship

The nurse-patient relationship may be described as having three phases: the initiation or orientation phase, the development or working phase, and the termination or closing phase [2, 3, 9]. Theoretically, each phase is discussed as a separate one, but in actual practice, boundaries are blurred and one phase merges into another.

Initiation or Orientation Phase

The relationship is initiated when the examining nurse orients the patient to her name, status, purpose of their meeting, and what they will be doing together. The approximate time she will spend with the patient should be indicated. Providing the patient with this information permits him the opportunity to develop realistic expectations [12] regarding the assessment interview and examination. This phase is a time for exploration and testing of each other, and the nurse needs to be alert to her own and the patient's feelings. It is the time when communication patterns are being formed and the nurse is establishing her role as a helper. The initiation or orientation phase is the crucial preliminary to progression of the relationship toward realizing positive outcomes (Fig. 5-1).

During this beginning phase, the nurse needs to make the clinical decision to proceed with the primary purpose, the assessment; or, if she observes highly anxious behavior, to reorder priorities and assist the patient in reducing his anxiety so that the assessment can be accomplished with his fullest participation and cooperation. In some instances, the assessment may have to be directed only to the most urgent needs of the patient, with complete assessment planned for a later time.

Development or Working Phase

This phase is the substantive body of the interaction, during which all aspects of the physical assessment are accomplished. The ease and facility with which this phase progresses is largely dependent on the nurse examiner's having skillful interview and examination practices. Inadequate attention to the orientation needs of the patient can, and often does, result in complicating or slowing this phase of the assessment process.

Figure 5-1.
During the initiation phase
mutual expectations are
clarified and observations
of the client's general
appearance and
responsiveness are made
that will guide the nurse's
conduct of the interview
and examination.
(Reproduced with
permission from R. D.
Judge, G. D. Zuidema, and
F. Fitzgerald (Eds.).
*Methods of Clinical
Examination* (4th ed.).
Boston: Little, Brown,
1982.)

Termination or Closing Phase

Preparation for the comfortable closure of the assessment session is begun during the orientation phase. Abrupt termination is avoided, and the patient is assured of a final opportunity to be informative or to question. As appropriate to the situation, the patient is told how to contact the nurse should he recollect information he thinks is important to share. Time is made available for discussion of findings and preliminary counsel regarding appropriate future care and referrals. What occurs during this time is likely to determine the patient's impression of the entire interaction and whether or not he follows through with recommendations made by the nurse.

NURSE-PATIENT COMMUNICATION

Communication is the essence of the helping relationship, and without the use of communication skills, helping relationships could not exist. Communication is generally understood to refer to verbal and nonverbal behavior within a social (human-to-human) context [15]. It includes a message that is sent by one individual and received by another. When the message sent is understood, the sender and receiver have a shared experience, which is fundamental to any relationship. The nurse performing the physical assessment must develop and demonstrate a working knowledge of the communication process, nonverbal and verbal, to ensure and expedite the collection and interpretation of information from and about the patient.

Nonverbal Communication

It is impossible for an individual *not* to communicate nonverbally at all times. Each person communicates by his gestures, facial expressions, body posturing and movement, tone and other characteristics of voice, and even by his mode of dress [6]. The nonverbal message may be accompanied by a verbal message, and these messages may or may not be contradictory. If the verbal and non-verbal messages are congruent, the receiver responds to the verbal message. However, when the nonverbal message contradicts the verbal one, the receiver usually believes the nonverbal rather than the verbal message. An example of this is illustrated by the patient who decides that something is wrong with his heart because the nurse auscultates one area longer or repetitively despite her later verbal reassurance to the contrary. Instances of this nature may be avoided or at least minimized by prior alerting of the patient to these possibilities.

Nonverbal communication is directly influenced by the beliefs we hold. An integral part of our personality, beliefs are expressed through our nonverbal as well as our verbal behavior. Becoming aware of beliefs, changing them, and acquiring new ones are part of the ongoing process of living. It is part of becoming the kind of person and professional we aspire to being. If a nurse's beliefs are similar to those of an effective helper, the establishment of helping relationships will be facilitated; if they are not, helping relationships will be more difficult to achieve, even though the nurse is familiar with communication techniques. Unfortunately, people's beliefs are not always in their immediate awareness. However, an experience may trigger into awareness a belief that the nurse never knew she had. Especially during the interview, the nurse needs to be sensitive to her own communication behavior to avoid conveying personal value judgments or negative emotional responses to information shared by the patient.

Listening   No single aspect of the communication process influences its effectiveness and success more than the quality of listening demonstrated by the nurse during the assessment interaction. Listening is an active rather than a passive phenomenon. It involves the nurse in directing a deliberative attention to hearing and understanding the patient's frame of reference and what he is saying. Maintaining eye contact and refraining from unnecessary and distracting involvement in other activities are two ways the nurse can convey active listening. It is a basic skill requiring continuous practice to develop expertise, and unless its priority is carefully guarded, active listening may be subjugated to the nurse examiner's pressures of time, interest, or need. When the nurse is an active listener, she demonstrates her interest in the patient, her desire to understand him, and her respect for him as an individual. This approach can be sustained only if the nurse actually has these feelings for the patient.

Silence   Periods of silence are necessary and useful, albeit intolerably uncomfortable at times. Hein [9] elaborates several functions served by silence:

Allows us to sift and sort the thoughts we have absorbed and file them for later use.

Gives us an opportunity to observe our patients unobtrusively.

Can be used for the reflection of our thoughts and the formulation of an alternate approach when the interview continues.

Invites a response . . . conveys an expectation to our patients that they can respond if given the needed time to formulate an answer.

Allows us to assess the level of anxiety in ourselves and our patients.

Recognizing these values in the use of silence and employing periods of silence in a planned way can do much to enhance communication and allay feelings of discomfort in both patient and nurse.

Skills and Techniques for Facilitating Verbal Communication

Words are the basic tools used in verbal communication. Words are symbols only and can mean different things to different people. Thus it is their meanings that must be understood and shared if successful communication is to occur. When meanings are shared, there is a feeling of understanding and being understood, and verbal exchange is a useful, productive experience.

Questioning

Multiple purposes are met by the use of questions in the assessment interview. Hein [8] clearly states these purposes as follows:

1. To describe and elaborate perceptions, ideas, and feelings.
2. To clarify perceptions, ideas, and feelings.
3. To validate observations.
4. To substantiate facts.
5. To assess the reliability of the information received.
6. To interpret the meaning of a group of facts.
7. To compare information with some predetermined criteria (e.g., nursing goals).
8. To formulate solutions based upon previous assessments and comparisons.
9. To evaluate the outcome of a plan or action [8].

How artfully these purposes are realized is materially influenced by the kinds of questions asked by the nurse. Knowledge of the type of response elicited by different kinds of questions helps the nurse to decide what kind of question to use.

Closed and Open-Ended Questions. Two of the most common formulations of questions are the closed and open-ended types. A *closed question* asks for specific factual data and can be answered simply by a yes or no with no other information. It is especially useful in eliciting explicit confirmation or negation of a particular point. When a patient needs to conserve strength and energy, answering closed questions is the least tiring. In selective circumstances, the nurse may use or modify the closed question to direct and circumscribe patient response choices deliberatively. If, as is frequently the case, the nurse overuses the closed question, the patient may see this as a pattern of interaction and offer little or no additional information. A nurse with this approach would have to maintain a large repertoire of questions.

An *open-ended question* is nonspecific in nature, cues the patient response only in a general way, and elicits expanded descriptive information. The open-ended form, exemplified by beginning a question with "what," allows the patient to express his thoughts, feelings, opinions, and experiences. The patient has the satisfaction of communicating what he feels is important and of doing so in his own way. The responses may furnish valuable data that otherwise would not have been solicited had the nurse utilized the more confining closed question. The latitude of response that the open-ended question permits provides the nurse with more data and clues to topics for needed exploration.

The nurse can use brief phrases and words to encourage the patient to continue and expand on the descriptive information he is giving. These phrases and words are referred to as *minimal encouragers* [9]. Here are some examples:

"Go on."
"Tell me more."
"Oh?"
"So?"
"What then?"
"Um . . . m."
"And?"

Minimal encouragers are useful in that they assist the patient responding to an open-ended question to elaborate a given point. They also elicit examples of specific behaviors, helping the nurse to comprehend better what the patient is saying and to influence the direction of the interview.

"Why" Questions. The nurse should use "why" questions selectively, recognizing that these questions call for formulations of rationale and reasons that the patient may not have worked out in his thought processes or have in mind at the time he is asked. As the patient verbalizes descriptive information during the interview, however, insights into "why" may evolve naturally, in both patient and nurse.

Benjamin [2] suggests that adult usage of the word *why* differs from that of the innocent inquiry of young children seeking information only and conveys learned negative connotations, e.g., disapproval, intimation of wrongdoing, displeasure. He postulates that "whatever the meaning intended by the interviewer, the effect on the interviewee will be predictably negative, for he will most probably have grown up in an environment in which *why* implied blame and condemnation" [2].

Clarification and Paraphrasing
Clarification of words and phrases is one of the most effective facilitators of verbal communication. Routinely, the nurse needs to request clarification of ambiguous terms, indefinite pronouns, and vague referents. The use of medical terminology by either patient or nurse can contribute significantly to ineffectual communication, and the user's meanings must be clarified. Identifying clearly "who, what, when, where, and how" will provide useful information and protect against erroneous interpretations.

Paraphrasing is the restatement of another's ideas in your own words. By paraphrasing the patient's words you indicate what you think the patient is saying. This technique may assist the patient in clarifying content that is confusing to him as well as to you and also serves to reassure him that you do, or are trying to, understand what he is saying.

Information-Giving and Feedback
A patient may request information during the data collection process, and it is appropriate to furnish such information, when possible, to satisfy his need. A satisfied patient is more amenable to continuing with the physical assessment and can be more cooperative than one kept in the dark and unduly concerned. Lengthy information-giving involvements can cut into the time available to the nurse, compromise the primary purposes, and should be avoided. Generally, brief informative statements are all the patient is interested in and will meet his need. The termination phase described earlier allows time for feedback and information-sharing to take place.

Reflection of Feelings   Often during physical assessment, the patient manifests verbal and nonverbal behaviors suggestive of particular feeling states, e.g., discouragement, fear, unhappiness, excitement, pleasure, worry, and relief. The tone of voice, and abrupt change in conversation or demeanor, sighing, and inappropriate laughter are a few examples of such verbal and nonverbal behavior. The nurse observing these behaviors must be cognizant that they provide only *clues* to the patient's feelings and that the nature of the feelings must be validated by the patient, since feeling states are private and personal. It is important that this validating be done by the nurse. She must accept what the patient communicates verbally and modify her assessment approach to work within his frame of reference.

Hazards of   The following are some hazards that may at times constitute definite barriers
Communication   to communication.

Asking Multiple Questions
When the nurse asks two or more questions in one sentence, the patient may attempt unsatisfactorily to answer all of them as one or, since the option is his,

may select the question he wishes to answer. Valuable interview time may be lost in clarifying avoidable confusions and repeating questions to recoup pertinent data.

Overuse of Open-ended or Closed Questions

If the nurse depends too heavily on the closed question, the interview is likely to assume the character of a one-sided interrogation. This practice usually limits the quality and quantity of useful information obtained and creates considerable discomfort for both the patient and nurse examiner.

Overdependence on the open-ended form of question may leave the control and direction of the interview with the patient rather than the nurse. Time may be lost with extraneous content and irrelevant detail. The inexperienced nurse may find it difficult to obtain the kinds of data needed and may react in a way that the patient views as negative—to the detriment of their relationship and communication.

Responding to Multiple Ideas

The descriptive information provided in the patient's response to an open-ended question usually encompasses multiple ideas and avenues for the nurse to explore. She may elect to encourage the patient to continue talking, judging that the topic he pursues is important to him and therefore has significance. An alternate course of action for the nurse is to respond to the topic she judges to be most clinically significant, thereby directing the interview to important data. The nurse must be alert to the hazard of not listening actively, or she will have difficulty making a deliberative choice among the options. Responding to the last idea mentioned is the tendency and should be guarded against.

An example illustrating this hazard involves a patient who responded to the nurse's request that she describe "what kinds of activities she engaged in routinely" by saying: "Up until about a year ago, I did a lot of sewing for my teenage daughter, managed my home, helped with my husband's books, and was very active in my church." The nurse might have inquired about the events of a year ago, or specifics of the patient's home management, or the meaning of helping with the husband's books. Instead, she responded to the last idea and elicited more precise data about the church activities. This information was useful, but more clinically significant data were obtained by later inquiry into what occurred a year ago.

Imposing Values and Providing Sanctions

Many people have a tendency to nod their heads in approval or say "Good" when another person is talking. This type of response arises from social amenities. When the nurse uses this response, she may view it as encouragement to the patient to continue. The patient, however, may construe this response as approval for what he is saying. Verbal and nonverbal mannerisms conveying approval or disapproval can, and often do, influence the kind of information the patient will share. Purposeful guarding against this is necessary, especially when the patient evidences values differing sharply from those held by the nurse.

FORMAT AND DATA-CATEGORY CONSIDERATIONS

Data collection during the interview and examination must be guided by some predetermined, organized framework to ensure that the assessment is thorough and the needed data are obtained. Various formats may be utilized to achieve these purposes and to provide a systematic framework for recording the data to facilitate analysis and reference use. Format decisions are influenced by the agency and setting in which the nurse practices and the particular needs of the patient population being served. Some uniform approach should be adopted which allows variable applications; e.g., for complete assessment on initial contact or periodically, or for partial assessment for follow-up purposes and specialized care needs.

The format should accommodate historical data, current findings, and nursing diagnoses. Information about the patient's perceptions of his health status in general and his specific concerns should be incorporated. Data about the patient as a person, his work, education, interests, family, and life-style form a category essential to include. These data permit the nurse to gain insight into the patient's real and potential health problems and the support systems available to him in dealing with these.

The succeeding chapters, which cover areas of system function and functional abilities important in physical assessment, convey no absolute prescription for format, but suggest some of the things nurses need to consider in deciding which format to use for the physical assessment process. Other useful categories of data to collect and ideas about the overall framework for the interview and examination can be found in varied nursing approaches described by Little and Carnevali [11], Mayers [13], and McCain [14]. Additional helpful perspectives may be gained by examining the medical models detailed in Judge and Zuidema [10] or in Weed's problem-oriented approach [16] (see Chap. 3).

ANXIETY

Numerous theoretic frameworks can be used to aid in understanding and responding to the behavior of individuals. The theoretic concept of anxiety [7, 12] is one of the most appropriate because it is generally useful in explaining much of the behavior the nurse observes. The theoretic concept also includes an operational definition of anxiety which offers additional assistance in determining the presence and level of anxiety.

The following are some specific ways in which an understanding of the concept of anxiety is helpful to the nurse during the process of patient assessment:

1. Aids in recognizing behavior indicating anxiety in her patients.
2. Aids in recognizing behavior indicating anxiety in herself.

3. Aids determining whether the physical findings are more likely to be a manifestation of the patient's anxiety or of an organic condition.
4. Aids recognizing the patient's inability to give accurate data because level of anxiety impairs function, e.g., decreases ability to concentrate and narrows perceptual abilities.
5. Aids in recognizing clues indicating behavior that is used to avoid feeling anxious.

Manaser and Werner's [12] operational definition of anxiety provides a useful guide in determining appropriate nursing actions to reduce severe anxiety. Their operational definition of anxiety states that an individual:

1. Has *expectations.*
2. These *expectations are not met.*
3. Experiences *extreme discomfort.*
4. Behaves in ways to *relieve* discomfort.
5. *Justifies* his behavior verbally.

Expectations   Expectations are expressed in terms of "wants, wishes, hopes, aspirations, and desires" [13]. Many of these are expressed verbally, whereas others are outside awareness but can be brought into awareness as the need arises. Whether conscious or not, they are operant in our behavior.

Expectations Not Met   Expectations held may or may not be met. When circumstances evolve in harmony with our expectations, no untoward effects on our sense of comfort and well-being are experienced. Impending unmet expectations, however, can be described as a threat to the individual, to his sense of himself as a person of worth, independence, and capability. Many times, unmet expectations are expressed as disguised communications, e.g., statements of inadequacy, uselessness, being unappreciated, or thwarted [12]. Frequently, when illness or the possibility of illness occurs, the patient's expectations of continuing his accustomed life-style are challenged. New questions related to the meaning of his illness, hospitalization, and recovery and their impact on his own and family's way of living press the patient to seek new answers. Questions posed by the patient during the interview must be regarded seriously and answered as truthfully as possible to facilitate his setting realistic expectations. When the patient's expectations are unmet, his anxiety increases, and he experiences extreme discomfort.

The Extreme   The extreme discomfort associated with increased anxiety usually is manifested
Discomfort of Anxiety   by feelings of helplessness and powerlessness. The patient often complains of weakness, nervousness, fatigue, tension, or apprehension and uneasiness. Other behaviors indicating anxiety which may be observed by the nurse include downcast eyes and difficulty in making eye contact, slowed or rapid speech,

Figure 5-2.
Organs affected by
stimulation of the
autonomic nervous system.

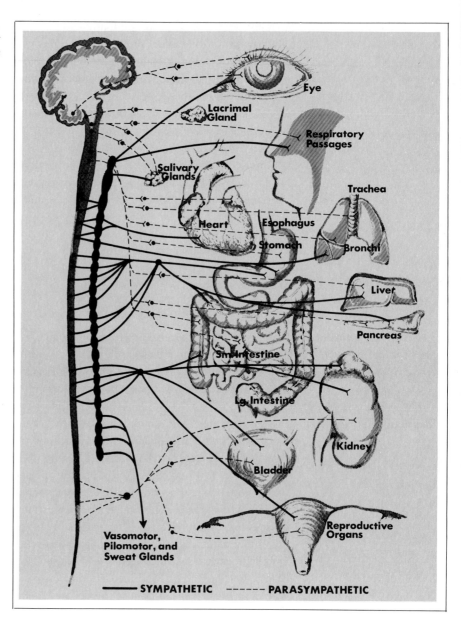

tone-of-voice change, purposeless and restless movements, chain smoking, nail-biting, pacing, and tensed posturing.

Physiologic responses to anxiety occur in the autonomic nervous system with varying effects on the body. Figure 5-2 provides an overview of the organs in which functioning may be affected by anxiety. It is imperative that the nurse be alert for behavioral indications that the patient is anxious and that she attempt to alleviate the discomfort during the interview and throughout the assessment. Since physiologic findings and their interpretations may be manifestations of anxiety rather than of organic dysfunction, these considerations must be incorporated into the nurse's assessment practices.

As anxiety increases, the patient has greater and greater difficulty in organizing his thought processes and may have trouble remembering, making relationships, and comprehending during the interview [7]. Questions may have to be repeated and rephrased and more time allowed the patient to respond. The very anxious patient may be unable to provide useful data, and the nurse may have to change her priorities from collecting data to therapeutic intervention to reduce the patient's anxiety.

Relief Behavior   When a person is unable to reduce his anxiety, his efforts (usually outside of awareness) will be directed toward converting the distressing feelings into other behaviors that make him feel more comfortable. This provides only temporary relief, and when anxiety is reexperienced, this same pattern repeats in cyclical fashion. Some of the more commonly encountered clues to relief behaviors are listed in Table 5-1. Individual instances of relief behavior do not have particular significance. It is the behavioral pattern that is important. Byrne [4] defines behavioral patterns as "a cluster of behaviors that appear to have a

Table 5-1.
Clues to Relief Behaviors

Relief Behavior	Clue
1. Acting out	Anger
	Annoyance
	Irritability
	Demanding
	Crying
	Inappropriate laughter, jokes, sarcasm
	Opposing actions and verbalizations
	Overdramatization and overreaction for the given situation
	Marked changes in patterns of daily activities: sleep, appetite, elimination
	Compulsive attention to details; extreme orderliness
2. Avoidance	Withdrawal, apathy, boredom, and unnaturally timed and prolonged silences
3. Somatization*	Pain syndromes
	Unusual fatigue in view of level of activity
	Headaches
	Paresthesias
	Weakness
	Paralysis
4. Verbalization	Repetitions: Reintroduces same topic repeatedly; asks same questions; gives exaggerated details about an event and/or person
	Significant omissions
	Blaming
	Self-excusing
	Intellectualizations
	Subject-changing

*Somatization is hypothesized if an organic basis is questionable and/or is contradicted by anatomic or physiologic facts, e.g., glove paralysis.

common drive or goal . . ." and states that there is "a degree of repetition." It is this clustering of behaviors into discernible repetitive patterns that is significant to note, as it will influence the planning and provision of nursing care.

Justification   The last concept in the operational definition of anxiety is justification, exemplified in the patient's effort to give rationale to substantiate his relief behavior. It is important for the examining nurse to recognize this step to avoid becoming involved in discussing this aspect of the patient's behavior with him. This involvement is counterproductive, as no useful outcome is likely, and time is wasted unnecessarily in a misdirected effort. Within the theoretic framework of anxiety presented, nurse efforts are more appropriately concentrated on helping the patient identify the expectations he holds that are compromised. Success in these efforts permits the nurse to help the patient to set more realistic expectations and to avoid the anxiety discomfort precipitating the relief behaviors and the need for their justification.

REFERENCES
1. Barrett-Lennard, G. T. Significant aspects of a helping relationship. *Ment. Hyg.* 47(2):223, 1963.
2. Benjamin, A. *The Helping Interview* (2nd ed.). Boston: Houghton Mifflin, 1974.
3. Brill, N. I. *Working with People* (2nd ed.). New York: Lippincott, 1978.
4. Byrne, M., and Thompson, L. F. *Key Concepts for the Study and Practice of Nursing* (2nd ed.). St. Louis: Mosby, 1978.
5. Coombs, A. W., Avila, D. L., and Purkey, W. W. *Helping Relationships, Basic Concepts for Helping Professions.* Boston: Allyn and Bacon, 1971.
6. Fast, J. *Body Language.* New York: Lippincott, 1970.
7. Hays, D. Teaching a concept of anxiety. *Nurs. Res.* 10(2):108, 1961.
8. Hein, E. C. *Communication in Nursing Practice* (2nd ed.). Boston: Little, Brown, 1980.
9. Ivey, A. E. *Microcounseling: Innovations in Interviewing Training.* Springfield, Ill.: Thomas, 1971.
10. Judge, R. D., and Zuidema, G. D. (Eds.). *Methods of Clinical Examination: A Physiologic Approach* (3rd ed.). Boston: Little, Brown, 1974.
11. Little, D. E., and Carnevali, D. L. *Nursing Care Planning* (2nd ed.). Philadelphia: Lippincott, 1976.
12. Manaser, J. C., and Werner, A. M. *Instruments for Study of Nurse-Patient Interaction.* New York: Macmillan, 1964.
13. Mayers, M. G. *A Systematic Approach to the Nursing Care Plan* (2nd ed.). New York: Appleton-Century-Crofts, 1978.
14. McCain, R. F. Nursing by assessment, not intuition. *Am. J. Nurs.* 65:82, 1965.
15. Satir, V. *Conjoint Family Therapy* (Revised ed.). Palo Alto, Calif.: Science and Behavior Books, 1967.
16. Weed, L. L. *Medical Records, Medical Education and Patient Care.* Cleveland Press of Case Western Reserve University, Year Book Medical Publishers, 1971.

SUGGESTED READINGS
Collins, M. *Communication in Health Care.* St. Louis: Mosby, 1977.
Froelich, R. E., and Bishop, F. M. *Clinical Interviewing Skills* (3rd ed.). St. Louis: Mosby, 1977.
Pluckhan, M. *Human Communication: The Matrix of Nursing.* New York: McGraw-Hill, 1978.
Sierra-Franco, M. *Therapeutic Communication in Nursing.* New York: McGraw-Hill, 1978.

Phyllis M. Coindreau Patterson
Linda K. Tanner Strodtman

6. General Appearance and Skin Behavior

GLOSSARY   **alopecia** Loss of hair.

canthus Angle at either end of slit between the eyelids.

ecchymosis Extravasation of blood under the skin (i.e., black-and-blue spots).

erythema Redness of skin, produced by capillary congestion.

excoriation Abraded skin area.

hirsutism State of increased amounts of body and facial hair, especially in the female.

induration Area of increased tissue firmness or hardness.

intertriginous Relating to chafing of apposing skin surfaces (i.e., deep fat folds seen under breasts and in obese states).

keloid Fibrous hyperplasia, usually at the site of a scar, rounded, white or pink, and most often seen on upper trunk or face.

melanin Dark brown, insoluble organic compound, produced by the melanocyte, giving the skin its characteristic shades of brown.

nevus In the general sense, a birthmark or mole.

parotid ducts Ducts found in the posterior mucosal surface of the cheek opposite the maxillary second molar.

petechiae Pinpoint-sized hemorrhages.

pruritus Itching, or term for conditions characterized by itching.

purpura Condition characterized by the presence of confluent petechiae or ecchymoses over any part of the body.

stippling Surface irregularities or indentations indicative of normal gingivae.

stomatitis Inflammation of the mouth.

stria Streak or line (e.g., white or colorless striae on abdomen, breasts, or thighs caused by mechanical stretching of skin).

submaxillary ducts Ducts located on the floor of the mouth on either side of the frenulum of the tongue which may be seen as dark spots.

telangiectasia Dilatation of a group of small blood vessels visible through skin, often with form of a medusa's head, spider, or woven mat.

turgor State of normal or other fullness of tissue.

urticaria Smooth, slightly elevated patches that are redder or paler than surrounding skin; often accompanied by severe itching.

> *The skin is an ecosystem, with a microscopic flora and fauna and diverse ecological niches: the desert of the forearm, the cool woods of the scalp and the tropical forest of the armpit.*
>
> Mary Marples [2]

PERCEPTIONS of human skin and its behavior are often narrowly focused. Skin is usually considered in terms of appearance and comfort, or as a defense mechanism, or both, with little or no attention given to it as a whole. In health it is a discrete world, or ecosystem, with its living and nonliving components all interacting with one another and existing in equilibrium. In bodily disequilibrium or dysfunction, the skin may be the cause or it may reflect the result.

Although the skin is a distinct area to assess, it is only a part of the person and thus the examiner usually forms an impression of the patient's general appearance before skin assessment is made. This composite picture gives a good indication of the individual's level of general health. After this initial impression, the character of the skin and specific areas, such as mucous membranes, scalp, and nails, are examined. It is the intent of this chapter to provide the nurse with the basic physical assessment knowledge for this examination with the understanding that in-depth knowledge and skill will be developed by each nurse through study and experience.

GENERAL APPEARANCE   General appearance is evaluated by a series of observations. It is not unusual for a nurse to observe a patient and, with little or no conversation, formulate a statement that sums up his current condition. Some typical summary statements are, "The patient looks ill," "is in no acute distress," or "must be moved nearer the nurses' station as soon as possible" (for closer observation). With experience the general features or characteristics of illness are learned by the nurse. Her ability to correlate these current observations with previous nursing care experiences and knowledge determines the validity of her conclusions. However, the development of acute observational skills augments the nurse's experiential knowledge and adds insight to her current and future practice.

Since observation involves *looking,* one must know how to look and what to look at. Observation is performed in an orderly cephalocaudal direction. Information regarding not only the patient's functional abilities, but also social and emotional data can be obtained by thorough visual observation. It is important to interview the patient for more detailed information, but very few questions are necessary during the general inspection. Since general inspection of an individual is all-inclusive, some guidelines for areas and features to observe are shown in the diagram in Figure 6-1. These guidelines are meant to offer a beginning outline for observation and to provide stimulating ideas upon which to expand.

Head and Face   Visual examination of the head will be used as an illustration of the interpretive process that occurs in the first few minutes of observation of a patient.

Beginning at the top of the head, the care of the hair is noted, since it is often indicative not only of personal hygiene, but also of the general feeling, tone, social status, body image, and identification with a social or age group (i.e., hair style may be reflective of current social trends). When feeling ill, many women may fail to continue keeping their hair well groomed. Nurses are aware of the "lipstick sign" and the "beard sign," using them as indications of medical or emotional improvement—women again become concerned with their appearance and apply cosmetics, and men want to shave. Occasionally, these may be signs of an attempt to mask true feelings and physical appearance. One differentiates between the two uses only by comparison with the baseline data.

When looking at the face in general, one notes its color (pasty, erythemic, pale, cyanotic), lines and wrinkles (age, expression of emotional state), nutri-

Figure 6-1.
Guidelines for assessment of
physical appearance.

EYES
Expression (dull, alert, blank)
Eye contact
Movement (coordinated, twitching)
Pupil size
Artificial lenses (glasses, contacts)
Cosmetics (false eyelashes, mascara,
eye shadow)
Conjunctiva color (red, pink, pale)
Symmetry (ptosis)

EARS
Position of head for hearing
Hearing aids
Adornments (earrings)

FACE
Color (sallow, pale, ashen, dusky)
Tone (wrinkled, smooth)
Symmetry
Complexion (oil, acne, dry)
Adornments (cosmetics,
appropriateness)
Hair (facial, chin, upper lip,
preauricular)
Mouth and lips
Expression (tense, pursed)
Speech (pitch, speed, tone)
Teeth (condition, absence)
Color (pale, cyanosis, stains)
Symmetry
Hydration (cracked, chapped)
Movement (paralysis, trembling)
Odors

LEGS
Color (varicosities)
Hair (amount, texture, distribution)
Symmetry (congenital or acute defects,
edema)
Musculature
Stockings (type)

HAIR
Color (dye, aging)
Style (cleanliness, neatness)
Amount
Lubrication (brilliantine, oily, dry)
Texture (coarse, fine)

TEETH CONDITION

NECK
Color
Symmetry (lymph nodes, goiter)
Musculature
Pulses (visibility)
Adornments (jewelry, perfume)

TORSO
Symmetry
Adornments
Dress
Style
Quality
Cleanliness

ARMS
Color
Hair (amount, texture)
Lesions (scars, tattoos, purpura)
Musculature
Axillary odor

HANDS
Movement (steady, tremulous, restricted fine)
Fingers (tapered, blunt, clubbed)
Adornments (jewelry)
Nails
Color (pallor, pink)
Length (bitten, manicured)
Ridges (horizontal, vertical)
Adornments (polish)
Cleanliness
Character of hands (nicotine
stains, rough, calluses, nervous
habits)

FEET
Shoes (type, style, fit)
Symmetry (edema)
Lesions (calluses, corns, ulcers)
Color
Toenails
Length
Texture (thick, thin)
Cleanliness
Adornment (polish)

Position or posture
Gait
Body movements
Speech
Breath and body odors
Nutrition
Stature and habitus

tion (fullness of cheeks), complexion (clear, mottled, scarred, moles, hair, lesions, cosmetics), symmetry, ability to use all facial muscles, general expression, and whether or not there is eye contact. The eyes are very expressive and can be evaluated as "dull," "alert," "blank," "active," and so on, to indicate the patient's state of health and emotional state. The ears are observed for color, texture, and presence of lesions. One notes the position in which the head is held for hearing. Does the person favor one ear? The nostrils may be flared, indicating respiratory distress. Distinct breath odors (acetone, fetid) should be noted. The appearance of the mouth is also indicative of a person's health, attitudes, and emotional state (set, smiling, corners down, expressionless.) The lips may demonstrate the state of health by their color (pale), texture (fissures, lesions), and movements (quivering, paralysis). Finally, one looks at the chin and observes the texture and quantity of hair and whether the movement is set or trembling. The ability to see and perceive a great deal about a person from looking at his face can be innate, but the subtleties of the face and its expression may be learned by experience.

Continue down the body, observing and interpreting data as you collect them. Of what use is this information to a nurse? Establishment of baseline data on physical impairments as well as reactions to stress are essential for comparison with future observations. These data allow one to anticipate patient behavior and plan his nursing care accordingly. In addition, by observing the important aspects of a person's appearance on admission, the nurse can help the patient and his family preserve or adapt to a new body image that may be necessitated by a change in functional ability.

Position or Posture What type of position does the patient assume? For example, is he stretched out in a relaxed manner, or upright and tense? Does he assume this for physical needs (e.g., curls up in a splinting position to decrease pain or needs to be propped up for easier breathing)? Can he move freely? Is he restless or still, fidgety or tremulous, round-shouldered or barrel-chested?

Gait In what manner does the patient walk, and with what aids? Possible abnormal gaits are the following:

1. Ataxic—staggering or reeling, resembling the walk of alcohol intoxication.
2. Slapping—walks on broad base with feet wide apart, raises leg high and then slaps feet on the ground. These patients fix their eyes on the ground to observe where they are going and to place their feet (e.g., as in tertiary syphilis).
3. Spastic—jerking uncoordinated movements (e.g., as in multiple sclerosis).
4. Scissors—characterized by walking with thighs close together, because of the rigidity of the abductor muscles (e.g., as in spastic paraplegia).
5. Parkinsonian—walks with the trunk and head bent forward and body held

rigid. These patients take short steps with the arms held rigid. They may suddenly run forward (propulsion) or backward (retropulsion).

Body Movements Body movements may be classified into voluntary (performs normal body activity) and involuntary (body moves in an abnormal pattern in either conscious or unconscious state). Does the patient have any of the following?

1. Tic—habit muscle spasm (usually appears in the eye, face, or neck under stress).
2. Tremor—trembling movement (often due to fatigue, parkinsonism).
3. Convulsive movements—series of violent involuntary contractions, either clonic (intermittent contraction and relaxation) or tonic (sustained contraction).

Speech Characterizing a patient's voice may be helpful in noting dysfunction (e.g., following laryngectomy) or planning for a change in status (e.g., when administering hormones such as androgens or estrogens). The voice is evaluated in terms of strength (weak or strong, soft or loud), tone (hoarse, whining, squeaky), enunciation, and resonance.

Three basic speech defects may be encountered: (1) *aphonia,* which is a loss of voice; (2) *anarthria* or *dysarthria,* the inability to articulate distinctly (e.g., stammering or stuttering); and (3) *aphasia,* a defect or loss of expressive powers in speech, writing, and/or signs, or of comprehending spoken or written language. In motor aphasia, the patient understands, but cannot repeat words or speak spontaneously. Receptive or sensory aphasia is characterized by a lack of understanding of the written or spoken word.

Breath and Body Odors Offensive breath odors are usually associated with poor oral hygiene, dental caries, and infections in the oral cavity. Putrefactive diseases of the lungs with infected sputum (e.g., lung abscesses, bronchiectasis) may cause accompanying fetid breath. In certain diseases or metabolic disorders accompanied by metabolic acidosis (e.g., diabetes mellitus) the breath may have the characteristic sweet fruity odor of acetone. Alcoholic odor of the breath usually indicates ingestion of alcohol, but one should not overlook the possible ingestion of alcohol-containing drugs. In some uremic patients, ammonia is detectable on the breath, and severe liver disease occasionally causes a musty breath odor.

Body odors are usually associated with personal hygiene practices, but may be dependent on cultural habits. Odors are also characteristic of certain types of conditions, including wound infections, advanced carcinoma, and gastrointestinal bleeding. It is difficult to describe these odors, but once the nurse has smelled the identified odor, she can easily recognize it on a subsequent occasion.

Nutrition   A person's nutritional state is frequently obvious and is usually evaluated in terms of overweight or underweight, to varying degrees.

Overweight, or obesity, is classified as exogenous or endogenous. The distribution of fat and its metabolic etiologies are the distinguishing characteristics. *Exogenous obesity,* usually caused by excessive caloric intake, is demonstrated by a generalized distribution of the excess fatty tissues. *Endogenous obesity,* a characteristic of certain endocrine diseases (e.g., Cushing's disease) in which fat distribution is localized to certain areas of predilection, commonly the girdle area, is not related to dietary intake (Fig. 6-2).

Obesity should be differentiated from edema. Edema is demonstrated by tissues that pit (indent) when pressed with a finger. This is not present in obesity. Ascites (fluid in the abdominal cavity) can easily be distinguished from fatty tissue by eliciting the fluid wave (for description of techniques, see Chap. 11).

An underweight condition may vary in degree from mild to severe, with the severely underweight person being referred to as cachectic or emaciated. The characteristic facial appearances are sharp nose, sunken eyes, and hollow temples and cheeks. Some people are naturally slender and are not necessarily ill. When one assesses nutrition, the patient's normal body weight and the rate at which he has either lost or gained weight should be ascertained. Weight loss can occur with wasting diseases (e.g., tuberculosis or carcinoma) or as a result of anorexia secondary to the "worry syndrome." Be sure to question the patient regarding weight change. The recent weight loss may be intentional and without consequence.

The concept of nutrition includes tissue turgor, tone, and volume of skeletal muscle. The volume or mass of the skeletal muscles can be surmised by observation and palpation (see Chap. 13).

Stature and Habitus   Stature is the height or tallness of a person when standing. There are normal variations in height dependent on age, sex, race, and heredity. Individuals whose height is excessive are referred to as giants. The physical characteristics of the giant are dependent on whether the growth hormone oversecretion occurs before or after fusion of the bony epiphysis. The former is refered to as eunuchoid gigantism and the latter as acromegaly.

Individuals whose height is far below normal for their age and race are called *dwarfs.* Included in this category is the *midget,* who has normal proportions but on a smaller scale. Dwarfism may be the result of systemic or nutritional disorders that occur in childhood. However, a large number of short-statured persons are normal since their parents are also short.

Habitus refers to body type or build. Normalcy covers a wide range of body types. The *asthenic type* is usually slender, active, and wiry and may appear to be underweight. The *sthenic type* is broad-shouldered, deep-chested, and athletic in appearance. The *pyknic type* is heavy, soft, and rounded due to an accumulation of body fat.

Figure 6-2.
The signs of Cushing's
Disease. Notice the
distribution of fat in the
girdle area.

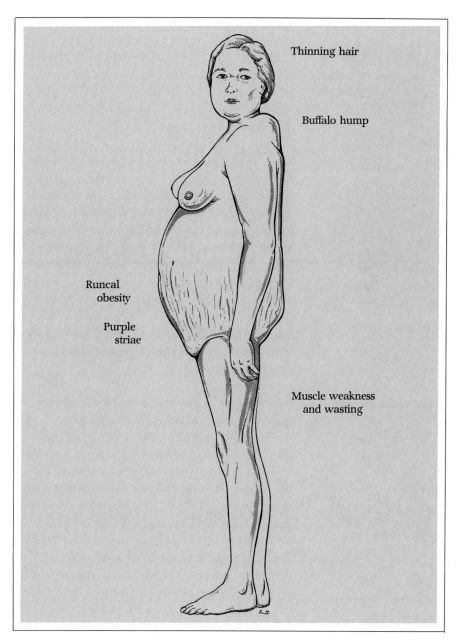

Thinning hair

Buffalo hump

Runcal
obesity

Purple
striae

Muscle weakness
and wasting

Body type is modified by secondary sexual characteristics. The masculine body is usually angular and rugged, with a well-muscled thorax and shoulders wider than hips. The feminine body characteristics are roundness and softness, with relatively more subcutaneous fat, ill-defined muscles, and hips wider than shoulders. In certain endocrine disorders, alterations in secondary sex characteristics occur, and the general habitus of an individual may resemble the opposite sex. Wide variations occur, for instance, the rugged "he-man" versus the effeminate type, or the mannish woman versus the ultrafeminine type.

Summary of General Appearance

A statement regarding general appearance is the end product of evaluation, interpretation, and integration of all the information gathered almost in a "blink of the eye." The amount and validity of the data and the conclusions drawn from them depend on the astuteness of the observer.

SKIN

The skin can be thought of as a mirror that often reflects a person's general health and well-being. The skin may sparkle and glow with vitality, or it may be dull and lifeless. Like the eye, it is important as a point of contact between the person's inner and outer worlds. It helps to regulate body temperature, transmit sensations, combat infections, and express emotions. Though this frontier of the human body is tough and resists the irritants and abrasions of daily living, the cliché "He is thin-skinned," with its numerous connotations, emphasizes the importance of skin reactions in revealing a person's true functional abilities (i.e., physical, social, and emotional). Accurate assessment of skin condition is dependent on the development of one's physical assessment skills and an underlying knowledge of skin physiology. Specifically, the two tools most often needed and utilized in assessing this vital mirror of function are inspection and palpation.

Skin Composition and Function

Before the technique and principles of physical assessment of the skin are discussed, its anatomy and physiology will be reviewed. When assessing the skin, one needs to know its basic structural components and understand their function. The skin is the largest body organ, comprising approximately 16 percent of the total body weight. It consists of three layers: the epidermis (outer layer), the dermis, or cutis (middle layer), and the subcutaneous tissue, or subcutis (inner layer) (Fig. 6-3). The epidermis is covered with a fine layer of horny protein called keratin, which forms the strateum corneum, or protective layer. Melanocytes, which produce melanin for shielding the body against the sun's rays, are present in the basal layer of the epidermis. From the epidermis the accessory appendages (hair, nails, sebaceous glands, apocrine glands, and eccrine glands) extend into the dermis. The dermal layer is composed of bundles of collagen fibers, which act as a supporting framework for the epidermis, and it contains blood vessels, nerves, and lymphatic vessels. The subcutaneous or fatty layer is innermost and is the principal area of fat storage. In brief, the functions of these three layers are protection, heat regulation, sensory control, synthesis of vitamin D and antibodies, and excretory control (Table 6-1).

Interview

The part of the nursing interview relating to the skin complements the general history. Questions are asked that elicit data on skin behavior and emphasize the following points:

Figure 6-3.
Structure of the skin.

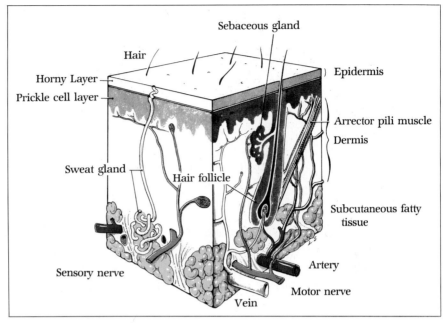

Figure 6-3.
Structure of the skin.

1. *Family history.* Some skin diseases are familial or hereditary. When this is ascertained, one may have the opportunity both to correct misconceptions and allay fears about the presence, absence, or prognosis of disease. What are the current familial dermatologic diseases?

2. *Personal history.* Age at onset of problem? How has the patient adjusted to the problem? By social withdrawal? Cosmetic cover-up? Withdrawal from school athletic activities that require showers (e.g., football, tennis)? Does the problem threaten patient's self-image of masculinity or femininity? What is race or ethnic origin? (Some skin diseases are more common in certain ethnic groups.)

3. *Geographic origin and present abode.* Length of time spent living in each area? (Some skin diseases are indigenous.) This may be important because of increased exposure. Occasionally, a contact of only five minutes is all that is necessary for acquisition of a disease.

4. *Season.* Seasonal occurrence of problem? Pollen? Sunlight?

5. *Occupation.* Type of work? Skin contact material, e.g., chemicals, dusts, gases; excessive heat and abnormal lighting; unhygienic surroundings; possible infected insects; other family members' occupational exposures?

6. *Leisure activities.* Does the problem occur only on weekends? After yard activities? Painting? Woodwork? Camping? Fishing? Hiking? Associated with children's play habits?

7. *Accompanying diseases.* Collagen disease? Drug therapy for collagen disease? Other diseases and their drug therapy?

Table 6-1.
Structure, Composition, and
Function of Skin

Structure and Composition	Function
Epidermis	
Keratinocytes	Protection from bacterial and foreign matter invasion
	Prevention of water and electrolyte loss
	Heat regulation
	Thickens with continual pressure or friction
Melanocytes	Pigmentation—protection from ultra-violet radiation
Epidermal or accessory organs	
Eccrine sweat glands	Heat regulation—evaporation
	Slight excretory function
Hair	Ornamentation
	Protection from dust and particulate matter
	Reduces surface area for heat conservation
Sebaceous glands	Sebum for lubrication of stratum corneum and hair
	Limits absorption and evaporation
Apocrine glands	Semivestigial
	Additional function of epidermis: vitamin D synthesis
Dermis (cutis)	
Collagen tissue	Supporting framework
Vasculature	Heat regulation
Lymphatics	Filters out antigens
Nerve endings	Sensory perception: heat, pain, touch, cold
Reticuloendothelial system	Antibody formation
Elastic fibers	Flexibility, elasticity, strength
	Additional function of dermis:
	Protection from gross physical trauma
	Storage of water and electrolytes
Subcutaneous (subcutis)	
Subcutaneous fatty layer	Fat storage; heat regulation

8. *Previous treatments.* Self-treatment? Other drugs prescribed?

9. *Special history.* Onset of skin lesion (abnormality)? Remissions, exacerbations, or recurrences? Site of onset? Character of lesions? Original character and subsequent changes? Course or extension? Symptoms? Itching? Ability to perform duties? Topical therapy? Self-treatment? Psychologic factors? What does the patient associate with exacerbations of the problem (e.g., stress of a family argument, tax time, report time)?

Physical Assessment Guidelines

Assessment of skin begins with inspection, the most important aspect of the physical assessment process. Palpation is used to verify and support the findings of inspection. Frequently, these two processes are interrelated and are performed simultaneously. Several basic principles valuable in assessment of the skin should be kept in mind. These principles, as modified from Judge and Zuidema [1], are:

1. Provide the patient with a comfortable environment and adequate room illumination. Nonglare (indirect) daylight is optimal. Flashlights and the usually dim lights over the bed are not adequate. Some of the newer lights that simulate daylight are acceptable. Observations made at night should be confirmed by the same person or another person in daylight.

2. Use metric measurements when possible. (A number of helpful aids are available from pharmaceutical companies for use in assessing the size of skin lesions.)

3. Compare each symmetrical or functional area with its opposite: for example, one side of the body against the other, or a sun-exposed area with an area not exposed to the sun.

4. Learn and use precise terminology and nomenclature when describing skin (see Glossary and Fig. 6-4).

5. Record the findings in the patient's record, and use this information as baseline data for determination of change. With each change in patient status, record progress notes.

6. Begin the examination by a brief careful survey of the entire skin, including the mucous membranes when possible. Start with the scalp and proceed to the toes. It is important to examine the entire skin, even though patients frequently deny the existence of skin changes. The expert nurse practitioner can usually list numerous examples of patients who denied any skin abnormalities, but in whom major alterations were uncovered on direct visualization. One such nurse discovered a thumbtack implanted in the sole of the patient's foot. The patient had diabetes mellitus with peripheral neuropathy and was unable to feel any abnormalities or to perform daily foot inspection to detect deviations. Often, patients are unwilling or hesitant to undress, which can be a hindrance to physical examination if the patient is not enlightened as to the importance of examining the whole integument even when he is "sure" there are no possible problems.

7. Proceed systematically, examining the smooth skin (back, chest, abdomen, and extremities); intertriginous areas (deep folds where skin surfaces are opposed); hair (scalp, facial, chest, axillary, and pubic); mucous membranes (buccal cavity and sclera); and nails.

8. When specific skin lesions (see Fig. 6-4) are noted, look first at their general distribution and then more closely at specific affected areas. Primary lesions appear first as a direct result of a causative factor (e.g., erythema following trauma such as a blow with a baseball). Secondary lesions are modifications of, or changes appearing after, the primary lesion (e.g., ecchymosis following the erythema of trauma). Later, the secondary lesion may undergo a series of

Figure 6-4.
(A) Primary and (B)
secondary skin lesions and
their characteristics.

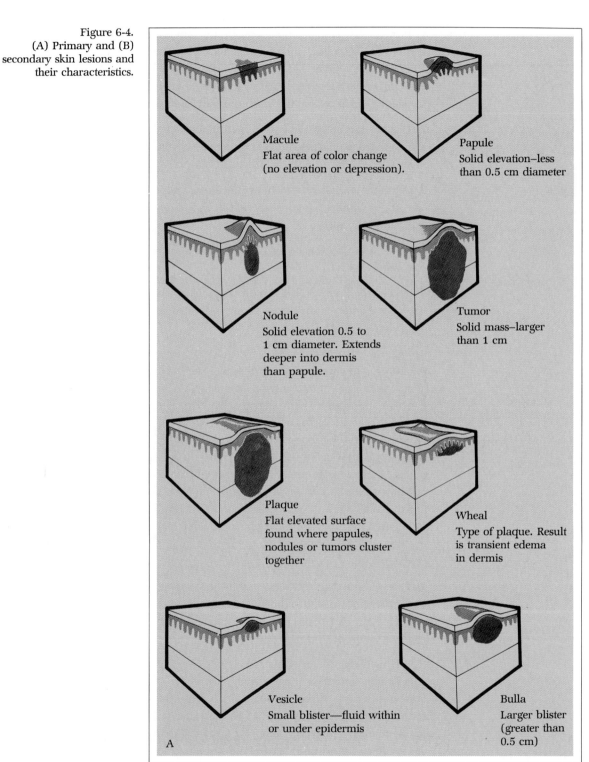

Macule
Flat area of color change
(no elevation or depression).

Papule
Solid elevation–less
than 0.5 cm diameter

Nodule
Solid elevation 0.5 to
1 cm diameter. Extends
deeper into dermis
than papule.

Tumor
Solid mass–larger
than 1 cm

Plaque
Flat elevated surface
found where papules,
nodules or tumors cluster
together

Wheal
Type of plaque. Result
is transient edema
in dermis

Vesicle
Small blister—fluid within
or under epidermis

Bulla
Larger blister
(greater than
0.5 cm)

A

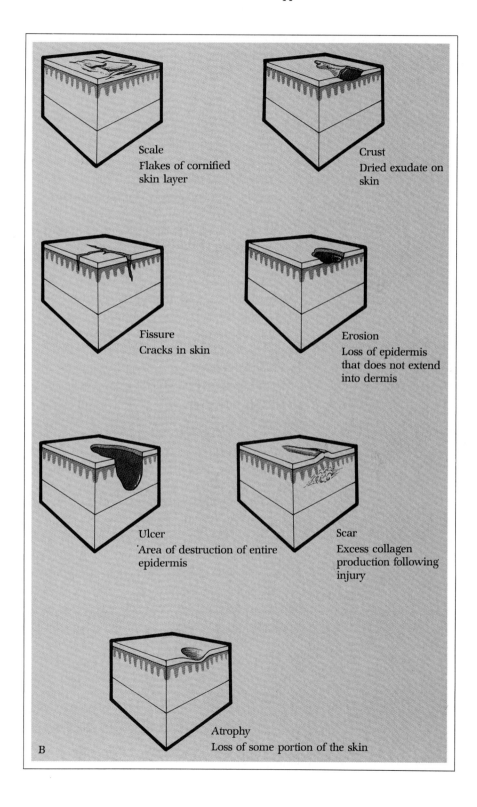

Scale
Flakes of cornified
skin layer

Crust
Dried exudate on
skin

Fissure
Cracks in skin

Erosion
Loss of epidermis
that does not extend
into dermis

Ulcer
Area of destruction of entire
epidermis

Scar
Excess collagen
production following
injury

Atrophy
Loss of some portion of the skin

B

characteristic changes until resolution of the lesion occurs (e.g., ecchymosis may change from its characteristic black-and-blue color to yellow and brown and then fade and disappear).

Assessment and Interpretation of Skin Findings

Color. An important but difficult element of skin inspection is assessment of color. There is great variability in skin color from person to person and in the same person. Heavily pigmented skin poses additional difficulties for the inexperienced eye, but with practice one sees few patients whose skin cannot be accurately evaluated.

The color of normal skin depends primarily on its content of melanin, carotene, oxyhemoglobin, or reduced hemoglobin. The melanin content of the keratinocytes and melanocytes determines the skin pigmentation. Contrary to popular belief, skin in all races has the same proportion of melanocytes. The variations in color are due to genetically determined and acquired differences in production of melanin and its transfer to the keratinocytes.

Both skin color and intensity (light or dark) are assessed. Areas of least pigmentation are best for assessing color (e.g., the sclera, conjunctiva, nail beds, lips, buccal mucosa, tongue, palms, and soles). Heavily calloused areas on the hands and feet usually have an opaque yellow color.

Skin color may be affected by position or gravity. For example, in a person with a peripheral vascular disorder, color changes of an extremity depend on whether it is elevated, level with the heart, or in a dependent position. A useful method for evaluating color of an extremity is to position it at all three levels: heart level, elevated at 15 degrees for at least five minutes, and finally lowered 30 to 90 degrees for at least five minutes [3].

Convolutions of the skin often distort the true coloration by intensifying the color. These areas, such as knees, elbows, nipple and areola of the female breast, and fat folds, should be smoothed or spread out when being assessed. Similarly, edema reduces skin color intensity by increasing the distance between the pigmented surface and its vasculature. These factors may lead to inaccurate appraisals if their significance is not considered.

The patient's activities immediately prior to assessment can influence skin color. Emotional factors such as anger and fright or embarrassment and self-consciousness may contribute to generalized pallor in the former two or superficial vasodilatation (blush) in the latter two. Since cigarette smoking causes vasoconstriction, it may affect correct assessment of nail bed color. Application of warm soaks, use of hypothermia, and other such treatment modalities can also alter color. Distortion of skin color may be externally induced by other agents such as lipstick, powders, tanning agents, and tattooing. Comprehensive history-taking helps to prevent observational mistakes. Recognition of these distorting factors and their influence on skin color is important. In cases of sudden or episodic skin color change, imaginative questioning might save time and testing later on. Recall the mysterious case of "red sweat," in which Eastern

Airlines attendants reported red spots on their skin after working on certain flights. Extensive testing and questioning finally revealed that fears of subcutaneous bleeding were unfounded. The red spots were attributed to the red ink marking on "demonstration only" vests worn by the attendants for passenger review of safety procedures. A few investigative questions and comparisons of the afflicted attendants' reports might have gotten to the source of the problem before diagnostic tests were carried out.

Normal color distribution patterns vary from person to person and race to race. For example, dark-skinned people like those of Mediterranean origin may have very blue lips, contributing to a mistaken judgment of cyanosis. Blotchy or bluish pigmentation of the gums and brown melanin deposits in the scleras, nail beds, or both are often normal findings in blacks who are very dark-skinned. In the dark-skinned person, the areas of lighter melanization (abdomen, buttocks, and volar surface of the forearm) allow for more accurate evaluation of pigmentation. Some types of skin abnormalities, such as erythema, are often visible in lighter-skinned persons, but not in those whose skin is dark; however, the affected part may become an even deeper shade of brown. When inflammation is suspected in the dark-skinned person, other parameters are assessed by palpation—increased skin temperature, tight skin suggestive of edema, induration of deep tissue or blood vessels, and tenderness. Since the dorsal skin surface of the fingers is more sensitive to subtle skin temperature differences than the palmar surface, use the dorsal portion of the fingers to move from one skin area to another for comparison. The patient's family and friends are also helpful in validating color change, particularly when it has occurred gradually.

The primary sites for assessing a patient's pallor are the nail beds, lips, and conjunctiva. When observing the inferior palpebral conjunctiva (lower eyelid) for pallor, the lid should be lowered sufficiently to see the conjunctiva near the temporal (outer) canthus in addition to the inner canthus, since the coloration of the former is often darker. When assessing the darkly pigmented individual for pallor, greater perception is necessary because the changes are subtle. There may be an absence of red tones; the brown-skinned person may appear more yellowish-brown; and the black-skinned person may appear ashen gray. This supports the need for accurate baseline data for comparison.

Jaundice and cyanosis are observed in the usual sites (e.g., mucous membranes, nail beds). Since many factors can alter these findings, one single positive finding should not be held as conclusive. Other parameters, such as environmental temperature, drugs, smoking, amount of hemoglobin, color of urine, stools, or both, can support a description of cyanosis or jaundice. Both in the dark-skinned and light-skinned person, yellow scleras may indicate jaundice, but other factors can cause yellow scleral pigmentation; fatty deposits that contain carotene are a common finding in dark-skinned people. To determine whether the yellow scleras signify jaundice, observe the hard palate in bright daylight. Jaundice can be detected there quite early, i.e., when serum bilirubin is 2 to 4 mg per 100 ml, if the palate does not have heavy melanin pigmentation [3]. If the hard palate does not show jaundice when the scleras are yellow, the pigmentation may be due to some other factor, such as carotene accumulation. All these factors support the importance of repeated observations and accurate descriptions of what is seen. As often as possible the same person should perform the entire examination and should confirm specific findings in one area with additional data from other areas.

Texture

Palpation is used to validate further the data that are gathered from inspection and to ascertain other qualities such as texture, temperature, hydration, and turgor. The character of the skin's surface (i.e., fineness, coarseness) and the feel of deeper portions are its texture. The presence or absence of such textures as rough, dry, smooth, or velvety is best ascertained by stroking the volar surface of the forearm with the dorsal side of the fingers. Feeling the deeper portions of the skin may reveal areas of induration such as those resulting from multiple intramuscular or subcutaneous administrations of medication. These lipodystrophies may consist of smooth, large depressions in the skin that indicate atrophy of the subcutaneous fat layer or marked hypertrophy of the subcutaneous fat layer, which is of a spongy consistency. Both of these conditions are often seen at sites of repeated insulin injections.

Surface Temperature

Another skin quality is its surface temperature. Although skin temperature is an inadequate measure of the body's internal temperature, it gives valuable data about the patient's functional status. If a febrile patient is warm and dry, the temperature is probably rising, since the thermoregulatory mechanism of sweating is not functioning. Likewise, if the skin is warm and wet, the temperature can be expected to fall, owing to the cooling mechanism of sweating. Since the skin temperature is dependent on the amount of blood circulating through the dermis, decreased localized blood flow, often to the feet, may indicate a peripheral vascular dysfunction. Generalized skin coolness may indicate decreased metabolism such as that occurring after general anesthesia. If the temperature is very low, signs of shock may be evident. An increase in skin temperature may indicate a hypermetabolic state, such as that occurring in hyperthyroidism and after sun exposure or sunburn.

  Of the total body heat produced, 85 percent is lost through the skin by conduction, convection, radiation, and evaporation. Cooling of the body by evaporation, through sweating, is of various types and has many etiologies. Identification of the type of sweating often helps in differentiating normal from abnormal body functioning. The exocrine sweat glands, which are found over the entire body, respond principally to thermal and emotional stimuli. Maximal sweating due to emotion occurs on the palms, soles, and axillae, whereas maximal thermal sweating is seen on the fingers, arms, forehead, and axillae. When evaluating thermal causes of sweating, factors that may raise body temperature and induce sweating must be sought. Has the patient been active, walking up and down stairs, for example, or has he been confined to bed? Is his room environment exceptionally warm? Has he just had a hot bath or shower? Is he receiving any medications that may induce sweating? Has he just eaten? After eating highly spiced foods, some people may exhibit gustatory sweating, indicated by sweat on the forehead, upper lip, scalp, and back of the neck. Sweating primarily of the palms and soles leads one to look for other evidence of fear or anxiety.

Sweating can also occur when there is a rapid fall in blood glucose, with resultant rise in the blood epinephrine level. This cause of sweating can usually be distinguished from the others because of the additional symptoms of weakness, tachycardia, hunger, headache, and "inward nervousness," or mental irritability or confusion.

The apocrine sweat glands are less numerous than the exocrine and are found in hair-bearing areas. They do not play a role in thermoregulation and respond only to emotional and sensory stimuli. These glands are responsible mainly for the sweat that produces "body odor," particularly in the axillae.

Hydration

Other skin qualities useful to the nurse in patient assessment are hydration and turgor. The state of hydration of skin and mucous membranes helps to indicate body fluid disturbances. A dry, leathery appearance of the tongue may not be a reliable indicator of negative water balance since mouth breathing frequently makes the tongue look dehydrated. A more reliable method of assessing hydration of the oral cavity is to palpate the mucous membranes along the area of the gum and cheek where the membranes approximate. If the membranes are dry and the finger does not slide easily, the patient may be water-deficient.

Turgor

Skin turgor can be assessed by picking up and releasing the skin, particularly on the dorsa of the hands or forearms. Normal skin usually snaps back immediately into its resting position. If the skin is loose and wrinkled or lacks tone, or both, the patient may be dehydrated. Remember, though, that with aging there is normally a loss of elasticity in subcutaneous tissue. If the skin over the hands, feet, ankles, and sacrum is firm and indents easily (pitting edema) on moderate pressure from the examiner's fingertips, fluid excess is present.

The Dermal Appendages

Hair. Some type of hair is found on all skin surfaces except the palms and soles, which have no hair follicles. There are two types of hair—terminal hair (long, coarse, thick hair that is easily visible on the scalp, beard, moustache, axillae, and pubis) and vellus hair (downy or lanugo hair, which is only visible on close inspection and covers the whole body, except the palms and soles) [4].

All hair has growth phases of both activity and rest. Hair in different regions has a different growth cycle. Scalp hair grows about 2 mm weekly, and the growing phase of any one hair is two to three years. Resting hairs make up 5 to 15 percent of the total of 100,000 hairs on the human scalp [4]. The resting phase occurs every few months to a few years. Terminal hairs elsewhere on the body have a shorter growing phase than those on the scalp. The high speed of growth of the scalp hair makes it more susceptible to damage from systemic disease, toxic drugs, and radiation [4]. The rate of growth varies with general health and age.

The distribution of hair over the body warrants careful observation. The scalp hair, eyebrows, eyelashes, and downy hair of the body are present in both sexes. After puberty, coarse body hair evolves in distinct male and female patterns of the axillary and genital areas (Fig. 6-5). Disturbances in body function are often reflected by changes in amount, texture, color, and growth pattern of the hair.

Alterations in amount of body hair can be extremely anxiety-provoking for both males and females. In the female with hirsutism, hair growth is intensified on the upper lip, chin, cheeks, chest, and from the pubic crest to the umbilicus (along the linea alba); and the downy hair on the arms, legs, and back becomes coarse. The pubic hair often takes on the upright triangular distribution typical of the male as opposed to the female's usual inverted triangle. An endocrine malfunction such as excess androgen production may sometimes be associated with hirsutism, but ethnic background (Mediterranean groups predominantly) may also be responsible for the excessive hair growth. This is especially true of the hair on the arms, legs, back, and face. Other ethnic group members such as the full-blooded black female and the male Indian rarely have facial hair or a beard. Distribution of the hair in family members and

Figure 6-5. Normal hair distribution in adult men and women. Changes may signal hormonal abnormalities. (Reproduced with permission from R. D. Judge, G. D. Zuidema, and F. Fitzgerald (Eds.). *Methods of Clinical Examination* (4th ed.). Boston: Little, Brown, 1982.)

Male escutcheon   Female escutcheon

Figure 6-6.
Alopecia areata.
(Reproduced with
permission from R. D.
Judge, G. D. Zuidema, and
F. Fitzgerald (Eds.).
*Methods of Clinical
Examination* (4th ed.).
Boston: Little, Brown,
1982.)

consideration of ethnic background are important in ascertaining the normalcy of hair growth.

Common disturbances of scalp hair involve its thickness. Baldness (alopecia) or thinning of the hair that is generalized or creates a receding hairline often is genetically determined (Fig. 6-6). Some rare genetic defects in the hair shaft itself may produce breaking of the hairs and be mistakenly diagnosed as alopecia. General and localized baldness may result from treatment modalities such as radiation or chemotherapy. In addition, various types of scalp diseases (e.g., fungal, lupus) and telogen effluvium (transient hair loss occurring two to three months after general anesthesia, febrile illness, or giving birth) can cause hair loss. Other traumatic types of hair loss may occur from pulling of the hair because of a nervous habit; hairstyles such as braiding or ponytails; or constrictive wearing apparel such as a hat. The normal scalp sheds about 20 to 100 hairs per day, so one needs to determine if hair loss is in excess of this amount [4]. To determine whether the complaint of hair loss is genuine, ask the patient to collect and count hairs on his comb or hairbrush the day before washing the head, after washing, and on two succeeding days—four days in all. An average daily loss of over 100 is abnormally high [4].

Since hair is essentially an adornment for many men and women, its loss or excess often provokes embarrassment and anxiety and conflict with the patient's self-image of masculinity or femininity. Awareness and sensitivity to the patient's need for personal expression of concerns and privacy is important in planning the care program.

Another pertinent feature relating to the hair is its amount of lubrication. Sebum from sebaceous glands anoints the hair and keeps it from drying and becoming brittle by limiting the amount of absorption and evaporation of water from the surface. The sebaceous glands are most numerous over the face and scalp. Assessing these areas gives one the best indication regarding the amount of skin oiliness. Hyperfunction of these glands is associated with androgen stimulation such as occurs with the excessive scalp oiliness and facial acne in adolescence. Dry, brittle hair is commonly the result of excessive washing or the application of chemical agents (coloring, bleach, or detergents) to the hair. In addition to the direct observation of the scalp and face, correlation of the findings with the data from the interview helps to determine dysfunctional states.

The Nails

The fingernails and toenails grow at a fairly constant rate, except when altered by generalized disease or injury. This makes them useful as an indicator of the person's general health; they should be examined closely (Fig. 6-7). The visible nail plate is a dead sheet of hard keratin, and changes seen in the nails reflect damage that occurred earlier. Fingernails normally grow at the rate of 0.1 mm

Figure 6-7. Fingernails are important indicators of a person's general health. They should be inspected carefully. (Reproduced with permission from R. D. Judge, G. D. Zuidema, and F. Fitzgerald (Eds.). *Methods of Clinical Examination* (4th ed.). Boston: Little, Brown, 1982.)

Figure 6-8.
Nail abnormalities.
(Reproduced with
permission from R. D.
Judge, G. D. Zuidema, and
F. Fitzgerald (Eds.).
*Methods of Clinical
Examination* (4th ed.).
Boston: Little, Brown,
1982.)

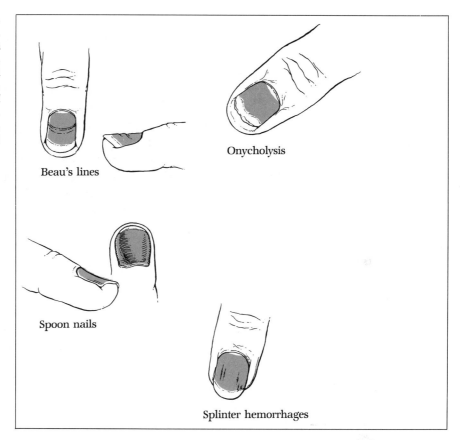

Beau's lines

Onycholysis

Spoon nails

Splinter hemorrhages

per day. By measuring the distance between abnormalities (pits, grooves, and lines) and the proximal nail border, one may estimate the time of initial illness.

Normal nails are transparent, with pink nail beds and translucent white tips at the point of separation of the nail from the nail bed. Surface longitudinal ridges and flecks of white spots in the nail are within normal limits. Transverse furrows *(Beau's lines)* in the nail indicate that nail growth has been disturbed. This can result from infection, systemic disease, or injury. Nails with concave curves are known as *spoon nails* or koilonychia. They may signal a form of iron deficiency anemia, and they are also associated with other disorders such as coronary disease, syphilis, or the use of strong soaps. Destruction of the nails *(onycholysis)* may accompany hyperthyroidism, fungal nail infection, or psoriasis. *Splinter hemorrhages* may be linked to bacterial endocarditis and trichinosis. These red or brown splinters or streaks run parallel to the finger in the nail bed. See Figure 6-8 for illustration of these nail signs. Clubbing of the fingers is characterized by a flattening of the angle of the base of the nail as in Figure 6-9. It may occur in association with cardiovascular disease, subacute bacterial endocarditis, and pulmonary disease.

Figure 6-9.
Clubbing. (Reproduced
with permission from R. D.
Judge, G. D. Zuidema, and
F. Fitzgerald (Eds.).
*Methods of Clinical
Examination* (4th ed.).
Boston: Little, Brown,
1982.)

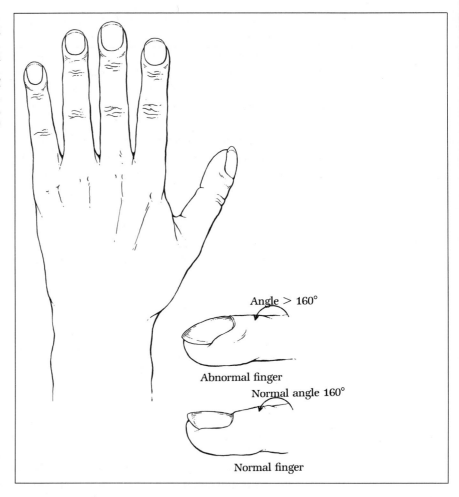

The nurse most often uses nail color as an indication of the amount of blood oxygenation. Bluish or purplish discoloration of the nail beds occurs with cyanosis, whereas pallor often indicates anemia. To compare color of the nail beds, apply slight pressure on the free edge of the second or third fingernail. The blanching that results is then compared to the normal color of the nail. The rate of color return also indicates the quality of peripheral vasomotor function.

Oral Mucous Membrane Examination

As with the skin, the mouth itself may reveal not only local but systemic disease and should be thoroughly examined. The recognition of poor oral hygiene early in hospitalization opens the path to immediate intervention, with the possibility of preventive nursing care. The purposes of a program of care are prevention, healing, and lessening of disease.

Repeated examination of the mouth provides a clinical knowledge base from which to recognize beginning and ongoing problems and to evaluate the effectiveness of prescribed care. The techniques used are inspection and palpation. The instruments needed are a tongue blade, bright mobile light source, and glove or finger cots. The patient may be sitting or recumbent. If both the examiner and patient are sitting, the examiner should face the patient at the same level.

The oral mucosal surface has a rich vascular supply. Normally the color of this surface is pale coral pink and is kept moist by numerous submucosal accessory salivary glands augmenting the major salivary gland secretion. Bright red surfaces usually indicate inflammation, while pallor indicates localized ischemia or generalized anemia. Cyanosis suggests hypoxemia, which may indicate local congestion or a systemic disease. The oral buccal cavity is pigmented with generalized and local melanin in accordance with racial background. Normally, the gums of pure blacks may be a bluish color, occurring either diffusely or in splotches; in other blacks, brown pigment is present in the gingival mucosa. On the tongue, brown pigmented dots, single or in groups, especially at the borders of the tongue, are not uncommon in blacks. Pigment changes in the oral mucous membrane may indicate many systemic conditions.

Begin the oral examination by explaining to the patient what is to occur. Observe the symmetry in form and function of the lips as the patient attempts to whistle. Observe the function and fit of dentures and then ask the patient to remove them. Always use direct lighting for the examination. Inspect the inner lip, cheek surfaces, and all the recesses of the gingivobuccal folds and gums by retracting the lips and cheeks with a tongue blade. Next ask the patient to open his mouth wide. Inspect the hard (anterior) and soft (posterior) palates. Depress the tongue with a tongue blade (being careful that the tongue is within the teeth) and request the "ah" phonation to observe midline uvula elevation and pharynx constriction (Fig. 6-10a). Have the patient protrude his tongue. Assess its size, symmetry, involuntary movements, and restricted protrusion, in addition to the dorsal surface characteristics. Finally, retract the patient's tongue laterally, and view the posterior surface of the floor of the mouth (Fig. 6-10c). Ask the patient to raise the tip of his tongue to the roof of his mouth while he keeps his mouth open. Inspect the ventral surface of the tongue and the anterior floor of the mouth (see Fig. 6-10b).

With the patient maintaining the open-mouth position, inspect the teeth for their form and support in the mouth. Using a probe, tap each tooth lightly for tenderness. Observe the movements of the mandible and occlusion of the teeth to evaluate their effectiveness during mastication.

Before proceeding with palpation of the oral mucosa, stop and explain the procedure to the patient. Ask the patient to protrude his tongue. The tongue can be controlled by grasping it between layers of gauze. The mucosa can now be adequately palpated. Using the index finger covered with a glove, gently

Figure 6-10.
Positions for mouth
examinations. *A.* View of
dorsum, palate, and
pharynx. *B.* Inspection of
ventral surface and floor of
the mouth. *C.* Inspection
and palpation of posterior
surface of floor of mouth.
(From Judge and Zuidema
[1].)

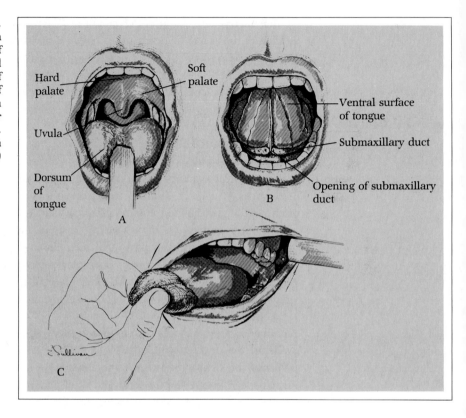

palpate the soft, smooth surfaces. Release the tongue and continue palpation to the floor of the mouth. Palpate this oral mucosa with the opposite hand, supporting external tissues. Continue this bimanual palpation in the cheek and lip region. Conclude by palpating the hard and soft palate areas. Note the flow and quality of secretions from the orifices of the submaxillary and parotid ducts [1].

Guidelines for examination of the mouth are presented in Table 6-2, p. 119.

LYMPH NODE EXAMINATION

When inspecting and palpating the skin, also examine the lymph nodes. The groups of nodes that are generally examined are the cervicofacial, supraclavicular, axillary, epitrochlear, inguinal, and femoral. The tools that are required for assessment of the lymph nodes are inspection and palpation. The description of each node should include:

1. Exact location.
2. Extent of enlargement (usually the diameter is expressed in centimeters or in some familiar size, e.g., split pea, bean, almond).
3. Presence or absence of tenderness.
4. Presence or absence of visible or palpable surrounding inflammation.

Table 6-2.
Regional Observations of
the Mouth

Regions	Functions	Normal Characteristics	Assessment Guidelines
Lips	Speech Oral intake Control of secretions Contribute to facial expression	Pink, smooth, soft Exposed portion: dry, vermilion, usually marked by slight superficial vertical wrinkling Inside lips: grayish red	Color, form, position, function, texture, asymmetry, chapping, cracking of the mucosa, irritations at the corners or angles of the mouth, congenital or acquired defects, lesions
Teeth	Mastication	White enamel surface; no debris, film, or hard deposits Number: 32 (full adult dentition) Number: 20 (deciduous)	Color, number, caries, size, discoloration, occlusion, notched or peglike, bridges, alveolar swelling
Gums	Supporting structure Mastication	Pale, coral-pink, firm, slightly stippled surface (like an orange), attached to teeth and projecting to fill interdental space as papillae	Color, form, density, retraction of gingival margin, pus in margins, inflammation, spongy or bleeding gums, localized gingival swelling
Tongue	Speech Mastication Taste Swallowing	*Dorsal:* moist, glistening coating, muscular; four types of papillae include: filiform (most important and numerous), fungiform (grayish-red), foliate (located along the lateral portion of the posterior of the tongue), vallate papillae (form a V near the back of the tongue) *Ventral:* pink, smooth, shows large veins	Color, size, texture, papillae cleanliness, moisture, voluntary or involuntary movements, deviation from midline, restricted protrusion, tenderness, position, lesions Varicose veins
Buccal mucosa (cheeks)	Mastication Houses parotid gland	Grayish-red color; may be crossed by fine grayish ridges where it settles between rows of teeth when the mouth is closed; the parotid gland emits a clear secretion	Color, texture, parotid gland, ulcer, melanin deposits, vesicles, neoplasms, cysts or swelling of parotid gland, ductal orifice

Table 6-2.
Continued.

Regions	Functions	Normal Characteristics	Assessment Guidelines
Hard palate	Mastication Houses mucous glands	Pale pink, immovable, moist underlying bony process of the maxilla; no debris; irregular; rugae running transversely; orifices of ducts of mucous glands in the posterior part of hard palate; midline, hard swelling is a common variation	Color, texture, glands, ductal orifices; ducts may look like red dots in heavy smokers (nicotine stomatitis); swelling; rugae
Soft palate	Swallowing Speech Houses mucous glands	Pink, muscular; has abundant submucosal accessory salivary glands; shows fine vessels under the mucosa	Color, texture, glands, ulcers, fungal infections, inflammation
Breath odors	Manifestation of condition of mouth, oral intake, systemic disease, lung disease	Absent or sweet	*Fetid:* infections of oral cavity, poor oral hygiene, putrefactive disease of the lung *Acetone:* diabetic acidosis *Ammonia:* renal failure *Musty:* liver disease
Floor of the mouth	Supporting structures Houses submaxillary gland, sublingual gland, lymph nodes	Pale, coral pink, loose tissue Submaxillary glands emit a clear mucous secretion Submental and submaxillary lymph nodes	Neoplasms here are sometimes detectable only by palpation; cysts of sublingual glands; sublingual and submaxillary ductal orifices; lymph nodes are palpated for swelling

5. Whether they are freely movable, adherent to the deeper structures, or matted together as a result of extensive inflammatory changes.
6. Texture (hard, soft, firm).

Inspect both sides and compare. Use the middle three fingers for palpation and notation of any visible lymphadenopathy. Movements should be slow and gentle; the fingers should move up and down, back and forth, and in a rotary motion. Palpation should be light or small nodes will be missed.

Figure 6-11.
Technique of examination
of cervicofacial lymph
nodes. *A.* Location of major
groups of nodes. *B.*
Anterior approach. *C.*
Posterior approach.
(Modified from Judge and
Zuidema [1] and R. D.
Judge, G. D. Zuidema, and
F. Fitzgerald (Eds.).
*Methods of Clinical
Examination* (4th ed.).
Boston: Little, Brown,
1982.)

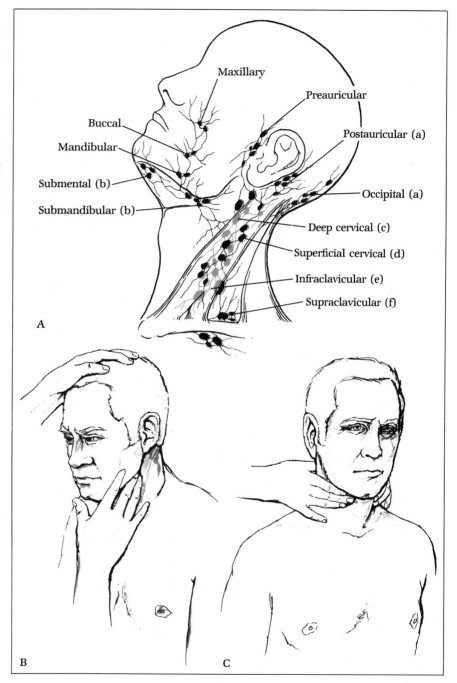

Figure 6-12.
Axillary nodes. *A.* Location
of major groups of nodes.
B. Technique of
examination of axillary
lymph nodes. *C.* Technique
of examination of
epitrochlear lymph nodes.
(From Judge and Zuidema
[1] and R. D. Judge, G. D.
Zuidema, and F. Fitzgerald
(Eds.). *Methods of Clinical
Examination* (4th ed.).
Boston: Little, Brown,
1982.)

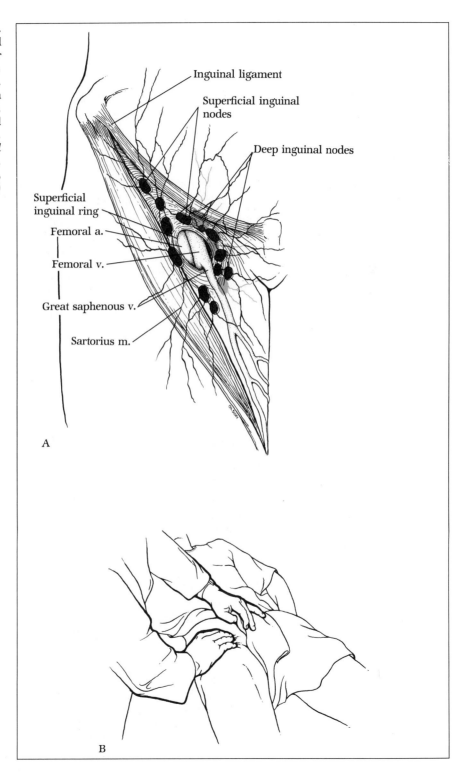

Figure 6-13. Inguinal and femoral nodes. *A.* Location of major groups of nodes. *B.* Technique for examination. (Reproduced with permission from R. D. Judge, G. D. Zuidema, and F. Fitzgerald (Eds.). *Methods of Clinical Examination* (4th ed.). Boston: Little, Brown, 1982.)

Inguinal ligament

Superficial inguinal nodes

Deep inguinal nodes

Superficial inguinal ring

Femoral a.

Femoral v.

Great saphenous v.

Sartorius m.

A

B

Cervicofacial and Supraclavicular Nodes

Proceed in an orderly fashion with the examination. Begin by examining the superior and posterior lymph nodes, proceeding downward as follows (Fig. 6-11A): (a) occipital and postauricular; (b) submandibular and submental; (c) anterior angle (upper end of deep cervical chain); (d) downward along the sternocleidomastoid muscle (superficial cervical nodes); (e) posterior triangle (lower end of deep cervical chain); (f) supraclavicular. The two approaches to examination of the nodes are shown in Figures 6-11B and C.

Axillary and Epitrochlear Nodes

For examination of the axillary and epitrochlear nodes the patient may be either sitting or supine. The axilla can be thoroughly assessed with one hand while the examiner's opposite hand holds the ipsilateral arm of the patient. The axilla should be thought of as having an apex and three walls: anterior or pectoral group, central group, and posterior group. Each of these areas should be palpated with the patient's arm at the side and again while the arm is moved through a full range of motion. This is done to uncover any lesions hidden under a muscle or in a fatty layer. Be aware of the patient's comfort and move the arm gently. Proceed by cupping the hand slightly and reach high into the apex of the axilla. Pull down, exerting gentle pressure with the fingertips against the thorax (see Fig. 6-12A and B).

Repeat this procedure, checking each group of nodes respectively.

The epitrochlear nodes are palpated as shown in Figure 6-12C. The nodes are located in the fossa above and behind the medial condyle of the humerus.

Inguinal Nodes

The superficial inguinal and *femoral nodes* (Fig. 6-13A) are palpated using the rotary motion described in Chapter 11 and shown in Fig. 6-13B.

Normal Findings

Lymph nodes are not normally palpable, but are frequently noted because of prior inflammation. If you note an enlarged or tender node, be sure to inspect the area that the node drains for possible infection. Cervical nodes are almost always felt in children under 12 years of age. These nodes are referred to as "shotty," which is generally interpreted as firm, freely movable, and nontender, and indicates a chronic inflammatory process. Palpable inguinal lymph nodes in the adolescent and the adult are a common finding [1]. Rarely, enlarged lymph nodes may interfere with body function (e.g., movement of the head, swallowing, adduction and abduction of the arm). Identification of these alterations in function requires that they be considered in the nursing care plan.

SKIN, HAIR, NAILS- ASSESSMENT GUIDE

A. History (Pertinent to Skin Function)
   1. Personal
   2. Family
   3. Geographic origin, present abode
   4. Season
   5. Occupation
   6. Leisure activities

Figure 6-14.
Characteristics of common
skin lesions.

Primary lesions	Secondary lesions
Macule Flat area of color change (no elevation or depression)	**Scales** Flakes of cornified skin layer
Papule Solid elevation—less than 0.5 cm diameter	**Crust** Dried exudate on skin
Nodule Solid elevation 0.5 to 1 cm diameter. Extends deeper into dermis than papule.	**Fissure** Cracks in skin
Tumor Solid mass—larger than 1 cm	**Erosion** Loss of epidermis that does not extend into dermis
Plaque Flat elevated surface found where papules, nodules or tumors cluster together	**Ulcer** Area of destruction of entire epidermis
Wheal Type of plaque. Result is transient edema in dermis	**Scar** Excess collagen production following injury
Vesicle Small blister—fluid within or under epidermis	**Atrophy** Loss of some portion of the skin
Bulla Larger blister (greater than 0.5 cm)	

        7. Accompanying diseases
        8. Previous treatments
    B. Physical Examination
        1. Skin: color, texture, temperature, hydration, turgor, lesions (Fig. 6-14)
        2. Hair: color/style, distribution, amount, thickness, texture, lubrication
        3. Nails: color, length, ridges, adornments, abnormalities—clubbing
        4. Mouth
            a. Inspection of lips
                i. Symmetry of form and function
                ii. Color and general physical appearance
            b. Inspection of oral mucosal surfaces
                i. Denture function and fit
                ii. Oral surfaces
                iii. Parotid duct
                iv. Gingiva
                v. Hard palate
                vi. Soft palate
                vii. Tongue—dorsal surface
                viii. Floor of the mouth
                ix. Tongue ventral surface
                x. Teeth
            c. Palpation of the oral mucosa
        5. Lymph Nodes
            a. Occipital and postauricular
            b. Submaxillary and submental
            c. Anterior angle (upper end of deep cervical chain)
            d. Downward along the sternocleidomastoid muscle (superficial cervical nodes)
            e. Posterior triangle (lower end of deep cervical chain)
            f. Supraclavicular
            g. Axillary
            h. Epitrochlear
            i. Describe each node according to the following characteristics: exact location; extent of enlargement (expressed in cm) or a familiar size, e.g., pea; tenderness, inflammation, mobility (freely movable or adherent to deeper structures)

REFERENCES

1. Judge, R. D., and Zuidema, G. D. (Eds.). *Methods of Clinical Examination: A Physiologic Approach* (3rd ed.). Boston: Little, Brown, 1974.
2. Marples, M. J. Life on the human skin. *Sci. Am.* 220:108, 1969.
3. Roach, L. B. Skin Changes: The Subtle and the Obvious. P. S. Chaney (Series Ed.). *Assessing Vital Functions Accurately.* Horsham, Pennsylvania: Nursing 77 Books Intermed Communications, 1977.
4. Sneddon, I. B. and Church, R. E. *Practical Dermatology.* London: Arnold, 1976.

SUGGESTED READINGS

Bates, B. *A Guide to Physical Examination* (2nd ed.). Philadelphia: Lippincott, 1979.
Davis, M. Getting to the root of the problem: Hair-grooming techniques for black patients. *Nursing '77* 7:4, 1977.
Derbes, V. J. Rashes: Recognition and management. *Nursing '78.* 78:3, 1978. Pp. 54–59.
Harmon, V. M. and Steele, S. M. *Nursing Care of the Skin: A Developmental Approach.* New York: Appleton-Century-Crofts, 1975.
McVan, B. Odors: What the nose knows. *Nursing '77,* 7:4, 1977.
Meissner, J. E. A simple guide for assessing oral health. *Nursing '80.* 10:4, 1980. Pp. 84–85.
Parrish, J. A. *Dermatology and Skin Care.* New York: McGraw-Hill, 1975.

Rook, A., Wilkinson, D. S., and Ebling, F. J. *Textbook of Dermatology* (vol. 1). Oxford, England: Blackwell, 1972.

Sauer, G. C. *Manual of Skin Diseases* (4th ed.). Philadelphia: Lippincott, 1980.

Schoen, L. A. *The AMA Book of Skin and Hair Care.* Philadelphia: Lippincott, 1976.

Schweiger, J. L. *et al.* Oral assessment: How to do it. *American Journal of Nursing,* 80:4. Pp. 654–657.

Solomons, B. *Lecture Notes on Dermatology* (4th ed.). Oxford, England: Blackwell, 1977.

Uhler, D. M. Common skin changes in the elderly. *American Journal of Nursing.* 78:8, pp. 1342–44.

Wilkinson, D. S. *The Nursing and Management of Skin Diseases* (4th ed.). London: Faber and Faber, 1977.

Black skin problems. *American Journal of Nursing.* 70:6. Pp. 1092–94.

Patricia Mitchell Butler

7. Physical Assessment of the Eye and Vision

GLOSSARY **abduction** Rotation of the eye temporally (outward).

accommodation Near focusing of the eye, accomplished by an increase in strength of the lens achieved by contractions of the ciliary muscle.

adduction Turning of the eye toward the nose (inward).

agnosia Cerebral inability to recognize the meaning of details seen or otherwise perceived.

amblyopia Reduced vision in an eye appearing normal to ophthalmoscopic examination (not due to refractive errors or organic defect).

aphakia Absence of the lens.

astigmatism Optical distortion usually caused by irregular corneal curvature which prevents a clear focus of light at any point.

aqueous humor Fluid produced in the ciliary body and occupying the anterior and posterior chambers.

arcus senilis Opaque white-gray ring around the corneal periphery from fatty degeneration, seen in older persons.

blepharitis Inflammation of the eyelid.

blepharospasm Twitching or spasmodic contraction of the orbicularis oculi muscle.

canthus Outer or inner angle formed by the eyelids.

color blindness Inability to differentiate normally between colors; the most common type causes confusion between red and green.

diplopia Double vision.

ectropion Eversion of the lid border.

emmetropia Normal condition of eye in refraction; with eye at rest, rays parallel to the optic axis are focused on the retina.

entropion Inversion, or the turning inward, of the margin of the eyelid.

epicanthus Congenital skin fold overlying the inner portion of the upper lid and the inner canthus; simulates the appearance of esotropia.

epiphoria Abnormal overflow of tears down the cheek.

esophoria A latent convergent deviation of the two eyes.

esotropia Convergent strabismus.

exophoria A latent divergent deviation of the two eyes.

exotropia Divergent strabismus.

extorsion Rotation of the organ (eye) outward (temporally).

floaters Opacities within the vitreous space that cause moving shadows on the retina.

fundoscopy Examination of the interior of the eyeball using an ophthalmoscope.

glaucoma Abnormally increased intraocular pressure that causes irreversible death of the optic nerve fibers if untreated.

hemianopia Loss of vision in approximately one half of the visual field.

hyperopia Eyeball is too short from front to back, and the retina lies in front of the posterior principal focus of the eye; farsightedness.

hyphema Blood in the anterior chamber of the eye in front of the iris.

hypopyon Presence of pus in the anterior chamber.

intorsion Rotation of the eye on an anterioposterior axis so that the upper portion of the eye moves toward the nose.

keratitis Corneal inflammation.

lagophthalmos Failure of the eyelids to close completely.

limbus Junction of the cornea and sclera.

miotic A medication causing the pupil to become constricted.

mydriatic A medication causing the pupil to become dilated.

myopia Eyeball is so long from front to back that the posterior principal focus of the eye lies in front of the retina; nearsightedness.

nystagmus Rapid involuntary eye movements.

O.D. Oculus dexter; right eye.

optic disc Area in retina for entrance of the optic nerve and blood vessels.

orthoptics Techniques used in diagnosis and treatment of strabismus.

O.S. Oculus sinister; left eye.

O.U. Oculi unitas (both eyes); oculus uterque (each eye).

palpebral Referring to the eyelid.

papilledema Ophthalmoscopically visible swelling of the optic disc, due to increased intracranial pressure or other cause of vascular stasis.

photophobia Abnormal intolerance of light.

presbyopia Decreased or weakened ability of the eye to accommodate, due to the loss of elasticity of the crystalline lens with advancing age.

ptosis Drooping of the upper lid.

refraction Clinical measurement of the error of focus in an eye.

scotoma Area of loss of vision within the visual field.

squint Synonym for strabismus.

strabismus Failure of eyes to straighten; one eye (fixing eye) looks directly at the object of attention, the other eye (deviating eye) does not.

sty (hordeolum) Infection of a gland of the eyelid margin.

trachoma A binding virus infection of the cornea and conjunctiva; widely prevalent throughout the world and probably the most common cause of blindness in under-developed countries.

uvea Vascular and pigmented layer of the eye, including the choroid, ciliary body, and iris.

zonule A system of fibers that suspend the lens.

THE role of the nurse in assessing eye function varies, depending on the patient's age and health, but includes an assessment of the functional status of the eyes, referral to an ophthalmologist or another specialist, and counseling of the individual for optimal visual functioning in his everyday life situation.

Assessment of the eye and vision includes both a history and physical examination. The examination should be done in a specific order according to an established system, so that no part is omitted. The complete examination in the following order encompasses:

1. Measurement of visual acuity
   a. Distance vision—Snellen Chart
   b. Near vision—Jaeger chart
   c. Color vision
2. Testing ocular mobility
   a. Ocular movement—8 diagnostic positions of gaze
   b. Cover test
   c. Alternating cover test
3. Evaluation of visual fields
4. Inspection of the external eye structures
5. Testing nerve reflexes
6. Gross measurement of intraocular pressure
7. Fundoscopic examination

A shortened version of the eye examination can be done when clients have a specific eye complaint. In these cases the shortened examination should also include tests that are indicated by the symptoms as well as the following determinations:

1. That vision is approximately normal and equal in each eye, measured separately, for near and distance.
2. That color vision of each eye, measured separately, is intact.
3. That the visual field of each eye is intact upon gross testing.
4. That pupillary reflexes are intact.
5. That the optic discs are flat and of normal color [7].

Equipment needed for the eye and vision examination includes:

1. Snellen chart
2. Jaeger chart
3. Color cards
4. Penlight
5. Cotton-tipped applicator
6. Cotton ball
7. Eye cover (occluder)
8. Ophthalmoscope

CULTURAL VARIABLES

It is important when doing an eye history and physical examination to remember that cultural, social, and climatic variables influence the type and incidence of eye disorders. Congenital anomalies depend on the level of social organization and security as well as inbreeding and isolation. They are rare where the struggle for existence is still fierce [6].

The United States has a mixture of cultural and racial types as well as wide variations in climate. For the most part, this country has a high level of social organization, and hereditary diseases are reflected in the statistics of eye disorders. There are, however, pockets of isolated culture that demonstrate widely differing eye disorders owing to their lower level of social organization. The American Indians and Eskimos are such groups. These populations, descended from the Mongolian race, exhibit hereditary eye disorders similar to those of the Japanese, Chinese, and other Mongolian peoples. These differ from the Caucasian and Negro types. Yet, because of cultural patterns and the generally low level of social organization, they share certain characteristic eye disorders, the most prominent of which is infection. As these groups become assimilated and become more highly organized the types of eye disorders they demonstrate will change. War, industrialization, and cultural aspects (such as toys) will cause eye disorders to be more or less prevalent in different societies. In the United States, 2 per 1,000 inhabitants are blind as contrasted with 40 per 1,000

Arabs living in the Middle East. Careful application of medical knowledge is the main reason for this [2].

HISTORY   The assessment of the eye is begun with a careful and detailed history. Throughout the history-taking and physical examination, observation is made of the physical appearance of the eye. Eye and head movements and facial expressions should be noted. These can provide clues both to systemic functional alterations of body systems and to alterations of the eye. Physical examination of the eye may also give clues to systemic disease, as many diseases manifest eye changes.

A familial history is necessary as many eye disorders are hereditary. Is there a family history of glaucoma, congenital cataracts, primary macular degenerations, squint, or retinoblastoma? In Negroes hereditary optic atrophy is common. In American Indians glaucoma is rare as are other congenital anomalies, but the rate of infectious diseases is high [6].

A past history of eye disorders must be elicited, including previous diagnoses, treatment, and results. When taking a child's history, determine what the parents or guardians perceive the child is able to see. Also, determine whether the infant or child looks at objects or reaches for people or for large or small objects, and whether any change in this behavior pattern has been noticed. The history should provide answers to the following:

A. Past history
   1. Familial history of eye disorders, hereditary and acquired
   2. Past eye disturbances, treatment and resolution
   3. Systemic disorders affecting the eye such as diabetes, hypertension, thyroid disorders
B. Present history
   1. Changes in visual acuity or visual field
   2. Signs and symptoms of eye disturbance
      a. Pain
      b. Photophobia
      c. Burning or itching
      d. Redness (red eye)
      e. Excessive tearing, crusting, or exudate
      f. Diplopia
      g. Blurring or veiling of vision; spider-web pattern in visual field; spots (suspect detached retina)
      h. Spots or flashing lights (vitreous floaters—suspect hemorrhage or detached retina)
      i. Blurring or fogging of vision or severe pain in an eye, especially after watching a movie or TV or exposure to prolonged darkness (suspect glaucoma)

j. Halos around lights (suspect glaucoma)
3. Are specific activities or body position associated with the occurrence of these symptoms?
4. When do the symptoms occur, what is their duration and how does the person obtain relief from them?
5. What does the client think is the problem?

MEASUREMENT OF VISUAL ACUITY

Measurement of visual acuity can be done first as it is an ideal screening test for most eye disorders. Eighty percent of eye disorders are accompanied by some type of decrease in visual acuity [2]. Visual acuity for distance should be measured in each eye separately and should be part of every complete physical examination [2].

Measurement of visual acuity for a complete eye examination includes the determination of:

1. Distance visual acuity—Snellen chart
2. Near visual acuity—Jaeger chart
3. Color vision—color cards
4. Dark adaptation—history

Distance Vision— Snellen Chart

The Snellen chart is the most readily available and easiest method to use for testing distant vision. There are many variations of this chart, but the most versatile is the block E chart, which can be used with children, illiterate persons, or those who do not read English. Cut-out block E's are available to familiarize the child with the "three-legged table." Children and other persons using this chart are asked to indicate the direction of the "legs" of the table, and the nurse must make certain that they clearly understand what they are to do and that they are capable of this activity. Children two years of age and older can be tested with this chart after some time is spent in teaching and game playing.

The letters or figures on the Snellen chart are specifically made to measure the form sense of the eye. The form sense of the eye is made up of the (1) resolving powers of the eye to discriminate two separate but adjacent stimuli (the smallest measurement of which is the minimum separable) and (2) the ability of the visual cortex to appreciate the nature of the stimulus by a perceptual process (the smallest measurement of which is minimum cognisible). Minimum separable is about a one-minute (1$'$) angle, and average measurement of the minimum cognisible is a five-minute (5$'$) angle [9]. The Snellen figures are constructed using the one-minute minimum separable pieces to make a five-minute cognisible angle of arc. Figure 7-1 demonstrates the 5$'$ angle of arc in the figures of the block E for 6 M, 30 M, and 60 M. The letters of different sizes in Figure 7-1 are constructed to subtend the angle of 5$'$ when they are placed at 6 M, 30 M, and 60 M.

Figure 7-1.
Visual acuity test using
Snellen chart. (From Judge
and Zuidema [3].)

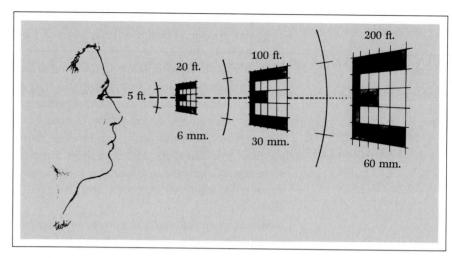

Figure 7-1.
Visual acuity test using Snellen chart. (From Judge and Zuidema [3].)

The numbers at the end of the row on the Snellen chart constitute the visual acuity measurement recorded for the client. These visual acuity numbers, e.g., 6/9 (20/30) are not fractions. The upper figure, 6 in this case, indicates the distance the person being tested is from the chart. The lower figure, 9 in this case, indicates the line being read. The lower figure also indicates the distance at which the normal eye would see the letter. For example, 6/9 (20/30) vision means that the person tested was 6 M (20 ft) from the chart and could read the line that those with normal vision can read at 9 M (30 ft), but could not read beyond this line.

Testing is begun with the person comfortably seated or standing 6 M from the chart. The chart must be at eye level and well illuminated. If the room where testing is done is not 6 M (20 ft) the distance the client is from the chart is used as the top number, e.g., 3 M (10 ft), 4.5 M (15 ft.). This means that the client with normal vision should be able to read better than the 6/6 line (20/20 line).

One eye should be tested at a time while the other eye is covered with an eye occluder. The patient's hand should not be used to cover his other eye. A tongue blade with a round piece of construction paper secured to it serves well as an eye cover. The nurse must make certain periodically that the person is unable to see with the covered eye, particularly when testing a child. Adults should be asked to read the line most comfortably read and should identify all the letters correctly. When testing the child, it is well to start at the top of the chart. Encourage the reading of as many letters as possible. If the person reads with the right eye the 6/9 line "missing" two letters, 6/9-2 O.D. is recorded. (See Table 7-1 for metric and foot conversions.) How the line was read is described also, i.e., "quickly and rhythmically," or "hesitantly, with great effort." The uncorrected vision is tested—first right eye, then left eye; then the corrected vision is tested—right eye, then left eye.

Table 7-1.
Metric Snellen Conversions

Metric*	Metric†	Feet
6M/60M	6.1M/61M	20ft/200 ft
6M/30M	6.1M/30.5M	20ft/100 ft
6M/20M	6.1M/21.7M	20 ft/70 ft
6M/15M	6.1M/15.2M	20 ft/50 ft
6M/12M	6.1M/12.2M	20 ft/40 ft
6M/9M	6.1M/9.1M	20 ft/30 ft
6M/6M	6.1M/6.1M	20 ft/20 ft—Normal vision
6M/4.5M	6.1M/4.6M	20 ft/15 ft
6M/3M	6.1M/3.05M	20 ft/10 ft

*Grossly, rounded numbers
†American Optical Co. Metric Conversion
The metric system is being used by many ophthalmologists. To convert from feet to meters, divide roughly by 3.3 or multiply by 0.3048. To convert meters to feet multiply by 3.281.

Normal visual acuity is 6/6 (20/20) in each eye. Many persons have visual acuity better than this uncorrected or corrected. Corrected vision is usually to 6/6. Any person with 6/12 (20/40) or less, corrected, should be referred to an ophthalmologist.

The person who cannot read the chart at 6/60 (top letter) is moved closer to the chart until able to read this top large letter. The distance and letter are recorded, e.g., 3/60 when the client can read it. If no chart letters can be read, a finger test is done. The nurse holds her hand in front of the client to determine whether variable numbers of fingers held up can be seen and accurately counted. One eye is tested at a time. If the finger count cannot be done, the nurse then determines whether hand movements (HM) can be identified or, finally, whether the client has light perception (LP). When an eye cannot perceive light, it is termed "blind" by the physician. Legal blindness is defined as less than 6/60 vision in the better eye with full correction, or less than 20 degrees field of vision [7]. Legal blindness should be established by a physician, as the patient is then entitled to tax and other benefits. Health professionals should be aware of services and agencies that promote the adjustment and independence of the blind. Information may be obtained from the American Foundation for the Blind, 15 West 16th Street, New York, New York, 10011. Each state has a state agency responsible for the Blind and Handicapped that would be listed in the phone book under State Agencies. Any local library can provide this type of information, as can local, state, and federal library services for the blind.

At birth, the visual acuity of infants is approximately 6/130 (20/700). There is no central fixation, and the eyes move randomly. Visual acuity increases gradually, and by one year, it is approximately 6/60 (20/200); by the second year, 6/20 (20/70), and at the end of the third year, 6/6 (20/20) [7]. Attempts to determine the visual acuity of children must be made as soon as possible as failure to use the eye interferes with normal development of visual acuity. The importance of testing visual acuity, particularly in children, cannot be stressed enough. Many children have defects in eyesight that may or may not be refractive errors. With one eye covered, children under 2 years of age can play games in which objects of varying sizes are picked up, permitting the nurse to make a gross estimate of visual acuity and functioning of each eye. Or the child can be taught to use the E chart and a gross estimate made of visual acuity in each eye in this way.

Visual acuity in Negroes appears to be better than in Caucasians. In a sample of recruits taken by Karpinos, 82 percent of Negros tested has an acuity of 6/6 or better compared to 69 percent of whites [6].

Near Visual Acuity— Jaeger Chart

This is a measure of the ability to read words composed of letters of different sizes at the normal reading distance of 34 cm (14 in). The Jaeger chart uses a random series of different sizes of printers' types—the smallest equals J 1 and the largest equals J 20. Sometimes common reading material is used with newsprint of varying sizes. Figure 7-2 illustrates both sides of a Near Vision Test Card. The client and the examiner should each have a card to facilitate the examination. This Near Vision Card (revised Jaeger cards also) have the Jaeger standard (see Fig. 7-2A), near Snellen notation, metric distance, distance Snellen approximation, and AMA near visual acuity efficiency.

The card (Jaeger or Near Vision) should be held 35 cm (14 in) from the eye. One eye is tested at a time while the other eye is covered. The client is asked to read the smallest print possible and as many lines as possible. The number of the line, the eye tested, and the way the line was read are recorded, e.g., Jaeger No. 3, O.D. and O.S., without hesitation.

Opinions in the literature vary concerning the accuracy and necessity for this test. Both near and distance visual acuity are measured for insurance compensation benefits. In industrial settings, near and distance acuity should be carefully measured at entrance and exit physical examinations. Occupational and educational demands place different requirements on near visual acuity. This author recommends measurement of near visual acuity with each complete eye examination.

This test is particularly useful for persons over 40 years of age who are beginning to experience presbyopia. Patients with hyperopia, astigmatism, and accommodation (cranial nerve III) impairment or other pathologic conditions may have poor near vision, and this test should be done routinely. In general, the inability to read the newspaper (or Jaeger No. 7) at 35 cm is an indicator that correction is needed for near vision. Testing games for children are available and recommended for the nurse who has many preschool children for visual screening. (The E Testing Game and Titmus Stereotests can be obtained

Figure 7-2. Front and reverse sides of Near Vision Test Card with matte finish. (Distributed by Guild Prescription Opticians of America, Washington, D.C. With permission of A. H. Keeney [5].)

NEAR VISION TEST CARD

UNIVERSITY OF LOUISVILLE

REVISED JAEGER STANDARD	NEAR SNELLEN NOTATION	METRIC DISTANCE	DISTANCE SNELLEN APPROXIMATION	DECIMAL NOTATION	A. M. A. 1955 NEAR VISUAL EFFICIENCY
12	14/89 (in.)	2.25 м.	20/130 (ft.)	0.15	10%

WHEN IN THE COURSE OF HUMAN EVENTS, IT BECOMES NECESSARY FOR

11	14/79	2.0	20/120	0.2	13%

ONE PEOPLE TO DISSOLVE THE POLITICAL BANDS WHICH HAVE CONNECTED THEM

9	14/60	1.5	20/85	0.22	20%

WITH ANOTHER, AND TO ASSUME AMONG THE POWERS OF THE EARTH, THE SEPARATE AND EQUAL STATION TO

7	14/42	1.05	20/60	0.35	40%

WHICH THE LAWS OF NATURE AND OF NATURE'S GOD ENTITLE THEM. A DECENT RESPECT TO THE OPINIONS OF MANKIND REQUIRES THAT THEY SHOULD DECLARE THE

6	14/35	.82	20/50	0.4	50%

CAUSES WHICH IMPEL THEM TO THE SEPARATION. WE HOLD THESE TRUTHS TO BE SELF-EVIDENT. THAT ALL MEN ARE CREATED EQUAL. THAT THEY ARE ENDOWED BY THEIR CREATOR WITH CERTAIN UNALIENABLE

5	14/28	.75	20/40	0.5	90%

RIGHTS, THAT AMONG THESE ARE LIFE, LIBERTY, AND THE PURSUIT OF HAPPINESS. THAT TO SECURE THESE RIGHTS, GOVERNMENTS ARE INSTITUTED AMONG MEN, DERIVING THEIR JUST POWERS FROM THE CONSENT OF THE GOVERNED,

3	14/21	.53	20/30	0.6	95%

THAT, WHENEVER ANY FORM OF GOVERNMENT BECOMES DESTRUCTIVE OF THESE ENDS, IT IS THE RIGHT OF THE PEOPLE TO ALTER OR TO ABOLISH IT, AND TO INSTITUTE NEW GOVERNMENT, LAYING ITS FOUNDATION ON SUCH PRINCIPLES AND ORGANIZING ITS POWERS IN SUCH FORM, AS TO THEM SHALL SEEM MOST LIKELY TO

1	14/14	.37	20/20	1.0	100%

EFFECT THEIR SAFETY AND HAPPINESS. PRUDENCE, INDEED, WILL DICTATE THAT GOVERNMENTS LONG ESTABLISHED SHOULD NOT BE CHANGED FOR LIGHT AND TRANSIENT CAUSES AND, ACCORDINGLY ALL EXPERIENCE HATH SHOWN, THAT MANKIND ARE MORE DISPOSED TO SUFFER, WHILE EVILS ARE SUFFERABLE, THAN TO RIGHT THEMSELVES BY ABOLISHING THE FORMS TO WHICH THEY ARE ACCUSTOMED. BUT WHEN A LONG TRAIN OF ABUSES AND USURPATIONS

CHART TO BE HELD 14 INCHES FROM EYE

ENGINEERED AND PRODUCED BY
COURIER-JOURNAL LITHO CO., LOUISVILLE 18, KY.

Figure 7-2.
Continued

NEAR VISION TEST CARD

UNIVERSITY OF LOUISVILLE

12

WHEN IN THE COURSE OF HUMAN
EVENTS, IT BECOMES NECESSARY FOR

11

ONE PEOPLE TO DISSOLVE THE POLITICAL
BANDS WHICH HAVE CONNECTED THEM

9

WITH ANOTHER, AND TO ASSUME AMONG THE POWERS
OF THE EARTH, THE SEPARATE AND EQUAL STATION TO

7

WHICH THE LAWS OF NATURE AND OF NATURE'S GOD ENTITLE THEM. A DECENT
RESPECT TO THE OPINIONS OF MANKIND REQUIRES THAT THEY SHOULD DECLARE THE

6

CAUSES WHICH IMPEL THEM TO THE SEPARATION. WE HOLD THESE TRUTHS TO BE SELF-EVIDENT, THAT ALL
MEN ARE CREATED EQUAL, THAT THEY ARE ENDOWED BY THEIR CREATOR WITH CERTAIN UNALIENABLE

5

RIGHTS, THAT AMONG THESE ARE LIFE, LIBERTY, AND THE PURSUIT OF HAPPINESS. THAT TO SECURE THESE RIGHTS,
GOVERNMENTS ARE INSTITUTED AMONG MEN, DERIVING THEIR JUST POWERS FROM THE CONSENT OF THE GOVERNED,

3

THAT, WHENEVER ANY FORM OF GOVERNMENT BECOMES DESTRUCTIVE OF THESE ENDS IT IS THE RIGHT OF THE PEOPLE TO ALTER OR TO ABOLISH IT, AND TO INSTITUTE
NEW GOVERNMENT, LAYING ITS FOUNDATION ON SUCH PRINCIPLES AND ORGANIZING ITS POWERS IN SUCH FORM, AS TO THEM SHALL SEEM MOST LIKELY TO

CHART TO BE HELD
14 INCHES FROM EYE

from the Benson Optical Co., 1812 Park Avenue, Box 679, Minneapolis, Minnesota, 55440.)

Refractive examination by ophthalmologists should be done for the client demonstrating poor distance or near visual acuity. "Good near acuity with poor distance acuity at any age suggests myopia and very little astigmatism (see Fig. 7-9). Good distance acuity with poor near acuity suggests moderate hyperopia (see Fig. 7-9) with little or no astigmatism, presbyopia, or accommodation (cranial nerve III) impairment. Comparatively poor acuity, both near and distance, suggests significant astigmatism or significant pathology" [5]. Myopia has a genetic basis and is more common in the Mongolian race, especially among the Chinese and Japanese. Many tranquilizers and antihypertension drugs are known to reduce accommodative amplitude, thereby causing blurred near vision [2].

Color Vision   Color vision is important in our society as color coding is frequently used in school, industry, and vehicle operation. Color testing is routinely done for certain job classifications, and a number of states now require color vision testing for drivers' licenses [8]. Unfortunately, color vision is not frequently tested. Approximately 8.4 percent of Caucasian males and 0.5 percent of Caucasian females in North America are color-blind. The American Negro male has a lower rate of color blindness, 3.9 percent. Color blindness is rare in the Eskimo male, 0.8 percent, and the Navajo Indian male has a rate of approximately 1.1 percent [6].

Besides inherited color blindness, there can be changes in color appreciation due to retrobulbar neuritis, chiasmal lesions, macular degeneration, optic nerve disease, and toxic amblyopia. It is necessary, therefore, to continue to test color vision throughout life [4,8].

The usual method of testing color vision is with color plates,* in which numbers or figures are outlined in the primary colors and surrounded by a confusion of color. The color vision deficient individual is unable to see these numbers/figures which are recognized quickly by a person with normal color vision. There are more sensitive tests which require specialized equipment. If color plates are not available, the client can be requested to match varying colors of yarn. Matching and grouping dyed skeins of yarn is a method well suited to test infants or small children, as this is a play pattern. It would be necessary to include skeins with the primary colors—red, green, and blue. This, however, is the least accurate test and should only be used if color plates are unavailable.

---

*Ishikara test plates are available, but have been found to be difficult for Spanish speaking groups and groups with low educational level to understand. It is imperative that the client have a good understanding of the test and what is expected of him or her before accurate results can be achieved. Ishikara plates—Tests for Color Blindness, Tokyo, Kanihara and Co. Also Color Charts, American Optical Company.

Several types of congenital color blindness involve either (1) deficiency or abnormality of cone pigment or (2) the complete absence of one of the cone pigments. These types are then designated according to the pigment involved: the red-sensitive pigment; the green-sensitive pigment; or the blue-sensitive pigment. The blue-sensitive defect is rare. Those persons who lack red and green pigment may see these colors as yellow. If yarn is used for testing, red, green, blue, and yellow should be tested.

Dark Adaptation   Clients should be questioned about their adaption to the dark. Dark adaptation is a function of the rods and is mediated by the build-up of rhodopsin in the rods. Dark adaptation is decreased with vitamin A deficiency in cirrhosis, optic nerve disease, glaucoma, and inadequate nutrition [7]. The client usually does not notice a decrease. The defect involves slow recovery of vision during night driving after the headlights of an oncoming car shine in the client's eyes. Normal dark adaptation is complete in 20 minutes when rhodopsin build-up is complete. The client will have to think about how his vision at night used to be, and how it is now. How long after the lights are turned out or dimmed does it take before he can see objects in the room or theater? How long does it take to recover from the effects of headlights on a dark road? Normally this is only seconds because all the rhodopsin in the rods has not been broken down. It is interesting to note that McFarland (in Keeney) has found that man, because of presbyopic changes, needs essentially doubled amounts of illumination every 13 years of life in order for objects to be seen [5]. Any detected abnormalities in dark adaptation responses should be referred to the ophthalmologist.

TESTING FOR OCULAR MOBILITY   Ocular muscles should be tested routinely from infancy through old age. In infants, the nurse observes particularly for muscle weakness, which may be too subtle to be detected easily. The nurse also observes for nerve impairment to the muscle. "The maintenance of parallel eyes (and therefore of corneal light reflexes that are equally centered) occurs in most persons because of the fusion reflex, which makes binocular vision possible" [3]. Man has learned to adapt to a certain degree of muscle weakness so that, despite it, he still achieves fusion and binocular vision, often to the detriment of one eye. When one eye is covered, this fusion is not possible, and one eye realigns to its visual axis to fixate the target on the fovea, i.e., it moves so that the object being looked at is centered on the fovea.

The client should be seated, looking directly at the nurse examiner, and asked to look straight ahead. The nurse shines the penlight on the client's cornea. The corneal light reflexes are the dots of reflected light on the cornea's shiny surface (see Fig. 7-3 and Fig. 7-8). If the pupil and iris are thought of as a clock, the corneal light reflex can be observed as a dot of light on a clock face, e.g., having a time position like that of 10 o'clock or 2 o'clock. The corneal light reflexes should be parallel. That is, if the corneal light reflex is at 10

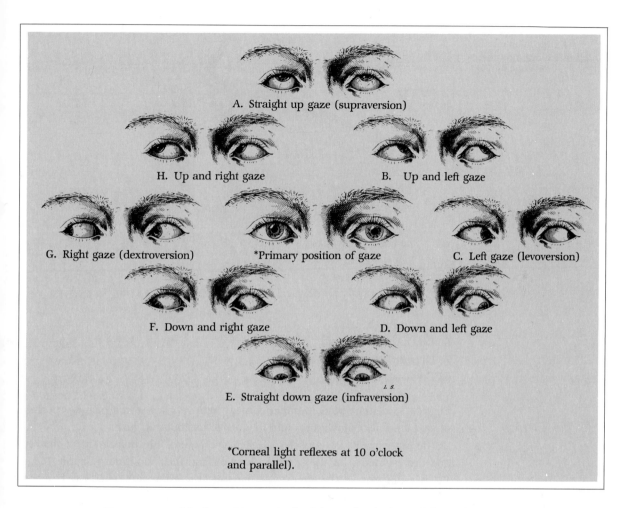

A. Straight up gaze (supraversion)

H. Up and right gaze   B. Up and left gaze

G. Right gaze (dextroversion)   *Primary position of gaze   C. Left gaze (levoversion)

F. Down and right gaze   D. Down and left gaze

E. Straight down gaze (infraversion)

*Corneal light reflexes at 10 o'clock
and parallel).

Figure 7-3.
Primary position of gaze
(note parallel light reflexes)
and right diagnostic
positions of gaze.

o'clock position over the iris on the cornea of the right eye, it should be at the 10 o'clock position over the iris on the cornea of the left eye.

Figure 7-3 demonstrates parallel corneal light reflexes. Parallel corneal light reflexes means that the client's eyes are parallel, and he is able to achieve fusion and binocular vision. Nonparallel corneal light reflexes are abnormal [3,5,8].

In muscle balance testing the corneal light reflexes are observed as the eyes are moved from the primary position of gaze (straight ahead) through the eight diagnostic positions of gaze. The corneal light reflexes should remain in a parallel position in each position of gaze. The eight diagnostic positions of gaze are:

1. Right gaze (detroversion)
2. Left gaze (levoversion)
3. Straight-up gaze (supraversion)
4. Straight-down gaze (infraversion)

Figure 7-4.
Extraocular muscles
controlling eye movements
(right eye).

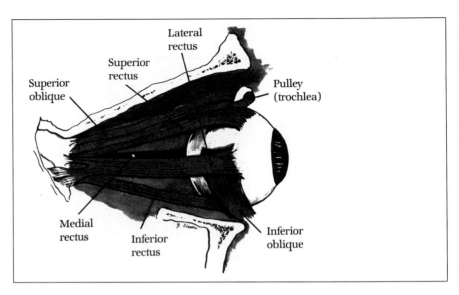

5. Up and right gaze
6. Down and right gaze
7. Up and left gaze
8. Down and left gaze

Figure 7-3 demonstrates parallel corneal light reflexes in the primary position of gaze and also shows the eight diagnostic positions of gaze.

The six extraocular muscles of each eye control the movement of that eye and are evaluated for the specific direction and their maximum action. Figure 7-4 is a diagram of the six extraocular muscles of the right eye. The functions of the 12 muscles of the eyes are listed, with their innervation, in Table 7-2.

The muscles of the same eye that act together to rotate the globe are termed agonist, e.g., the right superior rectus (RSR) and the right inferior oblique (RIO) are agonist in elevating the right globe. The muscles of the same eye that act in opposite directions and therefore require reciprocal inhibition of one while the other is contracting are termed antagonists. For example, when the left lateral rectus (LLR) is contracting to move the left eye to the left, its antagonist, the left medial rectus (LMR) is inhibited [8]. "Two antagonistic muscles may contract at the same time, but in one it may be with increasing intensity whereas in the other, with decreasing intensity. This phenomenon allows a finely graded response and steady movement" [8].

The yoke muscles are the muscles in the opposite eyes that work together to move the eyes to a given position of gaze; i.e., the right lateral rectus (RLR) and the left medial rectus (LMR) are yoke muscles in that they are the leading muscles in moving the gaze to the right [3].

Knowledge of agonist, antagonist, and yoke muscles and their innervation

Muscle	Movement Controlled	Innervation (Cranial Nerve)
Medial rectus		Oculomotor (III)
Right	Eye to left	
Left	Eye to right	
Lateral rectus		Abducens (VI)
Right	Eye to right	
Left	Eye to left	
Superior rectus	Elevates eye	Oculomotor (III)
(right and left)	Rotates eye upward and inward	
Inferior rectus	Depresses eyes	Oculomotor (III)
(right and left)	Rotates eye downward and inward	
Superior oblique	Depression	Trochlear (IV)
(right and left)	Intorsion	
	Abduction	
	Rotates eye downward and outward	
Inferior oblique	Elevation	Oculomotor (III)
(right and left)	Extorsion	
	Abduction	
	Rotates eye upward and outward	

and position of gaze is important for the nurse to effectively examine the ocular mobility of the client's eyes.

Using a penlight as a target and to create the corneal light reflexes, the nurse has the client fix her gaze on the light while she moves the light from the primary position of gaze through the eight diagnostic positions of gaze. Return to the primary position of gaze between each position, e.g., primary position of gaze to straight-up gaze, back to primary position, then to up and right gaze, and so on. When examining the down and right, down and left, and straight-down gazes, the nurse has to retract the client's eyelids in order to see the corneal light reflexes. Use the other hand or have the client hold her lids up. The nurse can also use an external light to elicit the corneal light reflexes and then have the client visually follow the examiner's finger through the positions of gaze.

The nurse watches closely the parallel position of the corneal light reflexes in all positions of gaze. Deviation of light reflexes is abnormal and requires further evaluation by an ophthalmologist. Nonparallel corneal reflexes are seen with squint, weakness of eye muscles, or defective innervation.

Other important tests for ocular mobility and the detection of squint are the cover test and the alternating cover test. These tests determine whether fixation of both eyes on the target is parallel. The eyes should be fixating the target on the fovea centralis of the retina.

To perform the cover test the client is asked to fix her vision on a target. The test should be done with a near target first, 33 cm (14 in) and then with a distant target, 6 M (20 ft). The right eye is covered with an occluder while the nurse observes the uncovered left eye for movement. Any movement means the uncovered eye was not fixating the target on the fovea and has realigned to achieve this target fixation on the fovea. When movement has ceased or if no movement occurs, the cover is removed from the right eye and is moved to the left eye. Now the uncovered right eye is observed for movement. This covering is done two or three times for each eye, first for near then for distant vision.

In the alternating cover test the client continues to watch the fixation target, first near then distant. The nurse alternately covers one eye, then the other. The eye that is *being* uncovered is observed for movement. If movement of the eye occurs, it is an indication of muscle imbalance.

Any vertical shifting (or movement) in the cover test is abnormal, as is diplopia. A slight horizontal shift of the visual axis may be seen with the alternating cover test. At the extreme of gaze, physiologic or end-point nystagmus may occur and is considered normal; any other nystagmus is considered abnormal. The nerve innervation for the ocular muscles listed in Table 7-2 will be helpful in the neurologic examination as well as in vision testing. Any abnormalities noted are indications for additional testing and referral to an ophthalmologist. Follow-up by the nurse is necessary to determine whether the client or family has proceeded as directed.

Parallel vision without deviation is normal from the age of six months throughout life. Movement of the eyes in the cover and alternating cover tests is abnormal after the age of six months, as are nonparallel corneal light reflexes. At birth, movement of the eyes does not appear to be coordinated. During the first three months, there is crossing of the eyes, with periods when the eyes are relatively parallel. At the age of three months, the eyes are parallel most of the time, and after six months, involuntary crossing of the eyes is abnormal.

Convergent squint is rare or absent in the Mongolian race. It appears to be increasing among Caucasians, possibly because early operation enhances marriageability and continuation of the trait. Some observers do not believe that it is genetically based. Divergent squint is universal, but does not have a high incidence [6].

Amblyopia is defined as reduction in visual acuity with proper correction in place in an eye that appears normal by ophthalmoscope examination. Approximately 1.5 to 2 percent of the young adult population in the United States has some form of amblyopia [8]. Although there are several types, the most frequently encountered is strabismic amblyopia (amblyopia resulting from constant macular suppression to prevent double vision resulting from strabismus). Careful examination of visual acuity using the Snellen chart and testing of ocular mobility can detect abnormalities before amblyopia has developed. The visual acuity and ocular mobility tests are extremely important in preschool children to ensure early detection and care of visual problems.

TESTING VISUAL FIELDS

The visual field and perimetry testing is done next. The visual field is that portion of the external world that the eye can encompass. The images formed on the retina are inverted and reversed representations of objects in the real world, but are subsequently inverted and reversed again by higher brain centers, so that we ultimately see objects as they really are.

Figure 7-5 shows the visual pathways. Lesions can occur in the retina, in the optic pathways, or in the brain. These lesions are described in terms of the field of vision they affect rather than the part of the retina affected by them [1]. Three visual field defects and the location of the lesion in the visual pathway are shown in Figure 7-5. Lesions can occur at other locations along the visual pathway causing a variety of patterns of visual field loss.

A lesion at *A*, such as optic neuritis, obliterates both the nasal and temporal field (superior and inferior) with total loss of vision of the right eye.

Lesions at the optic chiasm, *B*, such as pituitary tumors or bilateral aneurysms, cause loss of the temporal field of the right and left eye (bitemporal hemianopia). Lesions occurring at C or anywhere along the anterior optic tract will affect the nasal field of the right eye and the temporal field of the left eye

Figure 7-5. The visual pathway. On right and left are maps of visual fields with areas of blindness darkened to show the effects of lesions in each location. *(A)* Lesion of optic nerve (loss of vision, right eye). *(B)* Midline lesion of optic chiasm (bitemporal hemianopia). *(C)* Lesion of the right anterior optic tract; blindness for objects in left half of each field of vision (left homonymous hemianopia). Lesions can occur at other locations along the visual pathway causing a variety of patterns of visual field losses.

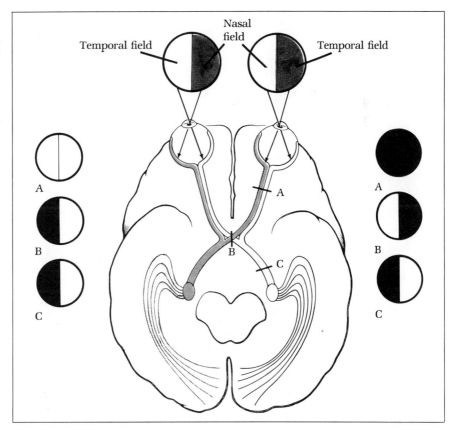

(homonymous hemianopia). This may be all of both fields or part of each, e.g., inferior fields only or superior fields only, depending on the location of the lesions. Interestingly, macular vision is commonly spared in homonymous hemianopia [1,8].

There is considerable separation of nerve pathways in the brain, and lesions in many areas of the central nervous system, the retina, or the optic tract may result in various patterns of visual field defects.

Glaucoma, elevated intraocular pressure, decreases peripheral vision because the increased intraocular pressure damages the optic nerve at its head or optic disc. Central vision, that vision in the central part of the retina, macula, and fovea, is unaffected until the disease has progressed.

The confrontation test is used for the *gross* measurement of visual fields and peripheral vision (Fig. 7-6). This test should be done at least yearly and whenever the client is having any eye or neurologic symptoms. Both the nurse and the client are seated facing each other 1 M (3 ft) apart. The right eye of the

Figure 7-6.
A. Testing the right temporal field of vision. *B.* Testing the right superior field of vision. *C.* Testing the right nasal field of vision.

client and the left eye of the nurse are each covered by an eye occluder. The nurse fixes her uncovered eye on that of the client, and vice versa. Then using her outstretched arm (which is midway between the client and herself), the nurse brings the test object, a wiggling finger, or a white ball at the end of a stick from the nonseeing periphery toward the center of the field of vision. Each quadrant (use the eight positions tested as in the ocular mobility test, but keep the client's eye on the examiner's eye) is successively tested. If an area is suspect, reduce the distance between points around the periphery, where the finger or ball is moved to the center. Both eyes are to be tested.

The confrontation test assumes (previously established) normal visual fields in the examiner. The test object should be seen simultaneously by the nurse and client if the fields are normal. If the examiner's arms are short, a wand with an object on it can be used so that the object can be extended beyond the visual field. If the client fails to see the test object in a given field (e.g., temporal field) or in the peripheral area (e.g., only sees the object when it is close to the eye), referral to an ophthalmologist or neurologist is indicated. This is an imprecise test; therefore any suspected defects require prompt referral for definitive diagnosis.

EXTERNAL OCULAR STRUCTURES

The *eyebrows* are normally symmetrical and are observed for loss of hair, seborrhea, and movement. Loss of hair may indicate hypothyroidism. Seborrhea of the eyebrows and scalp is often a cause of chronic marginal blepharitis (Fig. 7-7). Loss of movement of both eyebrows indicates the loss of integrity of

Figure 7-7. Blepharitis. Note scaling along lid margins (arrows). (From J. F. Smith and D. P. Nachazel, Jr. *Ophthalmologic Nursing.* Boston: Little, Brown, 1980. Photograph courtesy of Sally A. Rourke, Department of Ophthalmology, The University of Michigan Medical Center.)

the facial nerve (cranial nerve VII). Unilateral impairment of the eyebrow indicates peripheral impairment [3,7].

The appearance of the *eyelids* should be noted. The eyelid is subject to all the dermatologic conditions manifested by the other skin surfaces of the body. The color, texture, mobility, and position of the lids should be observed and the palpebral fissures examined. Differences other than normal racial differences in the upper lid folds should be described. The peoples of the Mongolian race have typical Mongolian eyelids. The lid folds are different and they demonstrate epicanthus. The Chinese have the most marked Mongolian lids and are subject to physiologic lagophthalmos. This is normal for this race. Localized swelling of the eyelid, inflammation, generalized periorbital edema, and scars from previous ocular injuries should be recorded. Any crusting, stys, or loss of eyelashes should also be noted, and further questioning of the client regarding these may be necessary.

The size of the palpebral fissures is altered by the position of the eyelids. The eyelids, when open, usually conceal the corneoscleral limbus in the 12 and 6 o'clock positions. Note in Figure 7-8 that the eyelid margins are at the corneoscleral limbus at 12 and 6 o'clock. Retraction of the upper lid in thyroid disorders is often manifest by exposure of a narrow rim of sclera at these positions. Frequent involuntary lid-blinking should be present. The lids should close easily by voluntary movement. Equal elevation and movement of the lids with the globe should occur in all positions of gaze. Motor innervation of the levator

Figure 7-8.
Diagrammatic structures of external eye. Note lacrimal gland, lacrimal ducts, and lacrimal sac are shown for position, but are covered by the eyelid, inner canthus, and nose respectively (right eye).

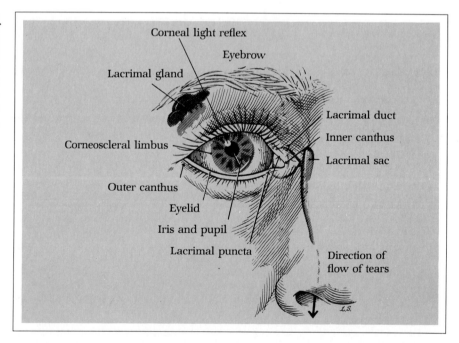

Table 7-3.
Muscles of the Eyelid and
Iris and Their Action and
Innervation

Muscles	Action	Innervation
Levator palpebrae superioris	Raises upper lid	Oculomotor (cranial nerve III)
Orbicularis oculi	Closes eyelids, acts as a sphincter (activates corneal reflex), wrinkles forehead, compresses lacrimal sac	Facial (cranial nerve VII)
Sphincter pupillae	Contracts pupil (miosis)	Oculomotor (cranial nerve III)
Dilator pupillae	Dilates pupil (mydriasis)	Sympathetic fibers

palpebrae superioris muscle, which raises the lid, is via the oculomotor (cranial nerve III) nerve (see Table 7-3). The lids should be in close approximation to the eyeball. Inverted (entropion) or everted (ectropion) lids are abnormal (Fig. 7-9). Protrusion of the eyeball is difficult to determine, but if it is suspected, the client should be sent to an ophthalmologist for instrument measurement [1,5,8].

The *conjunctiva* is the smooth transparent mucosal layers that unites the lids and globes. The palpebral conjunctiva lines the eyelids; the bulbar conjunctiva covers the exposed surface of the eyeball. The conjunctiva is an indicator of both systemic and local disease. The sclera should be seen through this transparent membrane and should be the color of white porcelain. There may be slight yellow pigmentation at the circumferential edge of the limbus. Normal conjunctiva contains a few large and tortuous visible episcleral vessels. Congestion of the conjunctiva may be distinguished from deeper diseases of the eye. In conjunctival congestion, vessels of the conjunctiva, both large and small, especially in the peripheral area, are engorged. Deeper diseases of the eye involve the cornea and deeper structures within the eye, and attention should be given to signs of corneal and iris involvement, to the pupillary reaction to light, and visual acuity [7,8].

Figure 7-9.
Entropion *A.* and ectropion
B. (Reproduced with
permission from R. D.
Judge, G. D. Zuidema, and
F. Fitzgerald (eds.).
*Methods of Clinical
Examination* (4th ed.).
Boston: Little, Brown,
1982.)

The bulbar and palpebral conjunctiva and the conjunctiva cul-de-sac (fold at junction of the two) should be inspected for edema congestion and pallor. The lower lid is everted by pulling downward with the index finger at the midpoint of the lid above the bone of the lower orbital rim. Have the client look upward. This position permits examination of the entire cul-de-sac of the lower lid.

To examine the palpebral conjunctiva of the upper eyelid, the lid must be everted. Even with the lid everted it is difficult to see the cul-de-sac. Visualization of the conjunctiva in this area is an important part of eye assessment, as this is an area where melanomas and lymphomas may go undetected by both client and examiner. The Mongolian upper eyelid is often difficult to evert. If some disorder is suspected, it may be necessary for an ophthalmologist to use a retractor to evert the eyelid.

To perform eversion of the upper eyelid, have the client look downward with the eye open, grasp the lashes of the upper lid between the index finger and thumb, pull the lid downward and away from the globe. With the other hand press a cotton-tipped applicator against the lid being pulled downward and outward. Fold the lid upward and over the applicator [8]. Figure 7-10 demonstrates the technique for eversion of the eyelid. Note especially the position of the applicator and that the client is looking downward. As long as the client

Figure 7-10. Eversion of lid for examination of the conjunctiva of upper lid and the area under the upper lid.

continues to look downward, the eyelid will remain everted. The lid may be manipulated by retraction on the eyelashes and slight movement of the applicator for better visualization. Imbedded sand or a hair can be removed from the everted lid with a sterile wet cotton ball or sterile wet applicator. The upper lid is returned to its normal position by directing the client to look upward. Palpation of the eyelid and eyebrows is essential.

A chalazion of either eyelid is not uncommon. A chalazion is a chronic inflammatory lipogranuloma of one of the meibomian glands (Fig. 7-11). It may be asymptomatic or cause discomfort upon lid movement. Upon palpation the swelling may feel like a small buck-shot-like substance within the eyelid. The distortion it causes from pressure on the globe may cause astigmatism. It is usually painless and shows no gross inflammatory signs. It should be excised by an ophthalmologist.

Yellowish pigmentation of the conjunctiva from excess pigment (carotene) may be seen and should be distinguished from jaundice. The conjunctiva, not the sclera, is stained with bilirubin in jaundice [7], reddened in infectious disease, and pale in anemia.

The *lacrimal gland,* which secretes the tears that flow across the eye and moisten the conjunctiva and cornea, is in the upper outer wall of the anterior portion of the orbit. There is a small palpebral portion located in the upper lid [8]. Figure 7-8 presents the location of the lacrimal gland and the direction of the flow of tears.

The lacrimal tissue sometimes can be seen when the upper lid is everted, particularly in the elderly. The lacrimal glands sometimes develop malignant and mixed cell tumors. The area should be examined for swelling, tenderness, redness, and pain. Infections and abscesses of the lacrimal gland occur, but are uncommon [5].

Figure 7-11. Chalazion (arrow). External appearance of lid. (From J. F. Smith and D. P. Nachazel, Jr. *Ophthalmologic Nursing.* Boston: Little, Brown, 1980. Photograph by Csaba Martonyi.)

Tears flow to the inner canthus, where they drain through the lacrimal puncta into the lacrimal duct, lacrimal sac, and nose. The lacrimal puncta are visible, on slight eversion of the lids, near the inner canthus. The inferior punctum turns slightly inward to dip into the lacrimal lake at the inner canthus (see Fig. 7-8). The lacrimal papilla, a small prominence surrounding the punctum, becomes more obvious with aging [7]. Regurgitation from the puncta following pressure on the lacrimal sac indicates blockage of the lacrimal duct. Infection of the sac is indicated when the material regurgitated is purulent. The client should be asked whether tears overflow the lower lid onto the cheek (epiphora) under conditions other than crying or tearing due to irritation [5].

The cornea is observed and examined for smoothness, clearness, and its reflective properties. Dullness in any area or irregularities are abnormal. The size and shape of one cornea is compared with that of the other. The iris pattern should be seen distinctly through the clear cornea. No blood vessels should be noted in the cornea [7]. A penlight is used for examination and reflection. The penlight is moved back and forth, up and down, so that it reflects off all surfaces of the cornea. The slit light on the ophthalmoscope can also be used for corneal examination. The light should be reflected in an even, smooth pattern. Irregularities in reflection must prompt referral, since corneal staining and use of a corneal microscope are necessary.* Any patient who has photophobia, dullness, irregularities of the cornea, opacity, blurring of vision, or blepharospasm should be referred to an ophthalmologist for diagnosis and treatment.

The anterior chamber is viewed for clearness of the aqueous humor and for a general impression of depth. Normal aqueous humor is acellular and transparent. Cloudiness of the aqueous, hyphema, or accumulation of any exudate is abnormal. A general impression of the depth of the chamber is achieved by directing a penlight beam across the iris from the temporal side. If the chamber is shallow, only the temporal side of the iris will be illuminated, because the iris is bowed forward and the nasal half will be shadowed [5]. Any bulging forward of the iris, or a shadow on the nasal half of the iris, would indicate narrow-angle anatomy, predisposing to glaucoma, and the client should be referred to an ophthalmologist for gonioscopic and tonometric examination [3].

Examination of the iris should include observation of color, texture, and pattern. Any unusual markings or growths should be noted. The iris pattern should be clearly visible. The inability to visualize iris patterns may be due to corneal opacity with cells in the aqueous or to iris inflammation. Changes in color of the iris are indicative of abnormal processes [7].

The lens of the eye is viewed and examined through the pupillary aperture. The lens normally is clear and transparent. Oblique illumination reveals opacities. The transparency of the lens decreases with age, and it may appear

*Neitz Hand Held Slit Lamp and Transformer. Order from Western Optical, 1200 Mercer Street, Seattle, Washington, 98109.

Figure 7-12.
Cataract. Note light reflex
on upper edge of pupil.
(From J. F. Smith and D. P.
Nachazel, Jr.
Ophthalmologic Nursing.
Boston: Little, Brown, 1980.
Photograph courtesy of
Frank Flanagin, Associated
Retinal Consultants,
Detroit.)

gray in elderly persons. Cataracts also may cause a gray, opaque appearance (Fig. 7-12).

TESTING NERVE
REFLEXES
Corneal Reflexes

The corneal reflex tests the sensitivity of the cornea to pain, touch, and pressure and is done as a part of the assessment. This is a test of an afferent sensory branch of the trigeminal nerve (cranial nerve V). The motor response is via the facial nerve and consists in activation of the orbicularis oculi muscle, which, among other functions, closes the eyelids [8]. In the reflex, both eyes are closed, owing to connecting fibers to the facial nuclei [8]. The response of the stimulated eye is called the "direct corneal reflex"; the response of the other eye is the "consensual corneal reflex" [6]. Both consensual and direct responses are obliterated by interruption of the trigeminal nerve pathways.

To test for the corneal reflex, the client is informed of what to expect and is seated opposite the nurse examiner. The client is asked to look to the right. A twisted wisp of cotton is lightly touched to the corneal surface of the client's left eye. An attempt should be made to approach the left eye with the cotton from the temporal side to prevent an avoidance response. To test the corneal reflex of the right eye, have the client look to the left and repeat the procedure as described for testing the left eye. The normal response is (1) closing and blinking of both eyes, that is, the direct and consensual corneal reflex, (2) increased lacrimation, and (3) a report of slight discomfort [3]. A consensual reflex, but no direct reflex, is obtained if the facial nerve on the same side is destroyed. However, there is still increased lacrimation [1].

The arcus senilis is seen at the corneoscleral limbus, but separated from it by a clear zone in most persons over the age of 50 or in persons with lipid disturbances [3].

Pupillary Reflexes   Compare and contrast the size, shape, and reaction of the pupils [7]. If the pupil is adherent to the cornea or to the lens, it is not circular [7]. Contraction of the pupil can be demonstrated by shining a penlight into the eye in a semi-darkened room. The direct pupillary light reflex is tested by shining the penlight into one eye (right) and observing that eye for the pupillary constriction that occurs. Move the light away and again shine the light into the right eye, this time watching the left eye, which should constrict with the "consensual" pupillary response. Now elicit the direct pupillary response of the left eye by shining the penlight into the left eye, watch the pupillary constriction, and the "consensual" response of the right eye. The consensual and direct responses should be equal. Abnormalities of the pupillary response may be due to any of a number of neurologic lesions or to the effect of drugs on the iris muscles. See Keeney [5] for a more extensive discussion of the neurologic implications.

The near-point pupillary reflex is tested by having the client look into the distance and then at an object 15 cm (6 in) from his nose at the nose level. Illumination should remain constant. The response evokes three reflexes: (1) convergence, (2) pupillary constriction, and (3) accommodation—not seen by the examiner [8]. Equality of response in both eyes is normal and is the important factor. Rapidity of response varies and tends to slow with age, particularly when accommodating for near-point reflex.

INTRAOCULAR PRESSURE   A rough estimation of intraocular pressure is done by using the finger tension test. The client is asked to close his eyes and look *down* while the nurse places two forefingers on the upper lid over the sclera of the eyeball. Pressure is exerted by alternating the forefingers in a back-and-forward movement. The globe should indent slightly with the pressure. The examiner must first learn what the "feel" of normal globe pressure is. Normal intraocular pressure is 12 to 22 mm Hg [3]. A comparison is made between the two eyes and between the client's eyes and those of the examiner (tested recently as normal). This estimation is made on all clients and is of particular importance for those over 40 years of age and those who have experienced eye trauma. Any suspected increased pressure or symptoms of glaucoma require the immediate referral of the client to the ophthalmologist.

Nurses can and do use the Schiötz tonometer, but this special test needs to be done in collaboration with the ophthalmologist, since medication of the eye is involved. Other tests may be required for clients with suspected or confirmed eye abnormalities, but are outside the scope of the general examination ordinarily done by nurses in most nonspecialized settings.

FUNDOSCOPIC EXAMINATION

Currently, the nurse's use of the ophthalmoscope is somewhat limited. Ophthalmoscopic examination is a necessary part of the eye examination, and as nurses gain the knowledge and skill in this area of assessment, it will become more and more a part of general nursing practice. Nurses working with hypertensive and diabetic clients are particularly encouraged to learn the fundoscopic examination. All infants and children should be examined with the ophthalmoscope to determine the red reflex (fundus reflex) to rule out congenital cataracts [7].

For basic ophthalmoscopy the direct ophthalmoscope is used. The ophthalmoscope has two dials (discs). One dial changes the image of light, of which there are five different patterns: (1) slit light, used to reflect off the cornea or when retinal detachments are suspected; (2) green light, actually a red filter to examine the macula; (3) the grid pattern, used for drawing on paper the precise point on the retina at which the lesion is located; (4) a pinpoint white light; (5) a larger white light. The larger white light is used for general fundoscopic examination.

The other dial, the lens selection disc, rotates clockwise or counterclockwise. Rotation of this disc changes the numbers that appear in the lighted diopter selection hole and changes the refractive power (measured in diopters) of the lenses in the key hole (the hole the examiner looks through). The lenses on the ophthalmoscope are convex or concave. The convex lenses are called "plus lenses" and are indicated by the black numbers in the diopter selection hole. The concave lenses are called "minus lenses" and are indicated as red numbers in the diopter selection hole (see Fig. 7-13). To become familiar with the ophthalmoscope, set the diopter setting at 0 (zero), now rotate the lens selection disc counterclockwise through the black numbers; return to zero; then rotate clockwise through the red numbers. Do this quickly and easily first with the right and then with left index finger.

Look through the key hole with the right eye, holding the scope in the right hand. Focus on a near object at 5 cm (2 in), such as the palm of the left hand. Change the distance and refocus. Learn to read the newspaper with the ophthalmoscope. Practice using the left eye with the left hand and index finger. Become proficient with handling and focusing the ophthalmoscope before using it to examine a person. The examiner closes the eye that is not looking through the scope.

The diopter setting varies with the refractive error of the client and examiner (see Fig. 7-13). The nurse examiner should wear her normal corrective lenses if she has any. Clients who have *severe* astigmatism should wear their contact lenses or glasses for the examination, as the distortion that occurs without them cannot be corrected by the lens of the ophthalmoscope. However, hyperopic and myopic conditions in the examiner and client are neutralized by the lenses of the ophthalmoscope. For the client with hyperopia, the nurse would start by

Figure 7-13.
Normal, myopic and
hyperopic eyeball
configurations. Depiction of
retinal visual image
position and shape of
corrective lenses.

A. Normal eye,
   image falls on fovea
   of eye

B. Myopic or nearsighted eye,
   image falls in front of retina

C. Concave correction for myopic eye.
   On ophthalmoscope use minus (red)
   diopter setting to visualize retina

D. Hyperopic or farsighted eye,
   image falls behind retina

E. Convex correction for hyperopic
   eye. On ophthalmoscope use
   plus (black) diopter setting to
   visualize retina

using the convex lens; with myopia, the concave lens. However, the combination of the examiner's eye and the client's eye determines the actual diopter setting.

The fundoscopic examination is done in a room with subdued light and minimum activity to eliminate reflections and distractions. The client and examiner both should be in a comfortable body alignment, with the eyes at the same height. The examiner uses her right eye with the ophthalmoscope in the right hand to examine the client's right eye. The left eye and hand of the examiner are used to examine the left eye of the client.

The index finger is positioned on the lens selection disc (the thumb does not allow the rapidity of the rotation allowed by the forefinger). The nurse examiner positions herself slightly to the right of the client's right eye, so that the ophthalmoscope is pointing slightly nasally rather than straight into the eye. The client is asked to fix his gaze straight ahead on a mark on the wall over the examiner's shoulder. The client should be able to see over the examiner's shoulder, and if he cannot, the examiner should move slightly so that he can (Fig. 7-14).

The ophthalmoscope is positioned immediately in front of the examiner's eye and approximately 15 cm (6 in) from the client's eye. Start the lens selection at 0 (zero); then move the lens selection disc until the cornea and iris are focused. Observe the iris for the iris pattern and muscle movements. Observe the cornea and lens for opacities, which appear as black areas against the reddish-orange background of the retina. The normal fundus is seen as a red reflex (circular, reddish-orange retinal reflection) also called the fundus reflex or red reflex. The opacities appear black on the red reflex because they prevent the reflected light from reaching the observer's eye. The ophthalmoscope is now moved 3.8 to 5 cm (1½ to 2 in) from the client's eye. The lens setting is then rotated counterclockwise and then clockwise to focus back toward the retina. The lens disc is rotated until a vessel is located on the retina and focused on. The vessel is followed as it grows progressively larger until the optic disc is located.

The optic disc, which is the site of entrance of the optic nerve and retinal blood vessels, may be oval or circular and is lighter than the retina in color, often described as reddish or pink (Fig. 7-15). The physiologic cup of the disc is a pale area of depression with a rim between the cup and the disc border. The border may be a clear-cut edge, may be demarcated by a white ring, or may merge gradually into the retina [8]. A black ring or crescent may be seen

Figure 7-15.
Structures seen in
examination of the fundus
by ophthalmoscope (as seen
with the pupil fully dilated
and wide-angle
photography).

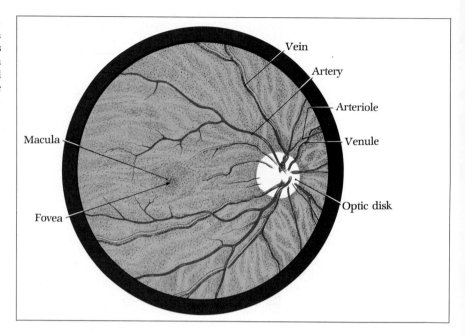

occasionally as a result of thickened pigmented retinal epithelium. In glaucoma, the rim and border are sharp, the physiologic cup is deep, and the disc is paler. A pale disc may indicate optic atrophy. When papilledema or papillitis is present, the disc borders may be blurry and the disc congested [8]. Elevation of the nerve head may also be present and is abnormal.

The optic disc is about 1.5 mm in diameter. The diameter of the disc is the standard unit of measurement in the fundus. The disc appears to be approximately the same size in most clients. Marked enlargement of the disc is abnormal and requires physician referral. With absence of the lens (aphakia), the disc appears smaller than normal [7]. It must be remembered that pictures of the retina are taken with the pupil dilated and by wide-angle photography. Normally nurses examine the fundus through undilated pupils. In this case only portions of the optic disc are visible, and to view its entirety the ophthalmoscope must be moved. It is difficult to view the fundus adequately without pupil dilatation. Any abnormality suspected from history or visualization must be referred for adequate examination by a doctor—preferably an ophthalmologist.

The central retinal artery enters at the optic disc and immediately bifurcates into the superior and inferior papillary arteries. After the second bifurcation, the vessels are arterioles (venules before the second major junction). The veins are larger and the column of blood is darker than in the arteries (see Fig. 7-15). A 3:2 vein-to-artery ratio is seen in normal persons [5]. Some sources give a ratio of 5:4 [8]. With arteriosclerotic and hypertensive changes, the arteries narrow (3:1 ratio), change color, become more opaque, show a copper-wire effect, and show changes at the arteriovenous crossings [8]. Indentation of the vein where the artery crosses, enlargement of the vein distal to the arterial crossing, and disappearance of the vein on either side of the artery indicate thickening of the arteriolar walls [3]. The entire fundus is examined by having the client rotate the globe or the examiner move the ophthalmoscope so that different areas can be examined. Avoid the center of the fundus (fovea) until all the periphery has been examined.

The fovea centralis is approximately 2 disc diameters temporally from the optic disc and is normally darker than the surrounding fundus (see Fig. 7-15). The darkness of the fovea varies with complexion. In blondes the fovea may not be differentiated by color, and location may be determined by relation to the optic disc and retinal vessels. Brunettes have a dark foveal area. Pigmented races have a darker fundus and the fovea is also darker. The pit of the fovea presents a bright dotlike reflex (foveal reflex in Fig. 7-15) owing to its concave surface. The fovea centralis is approximately 1.5 mm and is surrounded by the macula (3 mm in diameter). The macula butea (a yellow spot) has a yellowish pigmentation that can be seen when a red-free light (green light on ophthalmoscope) is used. This area is examined last as the client will become light-dazzled, her eyes will tear, and she will be unable to keep the eyelids open. The variations of normal are great. It takes considerable skill, knowledge, and practice to be able to identify more than the grossly abnormal. Yet, the nurse plays a significant role in preventive screening and early detection of potentially catastrophic eye problems.

THE EYE-ASSESSMENT GUIDE

A. History
  1. a. Past problems and resolutions
     b. Recent changes
  2. Photophobia
  3. Pain—duration, intensity, relief
  4. Itching or burning—seasonal?
  5. Tearing—when, how much, how long
  6. Redness
  7. Blurring or veiling
  8. Spots, flickering lights
B. Visual Acuity
  1. Snellen (distance)
     a. 6 M/20 ft. from chart
     b. Uncorrected, then corrected
     c. Encourage to try next line
     d. Record distance 6 M/ _____what client reads, describe line read—quickly
  2. Jaeger (near)
     a. 35 cm (14 in.) from card—watch they don't move card closer or farther away
     b. Encourage to read smallest possible print
  3. Color vision

C. Ocular Movements
   1. Corneal light reflexes parallel in primary and 8 diagnostic positions of gaze
   2. Cover test—observe eye not covered
   3. Alternating cover test—observe eye uncovered
D. Visual Fields
   1. Confrontation test
      a. Temporal fields
      b. Nasal fields
      c. Peripheral fields
E. External Ocular Structures
   1. Eyebrows
   2. Eyelids—epicanthal folds, movements, position
   3. Conjunctiva—eversion
   4. Lacrimal puncta—tearing
F. Cornea
   1. Clearness, reflectiveness
   2. Corneal reflexes—direct and consensual (cranial nerve V)
G. Anterior Chamber—fluid, depth
H. Pupillary Reflexes, Iris, Lens
   1. Iris—color, texture, pattern
   2. Pupillary reflexes—direct and consensual (cranial nerve III)
   3. Near point pupillary reflex
   4. Lens opacity reflections
I. Intraocular Pressure
J. Fundoscopic
   1. Black spots on red reflex
   2. Optic disc—disc borders, vein to artery ratio, depth, color, disc to cup ratio
   3. Retina—color, tortuosity of vessels
   4. Macula and fovea

REFERENCES
1. Gatz, A. J. *Manter's Essentials of Clinical Neuroanatomy and Neurophysiology* (5th ed.). Philadelphia: Davis, 1975.
2. Havener, W. H. *Synopsis of Ophthalmology* (5th ed.). St. Louis: Mosby, 1979.
3. Henderson, J. W. "Eye." In R. D. Judge and G. D. Zuidema (Eds.). *Methods of Clinical Examination: A Physiological Approach* (3rd ed.). Boston: Little, Brown, 1974.
4. Kalmus, H. *Diagnosis and Genetics of Defective Colour Vision.* New York: Pergamon, 1965.
5. Keeney, A. H. *Ocular Examination, Basis and Technique* (2nd ed.). St. Louis: Mosby, 1976.
6. Mann, I. C. *Culture, Race, Climate and Eye Diseases.* Springfield, Ill: Thomas, 1966.
7. Newell, F. W., and Ernst, J. T. *Ophthalmology, Principles and Concepts* (4th ed.). St. Louis: Mosby, 1978.
8. Scheie, H. G., and Albert, D. M. *Textbook of Ophthalmology* (9th ed.). Philadelphia: Saunders, 1977.
9. Wybar, K. C. *Ophthalmology.* London: Bailliére Tindall, 1974.

8. Physical Assessment of the Ear and Hearing

GLOSSARY

aerotitis See *barotrauma.*

annulus The ring structure at the edge of the tympanic membrane where it joins the tissue of the external ear canal. The tympanic membrane is supported around its periphery by the annulus.

auricle The external ear; pinna or flap.

barotrauma (aerotitis) A condition caused by exposure to differing atmospheric pressure.

atresia Pathologic closure of a normal anatomic opening or congenital absence of the same, used here in relation to external auditory canal.

cerumen Waxlike, soft, brown secretion found in the external auditory canal of the ear.

cholesteatoma An encysted putty-like mass (resulting from an accumulation of squamous epithelium and its products) in the middle ear and mastoid.

cochlea A winding cone-shaped tube forming the portion of the inner ear that contains the organ of Corti.

decibels Term used to measure intensity (See *intensity*).

dizziness Disturbed sense of relationship to space.

endolymph Fluid in the membranous labyrinth of the inner ear, continuous within semicircular canals and the cochlea.

frequency Number of vibrations per second made by a sound wave (expressed in cycles per second [cps] or Hertz [Hz]). Lowest audible tone to the human ear has a frequency of 20 cycles per second or Hertz (Hz). As frequency increases we perceive a rise in pitch. 256 Hz is the same pitch as middle C on the piano. If the frequency is doubled (512 Hz) it is one octave above middle C [2].

helix The superior and posterior free margin at the pinna of the ear.

injection Prominence and dilation of the normal vascular bed.

intensity Pressure exerted by a sound. The sensation of loudness depends on intensity (measure intensity in terms of decibels [2]). (See Table 8-2.)

labyrinth Intricate communicating canals in the inner ear. Consists of a bony capsule (bony labyrinth) and an inner membranous labyrinth.

meatus Opening of the external auditory canal at auricle.

nystagmus (labyrinthine or central) Slow movement of the eye in one direction followed by a rapid involuntary compensatory movement in the opposite direction (rhythmic).

ossicles The three small bones of the middle ear: malleus, incus, and stapes.

otalgia Pain in the ear.

otitis Inflammation of the ear.

    acute otitis media The name given to inflammation of the lining membrane in the middle ear cleft [6].

    chronic otitis media An infection of long standing in which there are no signs of acute inflammation. Caused by failure of an acute infection to resolve completely or by the infection of a cholesteatoma or of a serous effusion into the middle ear [6].

    purulent otitis media Acute otitis media with a pus discharge.

    otitis externa Inflammation of the external ear, usually the external auditory canal.

    secretory otitis media Sterile effusion into the middle ear, also called seromucinous otitis media, serous otitis media, exudative otitis media, glue ear, sterile otitis media, catarrhal otitis media [10], and chronic, nonsuppurative otitis media [6].

otosclerosis The formation of spongy bone in the inner ear; bones of middle ear, especially stapes, become fixed and do not pass on vibrations of sound [8].

ototoxicity The property of exerting damaging effects on the nerve cells of the inner ear.

pinna Projecting part of the external ear; auricle.

presbycusis Senile deafness, progressive sensorineural deafness, which occurs and advances, for no apparent reason, with age and is first noticed about age 66. Premature onset is associated with previous bouts of otitis media and exposure to loud noise throughout a working life [2].

recruitment Abnormally rapid increase in loudness with increasing sound intensity, which occurs in deafness of neural origin.

tinnitus Noise often of ringing, in the ears, originating within the body.

tragus Cartilaginous tongue-like projection in front of the external auditory meatus.

tympanic membrane Membrane serving as the lateral wall of the tympanic cavity and separating it from the external auditory meatus.

umbo of the tympanic membrane The point at which the handle (manubrium of the malleus) is attached to the inner surface of the tympanic membrane.

vertigo Sensation of whirling motion of oneself or of external objects. A hallucination of movement.

vestibule The middle part of the inner ear, behind the cochlea and in front of the semicircular canals.

HISTORY AND EXAMINATION

ASSESSMENT of the ear includes both physical and historic data collection by the nurse. The major objective is to determine the functional status of the ear and, if there is abnormality, to make the appropriate referral of the client to a specialist or an agency. The assessment of the ear and hearing includes the history, both past and present, testing for hearing, the physical assessment of the external ear, otoscopic examination of the external canal and tympanic membrane, and vestibular testing. Equipment needed for the otologic assessment includes:

1. List of spondee (bisyllabic) words and phonetically balanced (one syllable) words.
2. Tuning forks (512 cps or 1,024 or 2,000 cps).
3. Otoscope with pneumatic bulb attachment.
4. Masking device, i.e., paper, Barany noise box.

The history should begin with questions about hearing loss of family members and, insofar as possible, a determination of the type of loss. Next, a history of past ear diseases or surgery of the client is obtained. Specific inquiry is made regarding episodes of otalgia, drainage, stuffiness, fever, and decreased hearing. Occurrence and frequency of infections, treatment instituted, and response to therapy are determined also. An attempt is made to determine event-related and other potential causative factors, e.g., drainage and pain occurring after swimming, in cold weather, or when no hat or protective ear covering is worn. The client's occupation, leisure activities, and exposure to chemicals are also pertinent data.

In assessing infants and children unable to communicate verbally, behavioral changes are cardinal signs. Mothers should be asked about behavior changes observed and instructed to note these changes in the future. Explicit data about symptoms should be sought as indicated in the following:

1. *Otalgia.* Does the client have otalgia, and if so, when did it begin? Is it described as constant or intermittent? Is it associated with movement, activity, or noise, and is the pain sharp or dull? How has the individual attempted to relieve the pain and has the pain been relieved?

2. *Chills and fever.* Has the client had fever or chills? Did he take his temperature, and if so, what was it? Has he had a recent history of colds, influenza, or other systemic disease? Was medical treatment sought, and if so, what were the diagnosis and treatment? If medical treatment was not sought, what was the course of the fever? Was there self-treatment? What kind? What results were obtained?

3. *Drainage.* Is there drainage from the ears now and has there been drainage previously? What are the color, consistency, amount, and odor of the discharge? When was the drainage first noticed? Is the cerumen normally soft or hard? How are the ears normally cleaned? Has the drainage been separate from or associated with other symptoms?

4. *Medication history.* A medication history should be elicited. Is the client now taking ototoxic drugs? Has the client taken such medications recently, e.g., aspirin, quinine, streptomycin, kanamycin, gentamicin, neomycin, nitrofurantoin? (See Table 8-1) If ototoxic drugs have been taken, the extent to which the client has used the drug needs to be determined. Cytotoxic and diuretic drugs are also ototoxic. Clients with renal failure are more susceptible to the ototoxic effects of drugs cleared by the kidneys[11].

Table 8-1.
Ototoxic Drugs and
Chemicals

Chemicals	Drugs
Alcohol	Chloramphenical
Aniline dyes	Chloroquine
Arsenic	Dihydrostreptomycin
Lead	Ethacrynic acid (Edecrin)
Gold	Furosemide (Lasix)
Carbon monoxide	Gentamycin
Oil of chenopodium	Kanamycin
	Neomycin
	Nitrogen mustard (including cytoxan alberan)
	Polybrene
	Polymixin B
	Quinidine
	Quinine
	Ristocetin
	Salicylates
	Streptomycin
	Tobramycin
	Vancomycin
	Viomycin

Source: Adapted from G. L. Adams, L. R. Boies, and M. M. Paparella. *Boies's Fundamentals of Otolaryngology* (5th ed.). Philadelphia: Saunders, 1978.

5. *Tinnitus and vertigo.* It should be determined whether the client has or has had tinnitus, vertigo, or dizziness associated with the use of medications or with other diseases or symptoms. Evaluations of equilibrium, dizziness, and vertigo are made to determine the gross function of the vestibular portion of cranial nerve VIII. Vertigo can be a symptom of neurologic and systemic problems as well as of vestibular alterations. It is important to have the clients describe the sensation they feel. Does the vertigo occur only in one position (horizontal or vertical) or when bending over, standing, or changing position? Does the person feel he is moving, or does he feel that he is stationary and the room is moving? Are there other symptoms such as nausea, vomiting, a feeling of fullness in the ear, or fluctuations in hearing?

6. *Environmental noise.* A brief history of exposure to environmental noise in the work, home, and social settings should be taken. Determine whether the client is exposed to loud noise in the work setting and whether he utilizes protective devices provided. What is the extent of exposure?

7. *Stuffiness.* A history of the client's ability to equalize the pressure within the ear. Ask whether children have had frequent colds, sore throats, or tonsilitis, and whether a decreased ability to hear or a lack of attention has followed any of these episodes.

The ear examination is part of the complete physical examination. If this examination is done for a specific complaint without the complete physical examination, it is necessary to take a more detailed history, including the following additional questions:

1. Allergic disorders—severity, onset, treatment
2. Occurrence of head injury
3. Systemic disorders such as anemia (especially sudden, severe), renal disease, neurologic disorders, arteriosclerosis, syphilis, and hypertension.

Throughout the history-taking and physical examination the nurse can gain further information through nonverbal clues the client may give. Is the client's voice loud or soft? Is it proportional to the environmental noise? Do questions have to be repeated, or just certain words? Is body or head posture changed as if to facilitate hearing? Cultural, environmental, and age factors must be considered. Social organization of the country affects the level of ear health. In some areas mastoiditis is still prevalent because middle ear infections are not treated.

Secretory otitis media affects pre-school and early school age children. It is often undetected and leads to deafness if untreated. In one study an incidence of 3.6 percent was found in an otherwise healthy group of preschoolers [10]. In elderly persons, a recently identified phenomenon has been malignant external otitis. This occurs especially in elderly persons, with diabetes, with rapid changes in temperature and humidity. It was first reported in Florida [1].

TESTING HEARING ACUITY

Hearing acuity is tested to determine whether there is a hearing loss, and, if so, the degree and type of hearing loss. Nurses in industrial settings frequently do tone testing with an audiometer on admission and discharge employment physical examinations. In order to detect the V-shaped loss that frequently occurs from high frequency noise, it is necessary to use the audiometer. This test is not discussed here as it is quite specific, and if hearing impairment is detected by the following tests the client should be referred for audiometric and other more precise testing.

As noise becomes a greater problem in industrial settings and in the music and occupations of a country (e.g., dentists with high speed drills), more sensorineural hearing loss in the population can be expected. It is important to note that rock musicians suffer from hearing loss more often and to a greater degree than do classical orchestral musicians. Also, dentists who use high speed drills experience high frequency loss [2]. Presbycusis has been the "catch-all" term commonly used for most sensorineural hearing loss occurring in later life. There is, however, growing evidence that much of this sensorineural loss may be hereditary hearing loss that occurs in the later years [8]. The following hearing acuity tests are only gross measures of the client's hearing. If the history and results of these gross tests suggest a hearing impairment, the client must be referred to an otologist. Generally, the nurse tries to determine whether there is a hearing loss and, if so, the type of hearing loss.

The three types of hearing loss [9] are:

1. *Conductive hearing loss* occurs when there is interruption or attenuation of sound waves as they are conducted from the external meatus to the cochlea. (See Fig. 8-5B) This may occur in the external ear at the tympanic membrane or in the middle ear or its ossicles, and at the labyrinthine windows. Persons with conductive hearing loss speak softly, often hear better in a noisy environment (others speak above the noise), and are able to hear well on the telephone.

2. *Sensorineural* or *perceptive hearing loss* is an interruption or attenuation of impulses transmitted or interpreted at the level of the cochlea, auditory nerve, or hearing center of the cerebral cortex. (See Fig. 8-5B) Persons with a sensorineural hearing loss speak loudly, may hear sound but are unable to understand it (poor discrimination), and hear better in a quiet environment. These persons may also experience recruitment.

3. *Mixed hearing loss* is a combination of conductive and sensorineural hearing loss.

Table 8-2.
Voice Test Equivalent*

Voice Level and Decibel Equivalent	Clinical Equivalent
Inaudible whisper, 15–25 db	Normal hearing or very mild loss
Soft or just audible whisper, 25–35 db	Mild hearing loss (socially adequate for adults, inadequate for children)
Loud whisper, 35–45 db (mild masking, i.e., finger in opposite ear)	Moderate loss (borderline for conversational purposes)
Soft spoken voice, 45–55 db (mild masking, i.e., briskly moving finger in opposite ear)	Socially inadequate; needs some form of correction if best ear
Moderate spoken voice, 55–70 db (loud masking, i.e., rubbing paper, radio static or Bárány noise box in opposite ear)	Always involves some sensorineural loss, with or without associated conductive loss
Loud spoken voice, 70–90 db (very loud masking, i.e., Bárány noise box, white noise, or alarm from watch in opposite ear)	Severe loss with large sensorineural deficit, with or without associated conductive component

*Modified from R. Boles [3]. By permission of the author and publisher.

Tests for Conversational Hearing

Hearing for normal conversational purposes can be checked by the use of whisper and spoken-voice test [3] (see Table 8-2). The whisper and spoken voice should be several inches from the ear being tested. When testing is done by air conduction, the opposite ear from the one being tested must be masked. Masking is also important in the testing of bone conduction, particularly when the hearing difference between the two ears is greater than 30 db (the intensity level of the sounds normally heard in a quiet room). The greater the discrepancy in hearing between the ears, the greater the need for the better ear to be masked. A cellophane or "crackly paper" can be used, but a Bárány noise box is more effective. It is also possible to use an ear plug (the type used in industry) or ear covers.

Further testing can be done by determining the intensity level at which the individual can understand speech, called "sensitivity hearing." Magnetic phonographic and tape recordings are available for this test.* The live voice can be used, but has the disadvantage of not being standardized and thus can be used only for gross measurement of sensitivity. Spondee (spondaic) words are bisyllabic. The two syllables are equally stressed, such as airplane, oatmeal, daybreak, pancake (see Table 8-3). These are spoken to the client at normal conversational intensity and with increasing levels of intensity as needed (see Table 8-2). The words are spoken clearly, without exaggeration, one to two feet from the client's ear (with client and nurse comfortably seated, so that client cannot read the nurse's lips). The environment should be quiet and the ear not being tested should be masked. The client is asked to repeat the word after the nurse has stated it, e.g., "say the word _____." The level (in db) (see Table 8-2) at

*Techsonic Studios, 1201 South Brentwood Blvd., St. Louis, Missouri.

Table 8-3.
Spondaic (bisyllable) and
Phonetically Balanced
(monosyllable) Word Lists*

Spondaic Words		Phonetically Balanced Words	
airplane	pancake	an	you (ewe)
armchair	playground	yard	as
birthday	workshop	us	wet
daybreak	toothbrush	carve	chew
drawbridge	railroad	day	see (sea)
eardrum	school boy	toe	deaf
grandson	sidewalk	felt	them
hardware	sunset	stove	give
horseshoe	woodwork	hunt	true
hot dog	stairway	ran	isle (aisle)
iceberg	greyhound	knees	or (oar)
mousetrap	hothouse	not (knot)	law
northwest	doormat	low	me
padlock	cowboy	owl	none (nun)
oatmeal	baseball	it	jam
inkwell	headlight	she	poor
farewell	mushroom	high	him
whitewash		there (their)	skin
		earn (urn)	east
		twins	thing
		could	dad
Simple sentences		what	up
		bathe	bells
		ace	wire

*It is suggested that the nurse photocopy this table, circle the words missed and place with the client's record for future comparison.

which the person can correctly repeat 50 percent of the words is called his "speech reception threshold" (SRT).

Speech discrimination testing is another method the nurse can use for evaluation of hearing. Phonetically balanced (P-B), one-syllable words, phonetically difficult to understand, are presented at an optimal intensity for the client. The P-B words are presented to the client in the same manner as the spondee words (see Table 8-3).

The percentage of such words as knee, yard, carve, tin, and sin that are repeated correctly is used to give the nurse an idea of the client's discrimination ability. If less than 50 percent of the words are correct, or if the intensity level is greater than 55 to 70 db (moderate speech level), the client should be referred to an otologist. The threshold for monosyllabic words is different from that for bisyllabic words.

In sensorineural loss, both sensitivity and discrimination ability are decreased, and no matter how loudly the words are presented, the client is unable to correctly repeat some of them. If the intensity is raised too high, he understands less. With conductive loss, if the sound is made loud enough (intensity increased) the client is able to hear speech normally or almost normally [2].

Hearing testing in children is difficult, but it is imperative for early detection of loss. The presence or absence of the startle reflex can be used to test infants under 6 months of age. Testing the ability to localize sounds is another way of assessing hearing in infants and children. Or one can use toys that make varying noises at different intensities to test hearing levels. However, if this proves too difficult, gross measurement is better than none at all. Word games and play techniques can be used by the nurse or by the family for testing hearing.

Tuning Fork Tests

Tuning fork tests for hearing acuity are an important part of the otologic examination. It is nearly always possible, in adults, to distinguish a pure conductive deafness from a pure sensorineural deafness by careful performance of three simple tuning fork tests [2]. Tuning forks with the frequencies of 512 to 1,024 cps. (within the speech frequency range) should be used.

It must be possible to hold the tuning fork firmly by its stem without interfering with its vibrations, and its base must be flat and broad enough to be applied to the mastoid process. If the tuning fork is struck too forcibly, overtones may become prominent and the test invalidated [2]. If hair touches the tuning fork or is between the bone and fork, or between the fork and the ear, the vibrations are attenuated. Hearing by bone conduction can be regarded as a rough clinical measure of perceptive function, and provided this is normal, hearing by air conduction gives a rough guide to the integrity of the conducting mechanism [2].

Rinne's Test

Each ear is tested separately. The ear not being tested is masked. The tuning fork is struck lightly, and its base is held on the mastoid process of the ear being tested. After several seconds, it is transferred to the opening of the external auditory canal with the fork's acoustic axis in line with the axis of the canal. (The acoustic axis of the tuning fork is in an imaginary line drawn between the two tines of the tuning fork.) The tuning fork is held alternately with the base on the mastoid process and vibrating tinea at the external meatus until it is no longer heard by one or the other (Figs. 8-1 and 8-3). The sound vibrations are conducted via bone to the cochlea, activating hair cells that are connected to the fibers of the auditory nerve (cranial nerve VIII). When the still vibrating tuning fork is placed outside the external auditory meatus, conduction occurs via the air conduction. The normal ear hears the tuning fork twice as long by air conduction (AC) as by bone conduction (BC). When this occurs, the result is designated as a positive Rinne (AC > BC). This relationship is reversed in advanced conductive loss (negative Rinne) and is designated as a negative or equal Rinne (BC > or = AC). With sensorineural loss, the normal relationship is maintained (positive Rinne, AC > BC), but the length of time the fork is heard is reduced (see Table 8-4).

The nurse should be aware of false-negative Rinne, when only bone conduc-

Figure 8-1.
Rinne test for hearing loss.
A. Base of vibrating tuning
fork is placed on mastoid
process. *B.* Vibrating tinea
at the opening of the
external auditory canal. Be
sure the fork's acoustical
axis is correctly positioned,
as in B.

Figure 8-1.
Rinne test for hearing loss.
A. Base of vibrating tuning
fork is placed on mastoid
process. *B.* Vibrating tinea
at the opening of the
external auditory canal. Be
sure the fork's acoustical
axis is correctly positioned,
as in B.

tion is heard and is actually being heard by the ear not being tested. Masking of the nontested ear helps to prevent this. A false-negative Rinne may occur with an auditory nerve tumor, and it is imperative that it be identified early.

In the Weber test, a vibrating tuning fork is placed in the midline of the skull, usually the forehead, or, unless the client has dentures, on the maxillary incisors (Fig. 8-2). This test is useful in cases of unilateral deafness. The client is asked to say in which ear she hears the fork.

The person with conductive loss hears the sound in the impaired ear if the other ear has normal hearing. This is because the vibrations are being conducted through the skull bone and because the normal ear hears environmental

Table 8-4.
Results of Standard Tuning
Fork Tests

Hearing	Rinne's Test (AC and BC)	Weber's Test (BC only)	Schwabach's Test (BC only)
Normal	Positive Rinne (AC > BC)	Sound heard in midline of head—right ear hears same as left ear	Client's ear hears as long as examiner's ear
Conductive hearing loss	Negative Rinne (AC < BC; BC > AC)	BC referred to ear with conductive loss	Client hears longer than examiner
Sensorineural hearing loss	Positive Rinne (AC > BC)—both reduced in length False negative—BC only heard*	BC referred to normal ear	Examiner hears longer than client

*BC actually heard by ear not tested—see text.

Figure 8-2.
Weber test. *A.* Tuning fork
is placed at the midline of
the skull. *B.* Tuning fork is
placed on the maxillary
incisors.

noises that the impaired ear does not hear. (See Ballantyne [2] for a more extensive discussion of this phenomenon.)

If there is sensorineural loss in one ear with the other ear normal, the sound is heard louder in the normal ear. With normal hearing the sound is not lateralized (i.e., to the right or left ear), but is heard equally by both ears (as if in the midline). The nurse should indicate on the record the ear to which the sound is lateralized (see Table 8-4). Figure 8-3 summarizes the tuning fork positions for the Weber and Rinne tests.

The Schwabach test (bone conduction only) is a comparison of the client's and the examiner's bone conduction. The vibrating tuning fork is placed alternately on the client's mastoid process and on the examiner's mastoid process. When either stops hearing the tone, the number of seconds that elapse before

Figure 8-3.
Weber and Rinne tests. *A.*
Weber test on forehead or
maxillary incisors. *B.* Rinne
test on mastoid bone, and
C. beside external ear.

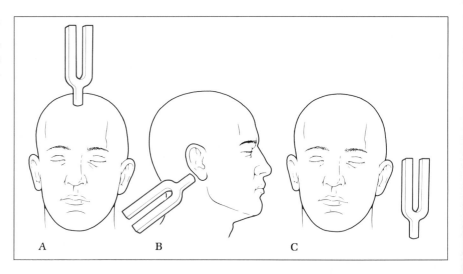

the tone can no longer be heard by the other person is recorded. The tone is not heard as long by the person with sensorineural loss as by the examiner. This test assumes recent testing of the examiner and normal hearing. The tone is heard longer by the client with a conductive hearing loss (provided the examiner's hearing is normal), which masks the environmental noises so that she hears the tone longer than the examiner (Table 8-4).

EXAMINATION OF THE EXTERNAL EAR

The physical assessment of the ear begins with the examination of the auricle. The size and shape are noted, and the auricle (pinna) is inspected for lesions or abnormal growths (Fig. 8-4). Figure 8-5A presents a drawing of the auricle and the names given to its various areas. These names can be used to identify and describe the location of a lesion. The outer edge, the helix, extends from the crus of the helix to the lobule. Note the anthelix, concha, and tragus. With swelling of the auricle or trauma these areas may not be clearly differentiated.

Movement of the auricle is normally not painful if the nurse examiner moves it gently. Pain on movement of the auricle or tragus is usually associated with abnormality, particularly with external otitis (otitis externa) or parotiditis.

Clients with deformities of the auricle such as macrotia (abnormal enlargement) or lop ears (projecting auricle) may be referred to a plastic surgeon if the cosmetic aspect is creating a problem and corrective surgery is desired. Gnarled, thickened cauliflower ears are indicative of repeated trauma. Persons with hematomas of the auricle and damage to the external structures should be referred to a physician for immediate care. Sebaceous cysts, nodules, and nonhealing sores may be seen on the auricle also, and these should be evaluated for medical diagnosis and treatment.

The mastoid process should be routinely examined and the area palpated for irregularities and tenderness.

Figure 8-4. Assessment of the ear begins with careful inspection of the auricle and external auditory meatus. (Reproduced with permission from R. D. Judge, G. D. Zuidema, and F. Fitzgerald (Eds.). *Methods of Clinical Examination* (4th ed.). Boston: Little, Brown, 1982.

Figure 8-5.
A. External ear. *B.* External
auditory meatus.

Helix

Auricular tubercle

Concha

External auditory meatus

Antihelix

Tragus

Antitragus

Lobe

A

Conductive hearing loss

Sensorineural hearing loss

External ear

Inner ear

Middle ear

Auricle

External
auditory
meatus

Semicircular canals

Cochlear
nerve

Auditory
- (8th cranial)
nerve

Ear canal

Cochlea

Cartilaginous
part of ear
canal

Cartilage

Mastoid process

Ossicles

Isthmus

Tympanic membrane

Bony part of ear canal

B

The external auditory meatus should be examined carefully noting the size of the opening, the presence of swelling, redness, discharge, cerumen, or any visible lesions (Figs. 8-5A, 8-5B). The external auditory meatus may be completely occluded by tumor or, as in external otitis, by swelling. It is important during history taking to determine whether the tumor is in fact a foreign body. With external otitis the swelling may extend to the tragus and auricle. This is very painful and the client may resist any examination of the ear. Systemic antibiotics are required and referral to a physician is necessary.

Loss of touch and pain sensation in the external auditory canal indicates functional alteration of the afferent glossopharyngeal (IX) and vagus (X) cranial nerves [5].

OTOSCOPIC EXAMINATION

After thorough examination of the auricle, mastoid, and external auditory meatus, the external auditory canal and tympanic membrane are then examined with an otoscope. The use of a head mirror and an appropriately sized aural speculum provides a better view of the ear and allows the examiner a free hand for instrumentation. This technique takes time and practice to learn to use safely and effectively. For most examinations the otoscope is used and provides excellent visualization. A pneumatic device consisting of a bulb and tube, attached to the otoscope, permits manipulation of the tympanic membrane. The largest-size speculum the ear will accommodate comfortably should be used on the otoscope for best visualization and to create a seal with the external canal for the use of the pneumatic device. *Slight* pressure on the pneumatic bulb causes the tympanic membrane to move, since the normal tympanic membrane is sensitive to slight changes of pressure. The use of the pneumatic bulb requires care and expertise and is described here, although it may not be within the general practice of the beginning nurse examiner (Fig.8-6).

As the otoscope is introduced into the external canal, the nurse must be very

Figure 8-6. Position of otoscope for examining right ear. Otoscope is inverted and held in right hand of examiner. Left thumb and index finger are retracting the pinna of ear upward and backward; and pneumatic bulb is held in left hand. Client (seen) and nurse are comfortably seated.

gentle, as the epithelial lining of the canal is extremely sensitive. Any pressure against the wall of the canal may be painful, and the tissue may be traumatized and bleed easily (Fig. 8-5B). The external auditory canal has only a thin epithelial lining over bone just inside the meatus and is easily traumatized (Fig. 8-5B). The otoscope should be held upside down, so that the hand holding it can be steadied against the client's head. This prevents the nurse from creating a lever-type movement against the canal with the tip of the speculum. If the person moves his head, the nurse's hand and otoscope move with it, preventing trauma and discomfort. The client should be instructed to indicate to the nurse any discomfort experienced during the examination. To facilitate the otoscope examination of adults, both client and nurse should be seated comfortably.

The small child or infant should be placed prone on an examining table with arms beside his body and head turned first to one side and then to the other for the otoscopic examination. The nurse can position her body over the child's and stabilize the child's head both with the left hand pulling the pinna (lower helix) back and with the right hand holding the otoscope or vice versa when examining the left ear (Figs. 8-7 and 15-5).

When examining the client's right ear, the otoscope should be held in the examiner's right hand and the auricle retracted with the left hand. When the left ear is examined, the otoscope is held in the left hand and the auricle retracted by the right hand. The pneumatic bulb is manipulated by the hand that is retracting the auricle.

The external canal may need to be cleaned if cerumen is excessive or if

Figure 8-7.
Positioning for otoscopic
examination of a child.

drainage is obscuring a suspected lesion. Determination of the intactness of the tympanic membrane must be made before any solution is instilled and can be made in two ways: first, by asking the client to create pressure to move the tympanic membrane by swallowing, or to equalize the pressure by yawning (the client can feel the change of pressure as this is done); second, by placing the otoscope into the external ear and gently squeezing the pneumatic bulb to create the feeling of pressure on the tympanic membrane. Solution *should not* be instilled if a ruptured tympanic membrane is suspected; rather, the client should be referred to an otologist without delay. If the tympanic membrane is intact, enough hydrogen peroxide (3 percent) *warmed* to body temperature is instilled to fill the canal. After instillation, the client should lie on the opposite side for 5 to 10 minutes while the cerumen softens. The ear is then irrigated with tap water *warmed* to body temperature. Either an ear bulb, an asepto syringe, or water pic can be used to irrigate. The force of the stream does not damage the tympanic membrane as long as water is allowed to escape via space around the syringe or bulb tip. The canal can then be dried with rolled tissue.

Once the canal is clean, or if the canal did not require cleaning, the otoscope can be introduced slowly while the nurse examines the canal. The scope is introduced by pointing it forward and upward. The color of the epithelial lining is noted. The "just cleaned" canal has a reddened epithelial lining. Persons who use Q-tips for periodic cleaning may have little or no cerumen and have a slightly reddened epithelial lining with a frequently reddened annulus. Q-tip cleansing may push wax back against the tympanic membrane. Any lesions, tumors, polyps, hematomas, exostoses, or chondromas (small, broad-based, cartilaginous lumps) observed are to be described in the record. Foreign bodies or insects in the ear may be seen in children. Drops of mineral or olive oil should be instilled to immobilize the insects if alive and facilitate their removal by irrigation. Any client with a foreign body in the ear requiring manipulation or instrumentation for its removal needs the immediate attention of a physician.

To visualize the tympanic membrane, the pinna is pulled backward and upward (in the child, only backward) to straighten the canal. It may be necessary to place the knuckles of the hand retracting the auricle against the mastoid process to get enough traction to straighten the canal. As a person ages the canal becomes more tortuous. In the presence of otitis externa this manipulation may be too painful.

The normal eardrum appears translucent or pearly gray. Landmarks to guide the nurse in her examination are seen in Figure 8-8. The tympanic membrane is on an inclined plane, which creates the light reflex anteroinferiorly from the umbo. The umbo is visualized in the center of the membrane, behind which is the lower end of the malleus. Ascending from the umbo, first is the manubrium (long process or handle) of the malleus and then its short process, which stands out like a tiny knob. Directly upward and outward from the short

Figure 8-8.
Landmarks of the tympanic
membrane, right ear. (See
discussion in text.)

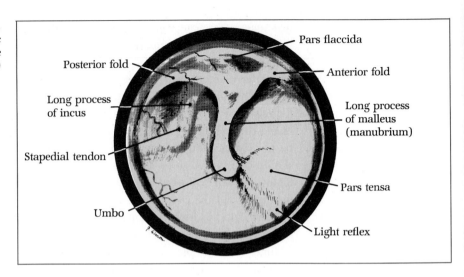

process of the malleus are the anterior and posterior malleolar folds of the tympanic membrane.

The pars tensa is the area of the tympanic membrane, which has a fibrous middle layer; the pars flaccida, above the anterior and posterior fold, does not. Through some eardrums the long process of the incus and the chorda tympani nerve may be seen posterior superiorly behind the malleus and high across the eardrum. The annulus is the thickened ring around the periphery of the tympanic membrane.

Vascularization of the eardrum varies significantly among individuals and is seen mainly along the manubrium, malleolar folds, and annulus. Injection of these vessels is abnormal. It may also be present after irrigation to cleanse the canal, or if daily self-cleaning measures are used by the client. Intense injection is seen with external otitis.

After clear identification of the landmarks, the nurse should gently squeeze the pneumatic bulb to cause movement of the tympanic membrane. If there is a good seal between the otoscope and the ear, gentle repeated squeezing of the bulb should move the membrane. Membrane movement is frequently best seen by watching the light reflex or pars flaccida. The inability to move the tympanic membrane (or the movement of air bubbles behind it) when the pneumatic bulb is used, along with evidence of retraction, or an amber color of the tympanic membrane, or both, may be signs of serous otitis media. Alterations of the color, position, and integrity of the tympanic membrane often reflect the presence of diseases of the middle ear. Clients with these alterations require referral to a physician.

The position of the eardrum may be altered in several ways. Retraction creates prominence of the landmarks. In a client in a sitting position, a fluid level or movement of air bubbles may be seen behind the eardrum. Bulging of the eardrum may occur from pressure within the middle ear. Then landmarks are faint or totally obscured. This is usually seen with purulent otitis media. With a cholesteatoma (extensive cystic mass associated with chronic middle ear infection) some bulging may occur, and the tympanic membrane may appear white.

The color and characteristics of the tympanic membrane vary with many disease processes. With acute external otitis it is injected and thickened and leathery [4]. Healed perforations may be present as flaccid areas that move more readily than the normal tympanic membrane on pneumatic stimulation. This results when the fibrous layer of the tympanic membrane fails to close after perforation. Dead white or ashen gray flecks or dense plaques may develop on the tympanic membrane as a result of cartilaginous deposits after inflammatory disease or after perforation. Blueness of the eardrum indicates bleeding into the tympanic membrane (ecchymosis) and may result from barotrauma (e.g., from too rapid descent during air travel).

Integrity of the eardrum may be altered by perforation, tearing, or surgical incision (myringotomy). Perforation is usually the result of purulent otitis media. Tears may result from concussion (explosions or hard slap on the ear), skull fracture, or the placement in the ear of any object that cuts or tears the membrane. Myringotomy is usually done posteriorly and inferiorly as a therapeutic measure to facilitate drainage of the middle ear.

The epithelial cells on the surface of the tympanic membrane move outward toward the annulus and into the auditory canal (epithelial migration) as opposed to the usual flaking off of dead epithelial tissue. This process takes approximately 30 days or more. Markings on the tympanic membrane thus appear to move outward and remain on the membrane or epithelial lining of the canal for at least 30 days. Because of this movement, the nurse working with a client who has had a previous pathologic condition of the tympanic membrane should draw a sketch of any markings on the eardrum for later reference. The lesions may appear not to have healed or to be just remaining there. With a diagram providing base line data the nurse can observe and record more accurately the progression of the healed or scabbed area.

TINNITUS Tinnitus is the name given to a sensation of sound in one or both ears, and it is a very common accompaniment to deafness [2]. The symptom of tinnitus, despite research efforts to date, is little understood and there is little known relief for it. Several facts are known however:

1. When tinnitus is present, there is nearly always some hearing loss.
2. We all experience head noise.
3. The pitch of a subjective tinnitus nearly always coincides with the frequency of the maximal hearing loss [2].
4. Tinnitus can usually be abolished by ambient noise.

5. Tinnitus often can be reduced or abolished by the restoration of normal or near normal hearing [2].

Tinnitus may be termed subjective (client experienced) or objective (heard by examiner as well as client) [2,4]. Tinnitus may be the first symptom associated with an acoustic neuroma, and further testing should be done of all clients who have this symptom. Ototoxicity, acoustic trauma, hypertension (rarely), and early Menieres disease also are known to cause tinnitus.

VESTIBULAR TESTING   In an examination of the ear, vestibular function must also be tested. The vestibular portion of the auditory (VIII) cranial nerve furnishes afferent fibers, ultimately influencing the coordination of the neck, eyes, and body necessary for maintaining equilibrium in relation to movement of the head and to posture [4]. Vestibular disorders are commonly characterized by objective, rotary vertigo and nonrotary hallucinations of movement, as well as by subjective swaying sensations. Symptoms of "lightheadedness, swimming sensations, faintness, and fear of falling" are not included under the term of vertigo [12].

When taking a history it is important to remember that the two most common causes of vertigo in Europe and North America are Menieres disorder and intermittent vertebrobasilar arterial insufficiency. The former is associated with unilateral sensorineural hearing loss, the latter with intermittent symptoms referable to the area of the brain supplied by this artery, e.g., diplopia, dysphagia, clouding of vision [12]. The history of all clients with vertigo is of the utmost importance. Divers, submariners, and flyers may suffer this as an occupational disorder. It may occur with hyperventilation or high blood pressure [12]. Auditory function adds clues to the vestibular examination.

Labyrinthine tests aim at the production of the aforementioned signs resulting from labyrinthine excitation. The tests stimulate the labyrinth in a controlled manner so that the reactions can be studied [6].

Past pointing is one measurement of labyrinth function. Past pointing occurs in the direction of the flow of the endolymphatic fluid in the labyrinth. The client should sit with eyes closed and two index fingers and arms extended in front of her. The nurse sits opposite the client and places her fingers on the client's fingers. The client is told to raise both hands and arms and then lower them to touch the nurse's fingers. The person with normal labyrinth function can do this, whereas the fingers of a person with abnormal labyrinth function deviate to the right or left of the nurse's fingers.

The functional vestibular test for falling can also be done. The client is requested to walk a straight line with feet tandem or to maintain an upright position with heels together (Romberg sign). A staggering, wide-based gait and excessive swaying motion or falling are abnormal [1]. This test should be done first with eyes open and then with eyes closed (Fig. 8-9). Be aware that the client may fall, and safeguard against this. The swaying motion of the client

Figure 8-9. Functional vestibular test for falling (Romberg sign). *A.* Feet together, eyes opened. *B.* Feet together, eyes closed. *C.* Feet placed tandem, eyes open. *D.* Feet placed tandem, eyes closed. (Photographs courtesy of Jerry Northern.)

A

B

C

D

when she stands with heels together eyes open is compared with that which occurs when her eyes are closed. Accentuation of swaying or loss of balance with eyes closed is a positive Romberg [5].

Another test is for nystagmus. Vestibular nystagmus is produced by disturbances of the labyrinth and sometimes by disturbances of the central nervous system. It should be distinguished from normal eye movements and from ocular nystagmus (in each of the above, both excursions of the eye are of equal amplitude) [4]. Vestibular nystagmus is a slow movement of the eyes in one direction until they reach a limit, followed by a rapid compensatory movement in the opposite direction. The movements are rhythmic. Vestibular nystagmus indicates presence of a disease process except when it occurs on extreme lateral gaze.

If the history given by the client suggests that movement of the head or body in a particular direction is associated with vertigo, then positional tests should be carried out. The client is first asked to sit erect on the examination table, then asked to lie flat with his head turned to the right and while in this position his eyes are observed for the presence of nystagmus. The nystagmus is observed until it decays (slows and then stops). The client is then asked to sit upright in the original position and again is observed for nystagmus. The test is repeated after a short rest with the client's head in left position and finally in the head-extended position. With each change of position the nurse observes the eyes for nystagmus. Any nystagmus detected is described according to its latent period, direction, duration, and fatigue ability [6]. Positional nystagmus may occur as a benign peripheral disorder in which case it is fatiguable and reversible [6]. Sometimes it is found associated with certain serious lesions of the brain stem and cerebellum, although with different nonfatiguing characteristics [6].

Nystagmus may be induced by use of the caloric test and the electro-nystagmogram. In the caloric test, either cold or hot water is used to douche the external auditory canal. Measurement of the resulting nystagmus gives important information on the location of the disease process. The electro-nystagmogram (ENG) is a refinement of the caloric test. Leads are placed around the eyes to record graphically the movements of the eye. These tests are usually done by nurses in the otologist's office or clinic.

The facial nerve (cranial nerve VII) passes through the posterior part of the middle ear and is enclosed in a bony canal (facial, or fallopian, canal). Chronic mastoiditis, skull fracture with damage to the middle ear, and trauma during middle ear surgery may result in temporary or permanent facial paralysis. The chorda tympani nerve (branch of the facial) passes immediately behind the tympanic membrane and is distributed to the taste receptors (sweet, salt, and sour) in the anterior two-thirds of the tongue. Chronic infection of the mastoid or middle ear surgery may cause temporary or permanent loss or decreased taste.

Nurses today are often called on to appraise the client's hearing and determine the presence or absence of many common ear problems. The data obtained from the examination guide the nurse in making responsible decisions regarding the care and counsel she can provide the client or the need for referral for medical evaluation and therapy.

The nurse's role in the appraisal of the ear is to determine its functional status. If any abnormalities are identified, the client must be referred to a physician, particularly to an otologist if one is available. The nurse should also refer persons with hearing loss to audiologists for further evaluation and as appropriate to centers and local agencies where classes in lipreading and correct use of hearing aids are offered.*

THE EAR-ASSESSMENT GUIDE

A. History
  1. Past problems and resolutions
  2. Hearing impairment—family, childhood, present
  3. Recent changes, stuffiness in ears
  4. Otalgia
  5. Chills and fever
  6. Drainage, odor
  7. Medication history, environmental noise history
  8. Tinnitus
  9. Vertigo
B. Hearing Acuity
  1. Conversational
    a. Sensitivity
    b. Speech discrimination
  2. Tuning fork tests
    a. Rinne
    b. Weber
    c. Schwabach
C. External Examination
  1. Auricle
  2. Tragus
  3. External auditory meatus
D. Otoscopic Examination
  1. External Auditory Canal
    a. Cerumen
    b. Tumors
    c. Epithelial lining
  2. Tympanic membrane
    a. Landmarks, prominence
    b. Color
    c. Movement
E. Vestibular Testing
  1. Past pointing
  2. Falling—Romberg sign
  3. Nystagmus

*Information on these classes can be obtained from the National Association of Hearing and Speech Agencies, 919 185th Street, N.W., Washington D.C., 20006.

REFERENCES

1. Adams, G. L., Boies, L. R., and Paparella, M. M. *Boies's Fundamentals of Otolaryngology* (5th ed.). Philadelphia: Saunders, 1978.
2. Ballantyne, J. D. *Deafness* (3rd ed.). New York: Churchill Livingstone, 1977.
3. Boles, R. Hearing test without an Audiometer. *University of Michigan Medical Center Journal* 37:156, 1971.
4. DeWeese, D. D., and Saunders, W. H. *Textbook of Otolaryngology* (5th ed.). St. Louis: Mosby, 1977.
5. Gatz, A. J. *Manter's Essentials of Clinical Neuroanatomy and Neurophysiology* (5th ed.). Philadelphia: Davis, 1975.
6. Hall, I. S., and Colman, B. H. *Diseases of the Nose, Throat and Ear.* New York: Churchill Livingstone 1975.
7. Konizsmark, B. W., and Gorlin, R. J. *Genetic and Metabolic Deafness.* Philadelphia: Saunders, 1976.
8. Miller, B. F., and Keane, C. B. *Encyclopedia and Dictionary of Medicine and Nursing* (2nd ed.). Philadelphia: Saunders, 1978.
9. Montgomery, W. W. Ears, Nose and Throat. In R. D. Judge and G. D. Zuidema (Eds.), *Methods of Clinical Examination: A Physiological Approach* (3rd ed.). Boston: Little, Brown, 1974.
10. Ransome, J. Secretory Otitis Media. In J. Ransome, H. Holden, and T. R. Bull (Eds.), *Recent Advances in Otolaryngology* (No. 4). London: Churchill Livingstone, 1973.
11. Ballantyne, J. D. Ototoxicity. In J. Ransome, H. Holden, T. R. Bull (Eds.), *Recent Advances in Otolaryngology* (No. 4). London: Churchill Livingstone, 1973.
12. Hinchcliffe, R. Investigation of Vertigo. In J. Ransome, H. Holden, T. R. Bull (Eds.), *Recent Advances in Otolaryngology* (No. 4). London: Churchill Livingstone, 1973.

9. Physical Assessment of Respiratory System Function

GLOSSARY

asthma Intermittent airway obstruction of small bronchioles, produced by bronchial secretions, mucosal edema, and bronchospasm; increased sensitivity to histamine and/or inhaled allergens.

atelectasis Incomplete expansion of the lung; a nonspecific term referring to partial or complete airlessness or reduction in lung volume, or both, with or without locally obstructed bronchi.

breath sounds Vibrations produced by movement of the bronchotracheal air column that may be perceived as sounds on auscultation.

bronchiectasis Chronic disease marked by dilatation of the bronchi or bronchioles and chronic suppuration.

bronchitis Acute or chronic inflammation of bronchial tubes.

collapse Reduction in lung volume, acute or chronic, due to any cause.

compression Mechanical reduction in lung volume by pressure.

congestion Excessive accumulation of blood in a part of the body. *pulmonary congestion* Excessive blood in the lungs.

consolidation Diffuse replacement of a large zone of pulmonary parenchyma with liquid and solid products of inflammation when the associated bronchus is patent.

crepitation Crackling; specifically, noise produced by pressure on subcutaneous tissue containing an abnormal amount of gas or air.

crepitant rale Rale of crackling quality, usually moist.

cyanosis Bluish coloration of the skin and mucous membranes due to severe insufficient oxygenation of the arterial blood.

emphysema Abnormal presence of, or increase in, air content. Most commonly, a disease associated with chronic bronchitis characterized by diffuse bronchial obstruction and breathlessness. *subcutaneous e.* Air or other gas in subcutaneous tissues.

empyema Accumulation of pus in the pleural cavity.

epistaxis Hemorrhage from the nose.

fremitus Palpable vibration. *friction f.* Vibrations due to friction rubs. *rhonchal f.* Vibrations due to passage of air through bronchial tubes filled with secretions. *tactile f.* Voice sound vibrations felt when applying hand to thorax; also called *vocal f.*

hemoptysis Expectoration of blood by coughing.

oropharynx Part of pharynx directly behind the oral cavity, extending from the inferior border of the soft palate to the lingual surface of the epiglottis.

paroxysmal Recurring suddenly or with suddenly increasing intensity.

pleural effusion Presence of fluid in the pleural space; the term includes bloody fluid (hemothorax), purulent fluid (empyema), and chylous fluid (chylothorax), which require thoracentesis for specific identification.

pneumonia Inflammation of the lungs due to infection.

pneumonitis Condition of localized acute inflammation of the lung without gross toxemia.

pneumothorax Accumulation of air or gas in the pleural cavity.

rhinorrhea Nasal discharge.

stridor Harsh, high-pitched crowing sounds during respiration.

suppuration Formation of pus.

voice sounds Vibrations of the spoken voice transmitted through the lungs and appreciated by auscultation; also called voice resonance and, rarely, vocal fremitus.

THE ability to perform a complete respiratory system assessment is a nursing skill that is crucial in the care of any person. The nurse encounters those with *acute* respiratory problems in the hospital, in clinics, or in their homes. She needs to use physical assessment skills to monitor their status and to detect the rapid changes that often occur. The incidence of *chronic* respiratory disease in our population continues to rise. These persons can be helped to maintain their alteration in the non-acute state, and to reach their optimal level of functioning. The nurse skilled in physical assessment can also help a client who is primarily worried about a respiratory symptom. She can sort out those symptoms that fall within the range of normal for that person and those that represent possible alterations.

Tools needed for the respiratory system assessment include a penlight, tongue blade, hand mirror, and stethoscope. The most important tool, however, is careful thought during the examination. The nurse must continuously be processing each bit of information, and comparing it to her knowledge base. She must attempt to synthesize a picture of physiologic interaction—adding pieces to the puzzle through each step of the examination—and at the same time being careful not to reach a conclusion until the examination is complete. Finally, the nurse must realize that her efforts will be fruitful only if she uses her physical assessment data in other components of the nursing process—in creating care plans, in making decisions about implementing her plans, and later, in obtaining more data to use in evaluating her plan.

GENERAL APPEARANCE

Posture provides many clues to respiratory system function. Clients with obstructive lung disease have an easily recognized posture, assumed in an effort to expand the thoracic cage and use all available thoracic space. Characteristically, the client is sitting, leaning forward, and attempting to prop his clavicles by placing his hands on his knees, or his elbows on the arms of a chair as seen in Figure 9-1. The sternocleidomastoid muscles, used as accessory muscles of respiration, are often prominent.

General color and facial expression are also indications of respiratory difficulty. A dusky or bluish coloration may be present, especially on the lips, and the cheeks may be ruddy. The facial expression is often drawn, because of exertion, and anxious, due to a feeling of air hunger. The client may be able to say only a few sentences before having to stop to catch his breath. Noting the number of words the client can say before having to gasp for breath is a useful measure for making future comparisons of the degree of respiratory distress.

Neurologic status is an important parameter to note and monitor, because changes in the alertness and personality of the client may reflect cerebral sensitivity to changes in oxygen, carbon dioxide, and hydrogen ion levels. As pulmonary decompensation and hypoxia progress, the neurologic picture changes from anxiety and restlessness to irritability, to drowsiness, and finally to coma.

Figure 9-1.
General appearance of
person with chronic
respiratory disease.
(©Copyright 1968 CIBA
Pharmaceutical Company,
Division of CIBA-GEIGY
Corporation. Reprinted with
permission from CLINICAL
SYMPOSIA, illustrated by
Frank H. Netter, M. D. All
rights reserved.)

Specific Findings   *Cyanosis*

Cyanosis is the blue color caused by an increased amount of reduced hemoglobin in the superficial capillaries. Cyanosis is often hard to detect in persons with dark skin, because their pigmentation either masks or mimics the cyanosis; it is therefore best detected in the nail beds of a darkly pigmented person, or under the tongue or inside the cheek. Cyanosis is also difficult to detect in the person who is anemic, since there is less hemoglobin, either oxygenated or reduced, to impart color to the skin. For this reason, a severely anemic person can die of hypoxia without becoming cyanotic. On the other hand, a client with polycythemia may appear more cyanotic than one with a normal hematocrit, but with the same arterial oxygen tension. This is because of the polycythemic client's inability to fully oxygenate the abnormally large mass of red blood cells, and usually does not represent inadequate oxygen delivery to the tissues. In this circumstance the presence of cyanosis cannot be given the same significance as cyanosis in a nonpolycythemic person (Fig. 9-2).

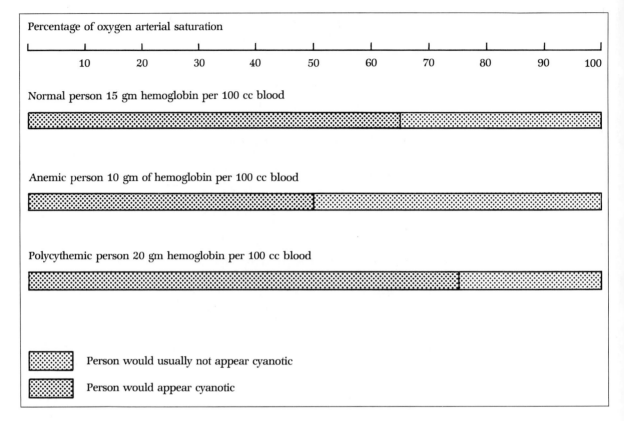

Percentage of oxygen arterial saturation

10   20   30   40   50   60   70   80   90   100

Normal person 15 gm hemoglobin per 100 cc blood

Anemic person 10 gm of hemoglobin per 100 cc blood

Polycythemic person 20 gm hemoglobin per 100 cc blood

Person would usually not appear cyanotic

Person would appear cyanotic

Figure 9-2.
Relationship of total body hemoglobin to appearance of cyanosis. Note that the normal person begins to appear cyanotic at an arterial oxygen saturation of about 65 percent. However, an anemic person (Hgb of 10 gm.) does not appear cyanotic until his arterial saturation drops to about 50 percent, while the polycythemic person appears cyanotic at a relatively high arterial saturation level (about 75 percent).

Cyanosis is a nonspecific sign, resulting from a number of cardiac and pulmonary problems. In a client with chronic obstructive pulmonary disease cyanosis is often of little help in assessing respiratory function because it appears so late—when the arterial P_{O_2} is 45 mm Hg or less (80 to 100 mm Hg is normal). However, any change—either the sudden onset of cyanosis or variance in its degree—is a sure indication of some important physiologic change.

Clubbing of Fingers

The condition of the fingers may be more reliable than cyanosis as an indicator of chronic hypoxia. Clubbing of the fingers is caused by a chronic decrease in the oxygen saturation of the blood supplying this area. This results in a bulbous enlargement of the tip of the finger, with convex overhanging of the nail and loss of the obtuse angle at the nail bed (see Fig. 10-13). A coarse vertical ridging in the fingernails may also reveal chronic pulmonary insufficiency.

Another sign the nurse may detect when observing the nails is their tendency to become periodically flushed and then return to their original color. This is evidence of excess blood supply, or hyperemia. As the carbon dioxide builds up in the capillaries, the arteries dilate, and the blood rushes through the area.

When more oxygen has been supplied to the area, the arteries return to their normal size and blood flow becomes normal.

Cough

The nurse needs to observe a client's cough for frequency, production or non-production of sputum, time of day during which it occurs, and changes with body position. The character of the cough can be described as hacking (frequent coughing, though not severe), paroxysmal (a sudden prolonged episode of forceful coughing), explosive, or brassy (harsh, unproductive, with a strident quality). In addition, the nurse should observe what measures the client uses to relieve the cough and their effectiveness.

Sputum Production

The nurse may want to ask the client to save his sputum to assist her in assessing it. Important characteristics of the sputum are its color, odor, consistency, and volume. Mucoid sputum, or sputum that is grayish-white, translucent, odorless, and slimy, is often seen with bronchitis. Purulent sputum may be green, yellow, or brown and often has a distinctive odor. Foul-smelling sputum is present with lung abscess, bronchiectasis, and other types of necrotizing infections, which also give the breath an offensive odor. The volume of sputum may range from a few teaspoons expectorated on arising to more than a pint daily. In acute pulmonary edema, the sputum is frothy and either white or pink.

Hemoptysis is often a serious sign that may occur in the course of pneumonia, tuberculosis, or cancer. Any description of hemoptysis must include the amount and color of the blood for the recording to be meaningful. The amount of blood may range from small streaks on the surface of the sputum to the red, frothy sputum seen with copious bleeding. The color should be described as bright or dark, since the brighter the blood, the fresher the bleeding. The presence of clots or pus should be noted. The nurse should try to estimate the amount of blood expectorated within a given period of time. Clients may or may not be helpful in providing this information because they are usually frightened and prone to overestimate the amount of blood. In this situation, it may be especially helpful to ask the client to save *all* of the sputum.

NOSE AND PARANASAL SINUSES
Technique of Examination

Following the cephalocaudal approach to physical assessment, a description of the respiratory system will begin with the nose and the paranasal sinuses.

First, inspect the contour of the external nose for asymmetry, and then palpate for any loss of structure or support. Test the patency of each nostril by occluding the other with digital compression while the client inhales with his mouth closed.

Position the client's head to examine the interior nose by placing the palm of one hand on his upper forehead, and then gently lift the bulbous portion of the

Figure 9-3.
Technique for examining
the interior of the nose and
septum with a penlight.

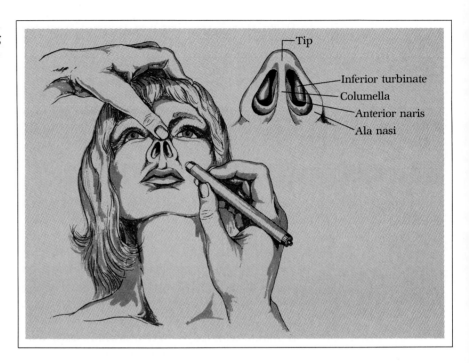

nose with the thumb, so that the interior can be seen. Holding a penlight in your other hand, examine the condition of the skin and the mucosa on the interior of the nose and the adequacy of each airway (Fig. 9-3).

Observe the septum for deviation and then perforation by shining a penlight into one naris and viewing the transilluminated septum through the open naris. The septal surface of the nasal chamber is normally planar and smooth. The lateral wall of the chamber, however, is made irregular by three projections, the superior, middle, and inferior *turbinates* (Fig. 9-4). In looking through the anterior chamber you will probably see the anterior two-thirds of the inferior turbinate and the anterior half of the middle turbinate; the superior turbinate is rarely visible.

The paranasal sinuses cannot be seen and therefore are indirectly examined by palpation. Palpate the frontal sinuses by pressing upward just below and behind the eyebrows. To detect tenderness of the maxillary sinuses, palpate along the ascending process of the maxilla and the canine fossa (Fig. 9-4). Placing pressure simultaneously on both sides often is more effective in demonstrating differences in tenderness.

Findings   The exterior nose may reveal chronic nasal obstruction and resultant mouth breathing, producing narrowing of the nose, described as adenoid facies. Tu-

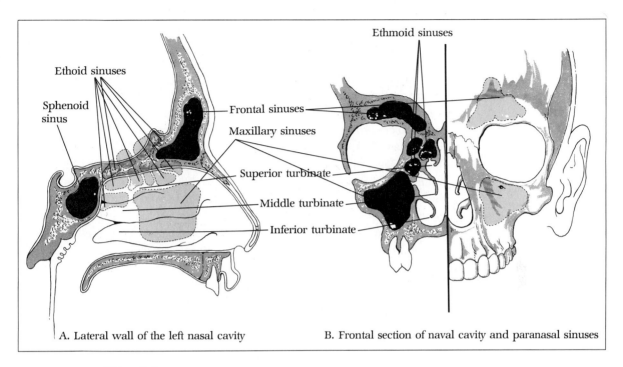

Ethoid sinuses

Sphenoid sinus

Ethmoid sinuses

Frontal sinuses

Maxillary sinuses

Superior turbinate

Middle turbinate

Inferior turbinate

A. Lateral wall of the left nasal cavity

B. Frontal section of naval cavity and paranasal sinuses

Figure 9-4.
The nasal cavity. *A.* Interior structures. *B.* Location of paranasal sinuses.

mors originating within the nose can cause marked deformity of its exterior. With increased respiratory effort, the nares may alternately dilate with inspiration and contract with expiration, in what is called a nasal flare.

Unilateral nasal obstruction may be caused by a foreign body, deviated septum, or neoplasm. An S-shaped deviation of the nasal septum may cause bilateral obstruction. Obstruction of both nares is most commonly due to rhinitis, but may also be due to the presence of nasal polyps.

The anterior chamber, or vestibule, of the naris is normally lined with skin, contains nasal hairs (vibrissae), and is the most common site for furuncles of the nose. The posterior vestibule is covered with nasal mucosa, which can be expected to be redder than oral mucosa. A blanket of mucus covers the entire interior nasal cavity and functions to collect bacteria and debris from inspired air. A nasal allergy produces stuffiness, sneezing, and a watery nasal discharge. The common cold begins with a discharge of clear, watery mucus, indicating the viral etiology; later, the discharge may become thick and purulent, as superimposed bacterial infection occurs. In acute and chronic infection of the paranasal sinuses the discharge is purulent, often viscid, and may tend to flow backward into the nasopharynx, causing a postnasal drip.

Epistaxis may be caused by trauma, but may also be a sign of serious local or generalized disease. A history of its repeated occurrence should always be reported to the physician. Many times the bleeding originates from a vascular network on the anterior nasal septum and is a result of repeated nose picking. Hypertension or polycythemia may also cause epistaxis once the small vessels have become eroded by increased pressure. Often a neoplasm produces a bloody discharge, in contrast to the brisk bleeding of real epistaxis.

In most people the septum is not perfectly straight. Irregularities normally cause no concern unless they are severe enough to interfere with the patency of the airway. Sharp projections, called "ridges" or "spurs," should be recorded. In some cases, the anterior end of the septum may be dislocated and project prominently into one nostril. Crusting often occurs at the site of nasal septum deviation, and evidence of some slight bleeding may also be found there. Perforation of the septum may be of traumatic, surgical, or infectious origin. Perforations commonly found in the anterior septum may be caused by chronic infection coupled with repeated trauma from picking off crusts.

Normally, the nasal turbinates have a deep pink color, similar to the rest of the nasal mucosa. However, with inflammation, the turbinates may become reddened and swell periodically. (This swelling may cause alternating nasal obstruction, which is especially noticeable at night. The individual turns from one side to the other to obtain decongestion of the previously dependent turbinate.) In allergic states the turbinates become pale and bluish and are often swollen or "boggy." When the septum is displaced to one side, the turbinates on the opposite side tend to swell and fill the cavity. *Nasal polyps* are overgrowths of mucosa that frequently may be seen as smooth, round pale masses protruding from between the turbinates.

Tenderness elicited by palpating over a paranasal sinus indicates disease in that area. Moist secretions seen in the interior of the nose or a stream of mucus on the posterior oropharynx may also indicate infection of the paranasal sinuses. Sinus disease often is accompanied by pain in the orbital area, diplopia, or swelling of the eyelids.

OROPHARYNX
Technique of
Examination

This segment of the respiratory system is usually done concurrently with the oral examinations (see Chap. 6), with both the examiner and client seated, facing each other. After inspecting the various parts of the oral cavity, ask the client to say "ah," and use the tongue blade to depress the dorsum of his tongue. As the client is doing this, observe for uvular elevation and coordinated pharyngeal construction. The tongue blade is best placed on the middle third of the tongue. If placed too far anteriorly, the blade causes the posterior part of the tongue to mound up so as to obscure rather than expose the pharynx. Most clients gag if the blade touches the posterior part of their tongue. While using the tongue blade, the nurse should be careful not to press the client's lower lip against his teeth (see Fig. 9-5).

Examine the palatine tonsils and estimate their size. Inspect these tonsils and the anterior and posterior tonsillar pillars for signs of inflammation. Examine

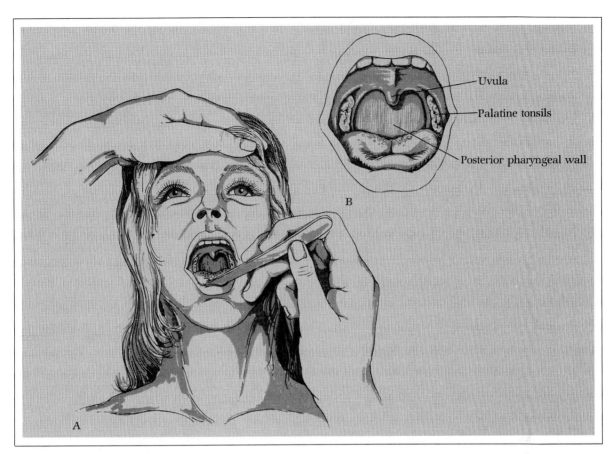

Figure 9-5.
Technique for examining
the *A.*, interior of the
mouth and pharynx with a
tongue blade, and tonsils, *B.*

the lingual tonsils by using a piece of gauze to pull the tongue forward, and looking at them with the hand mirror. Inspect the posterior wall of the oropharynx for color and for the presence of edema, ulceration, and mucopurulent material.

Findings

Uvula

The uvula is normally the same color or slightly pinker than the soft palate and varies greatly in length and thickness. With inflammation of the pharynx or the tonsils, the uvula becomes enlarged and erythematous. This pendulous uvula may fall forward and touch the base of the tongue where the person is lying down, producing an irritating, shallow cough.

Tonsils

The tonsils should be essentially the same color as the oral mucosa. Normally, the palatine, or faucial, tonsils do not project much beyond the tonsilar pillars. The glossopalatine fold, which connects the tongue to the palate, is known as the anterior tonsillar pillar. Behind it lies the posterior tonsillar pillar. It is sometimes helpful to retract the anterior pillar for a better view of the tonsils.

Following tonsillectomy, lymphoid nodules may remain in the tonsillar fossa and leave a tonsillar tag. The anterior and posterior pillars often also reveal evidence of changes occurring with healing following a tonsillectomy.

The surface of the normal tonsil is relatively smooth but contains indentations, or crypts, in which are found desquamated epithelial cells. If these crypts are deep, plugs of epithelial debris may be seen as white spots on the tonsils. A red zone surrounding the plug, however, suggests infection of the crypt.

Large tonsils are not necessarily diseased and may represent an alteration only if they interfere with respiration or swallowing. With acute tonsillitis, the entire tonsil is reddened and edematous, and displays white or yellow dots or streaks of exudate. Infection may also result in abscesses, forming a large grayish patch on the surface of the tonsils. Both malignant and benign tumors may arise from the tonsils. A physician should be asked to evaluate any alteration of the tonsils.

Posterior Pharyngeal Wall

The posterior pharyngeal wall is that part of the oropharynx visible through the open mouth, without using mirrors for examination. Small vessels can normally be seen here and on the soft palate and the tonsillar pillars; they usually do not represent inflammatory changes. Irregular spots of lymphoid tissue, pale pink and elevated, are also normal and frequently seen. Observe the posterior pharyngeal wall for soreness or acute pharyngitis, producing edema, redness, and possibly exudation of the mucosa or bleeding. Rhinitis or infection of the paranasal sinuses may cause a stream of mucopurulent material on the posterior pharyngeal wall.

TRACHEA
Technique of
Examination

With the client's head slightly flexed, the trachea may be palpated with the thumb and the index finger just above the suprasternal notch (Fig. 9-6). If the trachea is deviated, the examiner can easily insert his finger between the trachea and the sternocleidomastoid muscle on one side, but not on the other.

Findings

The trachea normally lies in midline, equidistant from the insertion of each sternocleidomastoid muscle. Deviation of the trachea indicates that the upper part of the mediastinum is displaced to one side. This may be due to various pathologic conditions, but should always be reported to the physician immediately. Aortic aneurysm, enlargement of the thyroid, a mediastinal mass, or gross thoracic asymmetry due to scoliosis may all cause displacement. Pressure produced by pleural effusion or pneumothorax causes deviation of the trachea away from the diseased side, whereas atelectasis pulls the trachea toward the diseased side (Fig. 9-7).

Figure 9-6.
Structures of the neck
identifiable by palpation.
(Reproduced with
permission from R. D.
Judge, G. D. Zuidema, and
F. Fitzgerald (Eds.).
*Methods of Clinical
Examination* (4th ed.).
Boston: Little, Brown,
1982.)

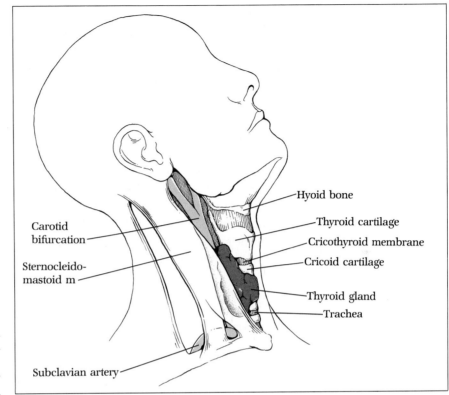

Figure 9-7.
Causes of tracheal
deviation. (Reproduced
with permission from R. D.
Judge, G. D. Zuidema, and
F. Fitzgerald (Eds.).
*Methods of Clinical
Examination* (4th ed.).
Boston: Little, Brown,
1982.)

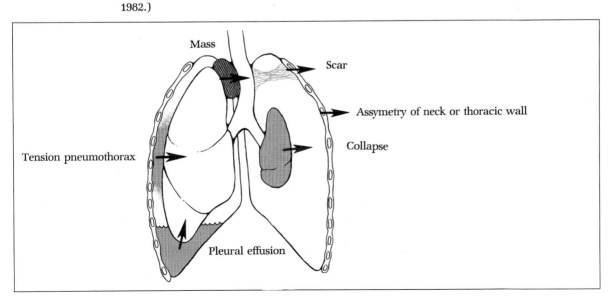

EXAMINATION OF THE THORAX
Landmarks of the Chest

Nurses must become familiar with landmarks of the chest. This information is needed to communicate effectively the exact position of abnormalities detected and to assist in locating and visualizing underlying anatomic structures of the thorax. Landmarks of the chest consist first of a series of imaginary lines and second, of anatomic topographic landmarks, such as bony prominences, ribs, and intercostal spaces.

Anterior Wall of the Chest

The locations of two commonly used vertical lines found on the anterior chest, the midsternal and midclavicular lines, are self-explanatory (Fig. 9-8A). Another important landmark, the sternal angle, or angle of Louis, is also found here (Fig. 9-8B). This is a visible projection of the sternum formed by the articulation of the first and second parts, the manubrium and the body, and is significant for several reasons. It is the location of the second chondrosternal junction and therefore facilitates identification of the second rib and serves as

Figure 9-8. Landmarks of the chest. *A.* Anterior thorax. *B.* Lateral thorax. *C.* Posterior thorax.

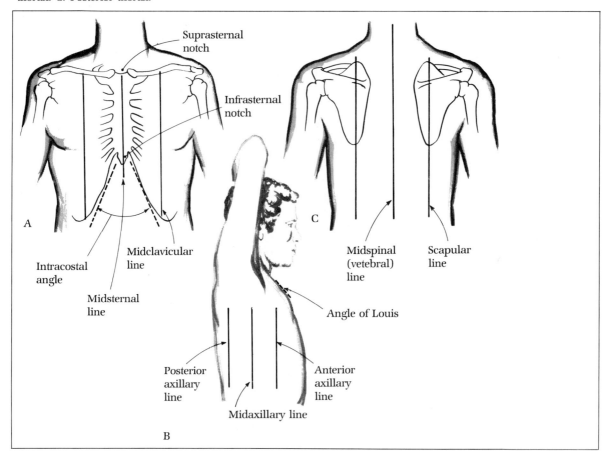

a convenient starting point for counting ribs. The angle of Louis also indicates the point of tracheal bifurcation forming the bronchi. Underneath it is the upper border of the atria of the heart. Finally, the fifth thoracic vertebra is located posteriorly at the same level.

After locating the second rib using the angle of Louis, the examiner should identify the other ribs and the intercostal spaces on the anterior chest. An intercostal space takes it name from the rib directly above it. To count ribs and intercostal spaces, first place the little finger of the left hand on the client's second right intercostal space, next to the sternum. Next, take the ring finger, place it on the third rib, and allow it to fall down into the third intercostal space. Proceed in the same manner with the remaining fingers. The index finger will be in the fifth intercostal space.

Lateral Wall of the Chest
Three commonly used lines are found on the lateral wall of the chest, namely, the anterior, posterior, and midaxillary lines (Fig. 9-8B). The anterior axillary line is a continuation of the anterior axillary fold, running downward along the anterolateral wall of the thorax. It begins at the insertion of the pectoralis major muscle. The posterior axillary line is drawn downward from the origin of the posterior axillary fold, which corresponds to the insertion of the latissimus dorsi muscle. The midaxillary line is midway between the other two and runs directly downward from the apex of the axilla. When the client is in the dorsal recumbent position, the midaxillary line is on the same horizontal plane as the level of the right atrium, and thus is often used as a landmark in measuring central venous pressure.

Care must be taken to see that the client is in the correct position when initially locating these lines. The arm must be abducted directly from the lateral chest, but not more than 90 degrees. It should not extend anteriorly or posteriorly. If the arm is not in the correct position, the relationship of the axilla to the chest wall becomes distorted, and these lines are then improperly located.

Posterior Wall of the Chest
On the posterior wall of the chest are found the midspinal or vertebral line, running down the spinous process of the vertebrae, and the scapular line, which runs parallel to the spine through the inferior angle of the scapula (Fig. 9-8C). The scapular line is considered a somewhat inconsistent reference because of the mobility of the scapula. For this reason it should be located only when the client is erect, with his arms at his sides.

Another landmark of the posterior chest is the vertebra prominens, or the prominent seventh cervical vertebra, found at the base of the neck. It can be used to assist in identifying the thoracic vertebrae and also indicates the highest point of lung tissue posteriorly.

Function of Lines and Landmarks

Lines and landmarks are most useful in communicating the exact position of detected abnormalities. Any alteration can be described as being so many centimeters medial or lateral to a line, or in a specific interspace or interspaces. Findings should be recorded in this manner. Nurses should be able to use these terms with ease, both verbally and in writing, and thus contribute to accurate diagnosis and monitoring of alterations.

Landmarks also assist in the location of anatomic structures that lie within the thorax. Anteriorly, the apices of the lungs extend for approximately $1^{1}/_{2}$ in. (about 4 cm) above the clavicle on each side and inferiorly to the sixth anterior rib or the sixth chondrosternal junction. Posteriorly, the lung superiorly reaches the seventh cervical vertebrae and inferiorly extends to the tenth or twelfth thoracic vertebra.

On the right side, the dome of the diaphragm is situated approximately at the level of the fifth rib at the midclavicular line. Beneath the right diaphragm is the liver, which extends down to the costal margin. The dome of the left part of the diaphragm is normally about an inch lower. It usually extends to the fifth interspace or the sixth rib at the midclavicular line. The stomach, splenic flexure of the colon, and the left kidney lie below the left diaphragm.

A further series of imaginary lines drawn on the chest help in anatomic interpretation of respiratory system findings. These lines, or fissures, delineate surface areas that generally correspond to findings from the upper, middle, and lower lobes of the lung. The actual lobes of the lungs may not be found exactly under those surface areas, but vibrations from them are transmitted to these corresponding areas of skin. The long fissure delimits the lower lobe from the others and extends posteriorly from the fourth thoracic vertebra, obliquely downward, crossing the fifth rib at the midaxilla to the sixth rib anteriorly. The posterior origin of the long fissure is also at the same level as the anterior sternal prominence, the angle of Louis. On the right side, the horizontal fissure separates the upper and middle lobes. It extends from the long fissure in the midaxilla to the third intercostal space anteriorly. Locate these fissures in Figure 9-9, and trace them on a friend or client.

The importance of visualizing the lobes of the lung soon becomes apparent. It is vital that the examiner be aware that findings from the upper lobes are principally located in the anterior chest and that those from the middle lobe are found only in the anterior chest on the right. It is also important to note that the lower lobes correspond to a large portion of the surface area of the posterior chest and that their superior segments extend fairly far upward.

The nurse should employ the anatomic interpretation of her physical assessment data in selecting the most effective nursing care. For example, with all this information in mind, she would plan positioning of the client, select a regimen for postural drainage, plan for other types of breathing exercises, and then later use physical assessment to evaluate the effectiveness of her nursing intervention.

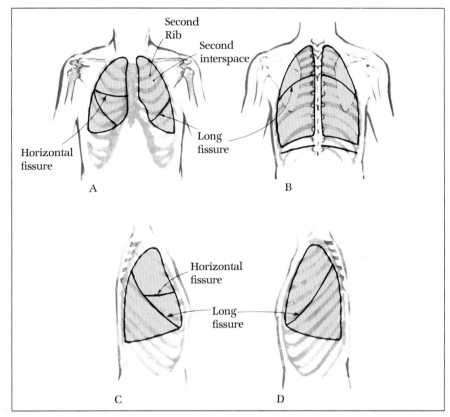

Figure 9-9. Topographic anatomy: location of lobes of the lung. *A.* Anterior thorax. *B.* Posterior thorax. *C.* Right lateral thorax. *D.* Left lateral thorax.

INSPECTION OF THE THORAX

Nurses have been using the tool of inspection extensively for many years and through its use have made valuable contributions to diagnosis and treatment of clients with respiratory alterations. However, nurses are often uncomfortable in just looking at the client without performing some concurrent motor activity. Yet initial inspection is most profitable in yielding valuable information when done by itself, with full concentration on the observation being made, as in Figure 9-10.

General Findings

Normal subjects present a wide range in size and shape of the chest. Posture and dominant use of one side of the body can create slight asymmetry, but general symmetry of the chest and its constituent parts is to be expected. Chest deformities or scars often provide the first clue to the nature of a respiratory difficulty.

The shoulders are usually at the same level, although one may be slightly higher than another. They generally have a convex shape from the neck to their lateral borders. Men usually have prominent clavicles, with depressed supra-clavicular spaces; in women the clavicles are frequently hidden by adipose tissue, and the supraclavicular spaces are full. Beneath the clavicles the chest wall

Figure 9-10.
Examination of the thorax
should begin with careful
inspection of both the
anterior, *A.,* and posterior,
B., thorax. (Reproduced
with permission from R. D.
Judge, G. D. Zuidema, and
F. Fitzgerald (Eds.).
*Methods of Clinical
Examination* (4th ed.).
Boston: Little, Brown,
1982.)

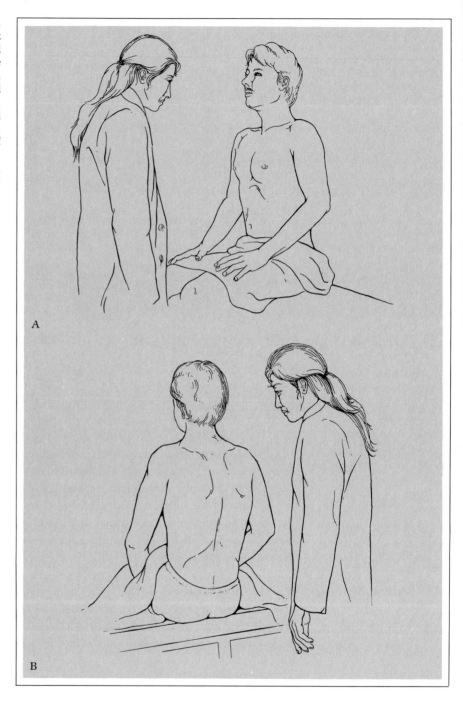

A

B

should be slightly convex and covered by subcutaneous tissue of moderate thickness. The intercostal spaces can be seen as slight depressions beneath the ribs, unless there is considerable adipose tissue. Because of the oblique downward angle of the ribs in traveling from the anterior chest to the posterior chest, the ribs and the intercostal spaces are highest posteriorly, lower laterally, and lowest anteriorly. Since the ribs have also progressively greater oblique angulation from top to bottom, the anterior intercostal spaces are wider than the posterior ones.

Anteriorly, each hemithorax projects further forward than the sternum, which actually represents some depression between the two sides of the thoracic wall. The lower part of the sternum is normally slightly further depressed from the chest wall. The subcostal angle, or the angle formed by the anterior margin of the ribs with the xyphoid at its apex, is normally about 90 degrees, although it can be slightly greater in females and less in males. During inspiration, this angle widens, as the thorax expands laterally.

In a normal adult the entire thorax should have a slightly elliptical shape, and the anteroposterior diameter should be definitely less than the transverse, or side-to-side, diameter. When looking at the posterior thoracic wall, the scapula should be symmetrically located and closely attached to the thoracic wall. Some depression exists between the medial scapular borders and the spine. The range of motion of the scapula should be evaluated. The spine should be straight, without lateral deviation. When viewed from the side, there is a slight anterior concavity of the thoracic spine and a similar but opposite curvature of the lumbar spine.

During inspiration, areas of the thorax should expand and relax synchronously and with equality of movement. Thoracic movement should be observed first as a whole, and then movement of one part in relation to another should be studied. Respirations in the male are usually diaphragmatic; female respirations tend to be more costal. Males also show less movement of the entire chest wall compared with females. Use of accessory muscles or retraction of intercostal spaces should not be detected in any normal client.

When observing a client with known emphysema, compare movement of the upper chest with the lower chest, and examine movement of the diaphragm to determine whether or not the client is concentrating on expanding the lower chest and is using his diaphragm to achieve maximum inspiration.

Specific Findings   *Increased Anteroposterior Diameter*

Clients with chronic obstructive pulmonary disease usually have a barrel chest, with an increased anteroposterior diameter, equal to or larger than the transverse diameter. This increase is most commonly due to overexpansion of the lungs with obstructive lung disease, but may also be caused by bone structure abnormalities in a client who has kyphosis (hunchback). Increased prominence of the angle of Louis often accompanies the barrel chest configuration.

Increased Horizontal Slope of Ribs

Posteriorly, the ribs are normally situated at a 45-degree angle in relation to the spine. However, in the client with chronic obstructive pulmonary disease, the ribs are more nearly horizontal, helping to establish the barrel chest configuration.

Use of Accessory Muscles

A client who is experiencing labored breathing ordinarily uses accessory muscles to aid respiration. These include the sternocleidomastoids, internal and external intercostals, abdominal muscles, anterior serratus, and scalene muscles. Over a period of time, enlargement and prominence of these muscles, especially of the muscles of the neck and shoulder girdle, develop in clients with chronic respiratory difficulty.

Increased Subcostal Angle

A widened subcostal angle and a fixed, expanded lower rib margin develop in clients with chronic pulmonary disease. For them, this angle widens little with each respiratory effort.

Unequal Expansion of the Thorax

Asymmetric expansion of the thorax has many causes. These include massive pleural effusion, atelectasis (especially caused by a mucous plug in a major bronchus), pneumothorax, or any cause of chest pain such as pulmonary embolus or fractured rib.

In the intensive care setting a client is occasionally seen who has unilateral diminished chest expansion due to an endotracheal or nasotracheal tube that has been inserted too far and extends beyond the trachea into one of the main-stem bronchi, usually the right. This causes diminished chest expansion in the unaerated side of the chest, and hypoxemia and atelectasis of that lung often result. The nurse who anticipates the possibility of this serious complication can examine the client with this in mind, and if it occurs, promptly secure medical attention for the client.

Some abnormalities of chest expansion may not be seen with quiet respirations, but become pronounced with forced inspiration. For this reason, inspection of the chest should be carried out during both quiet and deep breathing.

Retraction or Bulging of Interspaces

Intercostal retractions are seen when skin and muscle between the ribs are sucked in during inspiration. Retraction of the supraclavicular and substernal areas often occur at the same time. These findings are usually symptoms of obstruction to free inflow of air, causing a more strenuous inspiratory effort. Increased inspiratory effort may also occur when the lungs are less compliant (stiffer) than normal or as a result of excessive negativity of the pleural end-expiratory pressure, as seen in atelectasis.

Intercostal bulging may occur with massive pleural effusion or tension pneumothorax. It is occasionally seen on the thoracic wall when a tumor or aortic aneurysm is present. However, bulging is most frequently found with the forced and prolonged expirations of a client with asthma or emphysema.

Deformities of Bony Structure of Chest or Spine

The examiner should note any abnormalities of the thoracic bone structure, since these alterations often interfere with proper posture and adequate chest expansion and can be the cause of respiratory difficulty. Common bone deformities of the thorax and spine are illustrated in Figure 9-11.

Observation of Respirations

Respirations should be observed for three dimensions, namely, rate, rhythm, and amplitude of the respiratory excursion, and counted for a minimum of 15 seconds. The nurse should be aware of the hazards of estimating respirations rather than counting them.

The normal range for rate is 12 to 18 respirations per minute. Usually, the ratio of respiratory rate to pulse rate is 1:4. With fever, the respiratory rate increases with the pulse rate on an average of four additional respiratory cycles per minute for each 1 degree of elevation in temperature above normal.

The activity of respiratory cycles should occur rhythmically in the normal adult, and the interval between cycles should be equal. Normal respirations are usually two parts inspiration to three parts expiration, but in an adult with emphysema the expiratory time is often prolonged. The amplitude of respiration often reveals as much information as an assessment of the rate. Decreased amplitude may be caused by pain that is intensified with inspiratory effort, such as that occurring with fractured ribs, sprained muscles, or painful skin alteration. A decrease in amplitude may also result from dysfunction of either side or all of the diaphragm.

The common terms used to describe alterations in rate, rhythm, and depth of respiration are discussed next.

Dyspnea

Dyspnea can simply be described as "difficult respirations." It is primarily a subjective description, used to characterize the condition of a client who is experiencing obvious increased respiratory effort, often using accessory muscles. The client also describes experiencing an uncomfortable sensation of not being able to get enough air, which sometimes persists even with the increased respiratory effort.

Dyspnea naturally varies in degree. Some persons are dyspneic only with moderate amounts of exertion, such as climbing one or several flights of stairs; others become dyspneic with such simple activities as walking across the room,

Figure 9-11. Deformities of the bony structure of the chest or spine. *A. Pigeon breast.* Often seen with active rickets. Softening of the ribs causes the sternum to be pushed forward while the ribs slope away at either side. This causes an increase in the anteroposterior diameter at the expense of the width of the thorax. *B. Barrel chest.* Hyperinflation or augmented lung volume occurring with respiratory diseases such as emphysema or asthma cause the thorax to assume a permanent inspiratory position, with an increased anteroposterior diameter and increased horizontal slope of the ribs. The transverse diameter may remain the same or also may increase. *C. Funnel breast.* Seen in rickets and in some congenital disorders. In this case the softened ribs allow a depression of the lower portion the sternum. *D. Lordosis.* Curvature of the spinal column with anterior convexity, causing thoracic spine to be displaced posteriorly and the lower thorax to be held in expiratory position. *E. Scoliosis.* Lateral deviation of the spine. Deviation of the thoracic spine causes a compensating deviation of the lumbar region to the opposite side, resulting in an S-shaped curve. On the side of thoracic deviation the thorax is larger and convex, the ribs separated, and the lung emphysematous. On the concave side the ribs are close together and the chest small.

taking off a shirt, or carrying on a conversation. Those with severe respiratory dysfunction may experience dyspnea at rest. A notation of dyspnea is often useless information unless the amount of exertion needed to cause it is recorded, as well as the amount of rest needed to relieve it.

Dyspnea may be either inspiratory or expiratory. *Inspiratory dyspnea* occurs with obstruction to inflow of air, as with severe laryngitis, a foreign body, or a tumor causing exterior compression on the trachea or larger bronchi. It is often accompanied by intercostal retractions and by the crowing sound of inspiratory stridor. *Expiratory dyspnea* occurs with obstruction of the bronchioles or small bronchi and may be present in clients with asthma, bronchitis, and obstructive emphysema. Expiratory time is prolonged, and bulging of the intercostal spaces may occur.

Tachypnea

Tachypnea indicates increased respiratory rate, with or without a corresponding increase in depth. It is seen with increased metabolic activity (in fever, pneumonia), in states of alkalosis, and with pleurisy or respiratory insufficiency, either obstructive or restrictive.

Bradypnea, Apnea, and Hyperpnea

Bradypnea, an abnormal slowing of respirations, is the opposite of tachypnea. Agents that depress the respiratory center, such as opiates or brain tumors, produce respirations that are decreased in rate, but still uniform and regular in character. Alveolar hypoventilation (see below) can be expected in such a situation. *Apnea* is a temporary cessation of breathing. *Hyperpnea* indicates an increased depth of breathing.

Hyperventilation

Hyperventilation is an abnormal increase in both rate and depth of respiration. It is often present with fever, salicylate ingestion, hepatic coma, and lesions of the midbrain. If it results from acidosis, it is called *Kussmal's respiration.* Hyperventilation may also occur with fear, pain or anxiety.

Apneustic Respirations

Apneustic respirations are marked by maintained inspiratory activity unrelieved by expiration. Each inspiration is long and gasping, followed by a short expiratory period. This type of respiration usually follows damage to the pneumotaxic center of the pons.

Pleuritic, or Restrained, Breathing

As the term indicates, pleuritic breathing occurs during pleurisy, when pain abruptly halts the inspiratory phase of respiration. As a consequence, respirations are shallow, but often rapid.

Cyclic Respirations

Cyclic, or periodic, respirations display a patterned cycle of irregularities and are usually the result of central respiratory depression. Two common types of cyclic respirations, Cheyne-Stokes and Biot's, are differentiated by the rhythm of their cycles.

Cheyne-Stokes respirations are characterized by a repeating cycle of gradually increasing then decreasing rate and tidal volume. Each cycle is concluded by a period of quiet breathing or apnea. The client often lies quietly during the period of apnea, but becomes restless when respirations again resume. Cheyne-Stokes respirations are seen in a variety of disease states, including severe congestive heart failure, increased intracranial pressure, cerebral disease, and drug sensitivity. It is important to know that this type of respiratory pattern may also be seen occasionally in children and in adults as they sleep.

Biot's breathing is characterized by alternating periods of regular breathing and apnea, but without any consistent pattern of change. Biot's respirations are due to marked depression of the respiratory center and, though infrequently seen, may be observed occasionally with meningitis or other forms of central nervous system disease. This is a serious prognostic sign, indicating extensive damage to the respiratory control centers of the brain.

Stertorous Respirations

Stertorous respirations are noisy respirations (snoring sounds) produced by passage of air through secretions that have accumulated in the trachea and large bronchi as a result of the client's inability to clear them. These respirations are usually seen in a comatose patient whose cough reflex is severely depressed or absent and are often a terminal event. Hence, stertorous respirations are at times called the "death rattle."

Sighing Respirations

Sighing respirations are noted when a deep inspiration and then prolonged expiration interrupt the regular respiratory rhythm at frequent intervals. They are usually not a manifestation of organic disease, but of emotional tension.

Pursed Lip Breathing

Air trapping occurs in clients with emphysema or asthma during times when the flow of air both in and out of the thorax is impaired. Impairment of flow is usually more marked during expiration, making it easier to take in air than to let it out. Clients usually compensate for this by decreasing their velocity of expiration (prolonging expiratory time) and by exhaling through pursed lips.

PALPATION OF THE THORAX

Palpation of the thorax may reveal new findings or confirm or supplement findings from inspection. By simply moving the palm of the hand across the chest (Fig. 9-12), the examiner may detect lumps or masses. Pulsations or areas

Figure 9-12.
Technique for palpation of
the thorax. (Reproduced
with permission from R. D.
Judge, G. D. Zuidema, and
F. Fitzgerald (Eds.).
*Methods of Clinical
Examination* (4th ed.).
Boston: Little, Brown,
1982.)

of tenderness may also be noted. Some special techniques of palpation are also used in the chest examination.

1. *Thoracic excursion.* Hands are placed on different parts of the chest during the respiratory cycle to determine the amount of thoracic expansion.
2. *Fremitus.* Normal and abnormal vibrations felt on the surface of the chest are detected by palpation.
3. *Crepitation.* A coarse, crackling sensation palpated in the subcutaneous tissue.

Thoracic Excursion

Alterations in thoracic expansion may be first noted on inspection, but are often better detected by palpation. The examiner's hands are placed flat against the chest at several locations, and as the chest moves, the hands move also. The amount of excursion is then estimated, using two parameters: the velocity of movement and the distance the thumbs move from each other.

Technique of Examination
To first test excursion of the posterior lower chest, stand behind the client and place your hands on the lower portion of the rib cage, so that your thumbs are on the spine and your fingers point laterally. Press toward the spine, so that a

Figure 9-13.
Testing inspiratory
expansion. *A.* Testing
inspiratory expansion of the
posterior thorax. *B.* Testing
inspiratory expansion of the
lower anterior thorax. *C.*
Testing movement of the
costal margin.

small fold of skin is found between your thumbs (Fig. 9-13). Normally, a 3-in (7.6-cm) expansion of the thorax is found here as the client goes from maximum expiration to maximum inspiration. To test the anterosuperior thoracic wall, remain standing behind the client and place your hands on the anterior upper thorax, so that your thumbs are along the sternal border pointing toward the xyphoid process and your fingers are spread out over the anterolateral wall. Finally, to test the lower anterior thorax, position yourself to face the client and place your hands over the lower anterior thorax, thumbs again along the costal margin, but this time pointing upward toward the neck; your fingers should be pointing laterally. In each position, thoracic excursion should be tested with both a normal and maximum inspiration. Abnormalities in expansion are usually more readily detected on the anterior thoracic wall than posteriorly, since the anterolateral wall normally moves more than any other part of the chest. Although specific areas are tested separately, the entire thorax should be felt to move as a unit and not in several separate movements.

Findings

It is difficult to describe the correct feeling for normal thoracic excursion. Only by examining a variety of normal healthy people can the examiner acquire an appreciation for the range of normal and be able to detect abnormal findings outside that range. Alterations detected may have various causes; for example, pneumothorax, acute pleurisy, trauma, or thickening of the pleura.

Fremitus   Vocal fremitus, sometimes also called tactile fremitus, is the most common type of palpable vibration and is merely transmission of the vibration of air resulting from phonation. Sounds that are produced in the larynx are transmitted down the tracheobronchial tree to the smaller bronchioles and finally to the alveoli. This vibration is then transmitted to the thoracic wall and the examiner's hand on the chest wall.

Technique of Examination

To detect vocal fremitus, have the client speak in a soft voice, repeating phrases such as "99-99," or "1-2-3," or "blue moon," or "how now brown cow." The intensity of vocal fremitus varies with both the loudness and the frequency of the voice. If at first the vibration is slight, ask the client to speak a little louder. However, once you have begun comparing areas of the chest, the client should attempt to speak at the same level so as not to introduce an extraneous variable into the evaluation. In persons with a deep voice, the tactile sensation of fremitus is more distinct because of the lower frequency of voice vibrations. There are three commonly used methods of hand placement for detecting fremitus. The open palm may be placed flat against the chest wall. The narrow ulnar aspect of the hand may also be used either with the hand open or with the fingers closed in the palm.

Variations of fremitus normally occur in different areas of the thorax, but corresponding areas should have the same intensity of vibration. It is thus essential to compare corresponding areas consecutively, e.g., to compare the right apex with the left apex, the right middle anterior chest with the corresponding area on the left side (Fig. 9-14). Some prefer to place both hands on the chest at once; others find it best to use one hand and move from area to area. With the first method it is sometimes difficult to detect differences in vibratory levels while using both hands; however, with the second, one may lose the sense of level of vibration in moving from one area to another.

Findings

The intensity of vibrations felt at any point is dependent on the thickness of the subcutaneous tissue covering the wall of the thorax, and on the distance of the major bronchi from the chest wall at that area. Fremitus is most prominent in regions of the thorax where the major bronchi are closest to the chest wall and becomes less intense as one moves away from these bronchi. Fremitus is least

Figure 9-14. Three methods of hand position for testing vocal fremitus. Method of testing vocal fremitus, using ulnar aspect of hand and comparing contralateral areas sequentially.

noticeable at the bases of the lungs, an area separated from the bronchi by a large amount of aerated lung tissue. Fremitus of maximal intensity is found at the base of the neck, both anteriorly and posteriorly, at the first and second interspaces lateral to the sternum, at the right apex, and also between the scapulae. Tactile fremitus vibrations are more intense in the thin person than in the muscular or obese person because of the damping effect of the increased amount of subcutaneous tissue. The examiner should be looking for areas of increased intensity of fremitus, or decreased or absent fremitus. Only gross changes in the pleura and lungs give rise to significant changes in palpable fremitus; small areas of consolidation, tumors, and so on, cannot be expected to cause noticeable changes.

Anything that increases the density of the lung tissue also increases the transmission of vibrations through it. Solid or semisolid material of uniform structure conducts better than a porous structure of solid and air that is constantly undergoing changes in density, such as normal lung tissue. Increased vocal fremitus therefore occurs in conditions that are associated with consolidation of the lungs. However, to produce the increased intensity of fremitus the area of consolidation must be connected to a patent bronchus and must also extend to the surface of the lung, where vibrations travelling through it can set the thoracic wall in motion.

Decreased or absent fremitus results when something comes between the sound traveling down the tracheobronchial tree and the examining hand on the chest wall. Often, it is an upper airway blockage or an obstruction of a major bronchus. Air or fluid in the pleural space also dampens the vibrations or makes it impossible to feel them.

It is helpful to remember that one should always find a correlation between the intensity of fremitus and the intensity of auscultated breath sounds. In each case the examiner is evaluating a type of vibration in the bronchotracheal system. Also, in each case the degree of vibration is affected by the same physical factors. Therefore, one can expect to find decreased fremitus with diminished breath sounds, and increased fremitus with exaggerated breath sounds or bronchial breathing.

Vibrations felt on the surface of the chest can result from phenomena other than transmission of vibrations produced in the larynx. Tussive fremitus is the vibration of the chest wall produced by coughing. Pleural friction fremitus, as its name indicates, results when the inflamed pleural surfaces in acute pleurisy rub together, producing a grating sensation that can be detected by the hand on the chest wall. This sensation is usually felt during both phases of respiration and is most commonly noted on the anterolateral portion of the thoracic wall, where there is the greatest degree of respiratory movement. This palpable friction rub may also be heard on auscultation.

Rhonchal fremitus, in which palpable murmurs or vibrations are created during breathing by air moving through secretions or by an area of stenosis of the bronchi or trachea, is felt by palpating the client's chest during quiet breathing. Rhonchal fremitus can be differentiated from pleural friction rub fremitus, a more serious omen, by having the client cough. The rhonchal fremitus should disappear with movement of the exudate, but the palpatory and auscultatory evidence of the pleural friction rub remains.

Crepitation   Crepitation, the coarse, crackling sensation that is palpated when the subcutaneous tissues contain fine beads of air (also known as subcutaneous emphysema), results from leakage of air through traumatic or surgical wounds into the major airways or the alveoli. This sensation has been described as similar to rolling a lock of hair between the thumb and forefinger or crumpling a wad of plastic food wrap. The crackling sensation, like the "snap, crackle, and pop" of certain cereals, is sometimes actually audible. Immediate action must be taken when crepitation is detected, for it progresses quickly, causing rapid obstruction of the airway. In addition, the puffed subcutaneous tissues make it difficult to insert an endotracheal tube or perform a tracheostomy. This is an emergency situation and medical assistance must be sought at once.

PERCUSSION OF THE THORAX

In examining the thorax, percussion is used both to determine the relative amount of air or solid material in the underlying lung and to define the boundaries of portions of the lung that differ in structural density.

Technique of Examination

Indirect percussion is primarily used in examining the thorax, although direct percussion may be used for examining the area above the clavicles or for defining the cardiac borders. The palmar surface of the distal phalanx of the left middle finger serves as the pleximeter (i.e., receives the blow) and is firmly placed on the chest wall in an interspace, parallel to the ribs (Fig. 9-15). Only the distal phalanx of the pleximeter should rest on the chest wall. If the entire hand is touching the chest, the tone of the percussion note may be muffled. It has been estimated that a strong percussion stroke penetrates for about 6 cm (2.4 in) beneath the skin through 3 cm (1.2 in) of thoracic wall and 3 cm of lung tissue. For this reason a more forceful stroke is used to detect changes in density of lung tissue (sonorous percussion) and a lighter stroke to outline the borders of adjacent organs (definitive percussion).

Even when using the more forceful stroke to detect changes in density of lung tissue, many abnormalities may go unrecognized. Any deep-seated mass covered by aerated lung tissue does not cause an audible change in the percussion

Figure 9-15. Technique for indirect percussion of the thorax, posterior view. (Reproduced with permission from R. D. Judge, G. D. Zuidema, and F. Fitzgerald (Eds.). *Methods of Clinical Examination* (4th ed.). Boston: Little, Brown, 1982.)

note. A mass must also be as large as 2 to 3 cm (0.8 to 1.2 in) in diameter to be detected.

For ease in percussing, the client's thorax should be at least as high, if not higher, than the nurse's thorax. The room and examiner's hands should be warm. Before starting systematic percussion of the thorax, it is wise to attempt to establish a normal resonant percussion note for the person being examined; this can later be used as a basis for comparison of other notes. Select an area that has little muscular or subcutaneous tissue; the seventh or eighth posterolateral interspace well out toward the axilla gives a good percussion note and is an area usually free from disease.

Begin with the client in the supine position for percussion of the anterior chest (Fig. 9-16). His arms should be resting loosely at his sides. Start below the clavicles and use fairly heavy indirect percussion. Percuss downward, interspace by interspace, comparing the sound from each interspace sequentially

Figure 9-16. Quality of percussion note over the normal chest. *A.* Anterior chest. *B.* Posterior chest. *C.* Effect of lateral recumbent position on percussion note. *a.* Zone of relative dullness due to deadening effect of mattress. *b.* Zone of dullness due to compression of chest by weight of body. *c.* Zone of dullness due to crowding of ribs.

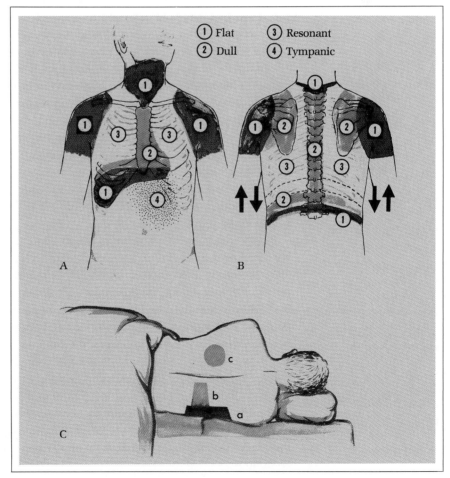

with that from the contralateral region. Continue downward to the region of hepatic dullness on the right and to the area of tympany, called *Traube's semilunar space,* on the left. The entire thorax should be resonant, with the exception of the area of cardiac dullness. On the right is the transition zone of hepatic dullness from about the fourth to sixth interspaces. This zone is a combination of resonance and dullness, as a portion of the liver lies over a portion of the lung. As you leave the area of the lung, the dullness becomes hepatic flatness. The upper tympanic border is somewhat lower on the left than the upper border of the liver on the right because the left diaphragm lies lower than the right.

Percussion of the other areas of the thorax, such as the anterior apices, the lateral thorax, and the posterior thorax, is most easily done with the client sitting on a stool. The apices of the lung extend above the clavicle, producing a band of resonance that widens at the scapular and clavicular ends. The upper narrow part of this band of resonance is called *Krönig's isthmus.* Percuss the supraclavicular spaces, using indirect percussion. The right apex is best percussed by using your left thumb as the pleximeter while facing the client. To percuss the left apex, reach around the client's back with your left arm and use your left middle finger, pointing downward, as the pleximeter.

Percuss the lateral aspects of the thorax by having the client rest his forearm on top of his head, and percuss downward from the axilla.

Next, percuss the posterior thorax with the client sitting, head and shoulders bent slightly forward in a hunchback position and arms folded in his lap. This position moves the scapulae laterally, since they interfere with percussion of the lung areas they cover. Again percuss downward, interspace by interspace, always immediately comparing the percussion note on the contralateral side. Use lighter percussion for the posterior thorax. During quiet respirations you should find the border of resonance at the ninth rib on the left and the eighth interspace on the right.

Finally, determine the amount of diaphragmatic excursion by comparing the border of resonance at maximum expiration with that at maximum inspiration. Have the client inhale deeply and hold his breath. Percuss downward on the posterior thorax, noting the line between resonant lung and dullness of abdominal viscera. Now tell the client to exhale as far as possible and hold. Again percuss downward to determine the lower border of resonance. The distance between these two points indicates the amount of diaphragmatic excursion, which is normally 5 to 6 cm (2 to 2.4 in). Diaphragmatic excursion is limited by pleurisy and severe emphysema. In emphysema, the level of the diaphragm is lower than normal, but with any condition that causes an increase in intra-abdominal pressure, such as pregnancy or ascites, the diaphragm is higher than normal. If there is phrenic nerve damage and diaphragmatic paralysis, the involved side of the diaphragm moves paradoxically upward with each respiration.

Whenever possible, posterior percussion should be carried out with the client sitting upright. However, where the client cannot sit up, posterior percussion can be performed in the lateral decubitus position if the examiner is aware of the resulting changes in body structure and percussion notes (Fig. 9-16C). The dependent lung is generally somewhat duller. The surface of the bed pressing against the thorax has a damping effect in that immediate area and causes a band of dullness along the chest wall next to the bed. Directly above this is another area of dullness caused by the body weight compressing the downward lung. In addition, body weight on the mattress causes some degree of sagging, which curves the spine, causing compression of the thoracic wall on the upward side and a similar compression of the underlying upward lung. This results in an area of relative dullness at approximately the tip of the upward scapula. The flexing of the spine also causes the upward intercostal spaces to widen and the downward ones to become more narrow. Curvature of the spine can be relieved to some degree if the pillow is taken away and the head rests directly on the bed.

Findings The full range of percussion notes that may be heard over the thorax include resonance, tympany, hyperresonance, dullness, and flatness.

Resonance

Resonance is the clear hollow percussion note heard on the thorax over healthy lung tissue. The normal resonant note varies in pitch and amplitude from person to person and across the individual chest; a very bony, muscular thorax has a less resonant note because of the greater amount of solid tissue. Changes in the ratio of air to solid tissue also explain why females often have a lighter, less resonant note (proportionately less aerated lung tissue to solid tissue) and children, a more resonant note.

The resonant note is also affected by structures overlying the lung tissue. The apical or superior segments of the lung are covered by fairly thick muscle and bone, resulting in a duller percussion note. However, the base of the thorax has a relatively greater proportion of lung and relatively less muscle and bone—hence a more resonant note. The denser tissues of the scapula, the pectoral and back muscles, and the breasts all tend to dull the resonant percussion note. Therefore, in clients with thick subcutaneous tissues, as in obesity, a more forceful percussion stroke must be used to obtain an adequate diagnostic sound.

In percussing the thorax it is important to note that percussion produces not only a sound, but also varying degrees of resistance and vibration, which can be sensed by the pleximeter finger. Vibration of the underlying tissues, such as occurs in the thorax, produces less resistance and more elasticity detected by the pleximeter finger. In percussing the thigh, which has little vibration, there is a sense of increased resistance. Percussing the air-filled lung, on the other hand, causes much vibration and decreased resistance. The perimeter finger can also sense changes in relative pitch and duration of the percussion note.

Tympany

Tympany often is found physiologically in the lower left hemithorax and the left upper abdomen. Here, it results from air in the stomach, the upper portion of which lies beneath the lower ribs, and possibly from air in the splenic flexure of the colon. Tympany is abnormal when heard anywhere in the thorax other than in Traube's semilunar space, in the left anterior hemithorax, and in the left upper abdomen. Abnormal areas of tympany may be caused by large emphysematous bullae or collapse of the lung due to pneumothorax.

Hyperresonance

Hyperresonance is usually pathologic in the thorax. It is most often caused by the emphysematous lung filled with small air sacs. It may be present also with a small pneumothorax with minimal collapse of the lung, where a combination of resonance and tympany produces it. Physiologically, hyperresonance may occasionally be found in the base of the left lung, due to the same combination of tympany (small amount of air in the stomach) and resonance (lung).

Dullness

Dullness is obtained in percussion over the heart when it is not covered by inflated lung. As indicated in Chapter 2, it is a high-pitched sound, short, and thudlike and does not create a vibrating sensation in the pleximeter finger as does resonance or hyperresonance. These notes are normally elicited over the scapula, areas of the thorax that are covered by thick musculature, the mediastinum, or the upper portion of the liver and spleen—solid organs adjacent to air-containing lung.

Flatness

Flatness or absolute dullness is never normal in the thorax and, when present, indicates massive pleural effusion in which air-containing lung is displaced toward the interior and out of range of the percussion stroke.

AUSCULTATION OF THE LUNGS

Auscultation of the lungs is used to detect and study sounds from the lungs to determine both deviation from normal breath and voice sounds and the presence of abnormal additional or adventitious sounds. Auscultation may elicit new findings or may provide information to supplement or confirm previous observations.

Auscultation is used to detect three different types of sounds.

1. Breath sounds normally present are auscultated for variations and deviations from their visual characteristics.

2. Sound vibrations produced from the spoken voice are auscultated on the chest wall.
3. An attempt is made to detect adventitious sounds, or sounds not normally heard across the chest.

Technique of Examination

Since breath sounds are generally high-pitched, one should use the closed chestpiece of the stethoscope in auscultating the chest. The chestpiece should be held so that the diaphragm is placed firmly against the skin, while the rim of the chestpiece touches the skin lightly. If the chestpiece is held too tightly, the skin is stretched, itself becoming a diaphragm and excluding lower-pitched sounds. For narrower spaces, such as the intercostal spaces or the supraclavicular fossa, the smaller open bell chestpieces may be used, but held tightly against the skin so that the skin can become a diaphragm.

Remember that if the entire rim of the chestpiece does not touch the skin and a leak occurs, extraneous noise in the form of a roaring sound is heard by the examiner. If the chestpiece is not held firmly, sounds of respiratory excursion, such as movement of intercostal muscles, joints, or skin, are heard and may mimic a friction rub. Movement of the chestpiece over hair on the chest can produce a sound that resembles rales. This can be eliminated by wetting the hair. Breathing on the tubing or sliding one's fingers over the chestpiece may also cause confusing sounds. The examiner should purposely produce all these sounds and become familiar with them so that they can be recognized and eliminated during the chest examination.

Auscultation of the chest must be done in a quiet room. The level of background noise may not seem high, but very little noise will be sufficient to interfere with the low-intensity sounds important to detect on auscultation.

Preferably the client should be sitting for chest auscultation. If he must remain recumbent, have him turn from side to side to allow auscultation of all areas of the chest. Demonstrate to the client how to breathe while you are auscultating, having him breathe more deeply than normal and with his mouth open. Keeping his mouth open reduces the noise caused by the turbulence of air passing through the nose and mouth. Respirations slightly deeper than normal make breath sounds more audible, but very deep, strenuous respirations may result in the introduction of sounds actually caused by muscle movement. The examiner needs to be aware that there is normally a fourfold increase in the intensity of breath sounds with deep breathing over that in quiet breathing.

Begin auscultation with the anterior chest, first auscultating the apices and then proceeding downward. As with percussion, compare contralateral points sequentially. Auscultate the posterior chest in a similar manner, again comparing contralateral areas as you move downward (Fig. 9-17). When auscultating the back, note where the breath sounds disappear and compare these data with data obtained from palpation of vocal fremitus and percussion to determine where the lung bases lie.

Figure 9-17. Technique for auscultation of the chest, posterior view. (Reproduced with permission from R. D. Judge, G. D. Zuidema, and F. Fitzgerald (Eds.). *Methods of Clinical Examination* (4th ed.). Boston: Little, Brown, 1982.)

As the nurse listens to breath sounds, she must discipline herself to note systematically the duration of inspiration and expiration, and the quality and pitch of sounds in each area. Particular attention to the expiratory phase is important, since most abnormalities of breath sounds are characterized by changes here. The nurse should identify the breath sounds as vesicular, bronchovesicular, bronchial, asthmatic, cavernous, or absent. Next, she should listen for adventitious sounds such as rales or rhonchi, noting whether rales clear after a few deep breaths or cough. Both the anterior and posterior chest should be auscultated a second time while the client whispers a phrase the examiner suggests in order to determine the presence or absence of whispered pectoriloquy. The nurse should have the client speak, to test for bronchophony. Finally, she should listen for friction rubs and other types of abnormal sounds.

Breath Sounds   Breath sounds are essentially the vibrations produced by movement of air through the tracheobronchial tree. What is heard through the stethoscope depends on the place of auscultation on the chest wall, and on the resonating and conducting properties of the lung and other tissues between the larger airways.

In listening to breath sounds, four characteristics should be considered:

1. *Pitch.* Normal breath sounds have a rising pitch during inspiration and falling pitch during expiration. In describing pitch of breath sounds, *high* and *low* are used in relation to the pitch of other breath sounds.
2. *Duration.* Ratio of the duration of the two phases of respiration is a distinguishing factor in determining various abnormal breath sounds and should always be noted.
3. *Intensity.* Breath sounds are described as loud or soft in relation to other breath sounds, or inspiration and expiration may be contrasted with one another in loudness. Usually, the longer the phase of respiration, the louder the sound in that phase.
4. *Quality.* This is difficult to describe, but various terms such as *honking* and *wheezing* have been used to indicate quality of breath sounds.

Normal Breath Sounds

There are only two types of normal breath sounds heard over the thorax, vesicular and bronchovesicular (Table 9-1).

Vesicular. The normal breath sounds heard over most of the lungs are the vesicular breath sounds. They are caused by air moving through the bronchioles and the alveoli and are a result of the turbulence of air as it is distributed to the individual alveoli. Because of the wide distribution of alveoli beneath the chest wall, this respiratory sound is heard over almost all of the chest surface. An expiratory component of the vesicular sound is normally heard over some areas of the chest and originates as the expired air moves out through the bifurcations of the large airways. It is more clearly heard in areas where the

Table 9-1.
Characteristics of Breath
Sounds

Type	Description	Schematic Representation	Normal Location
Vesicular	Soft, low-pitched Inspiration longer, louder, and higher pitched than expiration		Heard over most of chest surface
Bronchovesicular	Higher pitched Inspiration and expiration have very similar pitch, duration, intensity		Anterior—on either side of sternum around first and second interspaces Posterior—between scapula
Bronchial	Blowing, hollow and high-pitched Expiration longer, louder, high-pitched tubular		Not heard on normal chest

tracheobronchial tree lies close to the chest surface, such as in the upper mid-thorax, anteriorly and posteriorly. Over other areas of the chest the porous lung tissue greatly dampens the expiratory sound. Breath sounds in the normal person are therefore mainly inspiratory and low-pitched. The ratio of inspiratory sound to expiratory sound is 3 to 1.

The vesicular breath sound is a soft, relatively low-pitched sound and has been likened to the gentle rustling of leaves as the air moves through the trees. The inspiratory sound is louder than the expiratory sound, but there is no noticeable pause between inspiration and expiration. Generally, the inspiratory sound lasts three times as long as the audible expiratory sound. As always, great individual variation can be expected both in the intensity and in the relative duration of the two phases.

Bronchovesicular. The bronchovesicular breath sound is heard where the tracheobronchial tree is close to the chest surface. This sound is caused by a mixture of vesicular sounds and the sound produced as air travels in and out through the tracheobronchial tree.

Bronchovesicular sounds are normally heard on either side of the sternum in the first and second interspaces anteriorly and between the scapulae posteriorly. They may be heard over the apices, often the right more than the left. Their inspiratory phase resembles normal vesicular breathing, but is slightly longer and higher pitched. The expiratory phase is also higher in pitch and increased in duration to the point where it may be longer than inspiration. The expiratory phase may have a slightly tubular quality as compared with the vesicular sound. Actually, the inspiratory and expiratory phases are much alike in duration, pitch, intensity, and quality. Again, there should be little if any pause between phases.

Because of their thinner chest wall, slender adults or children often have louder breath sounds than does the average adult. These sounds have been called "puerile" or "exaggerated" breath sounds and often resemble bronchovesicular sounds in the normal adult.

Abnormal Breath Sounds

Abnormal breath sounds are most frequently characterized by changes in the expiratory phase, although changes in the inspiratory phase may occur.

Bronchial Breath Sounds. Bronchial breathing is a blowing, hollow, high-pitched breath sound, also sometimes called *tubular breathing.* The inspiratory phase is relatively short, but the expiratory phase is prolonged. The expiratory phase is also louder and higher in pitch than the inspiratory phase, perhaps even rising in pitch. There is a definite short pause between the two phases. A distinguishing characteristic of the sound is that it seems to originate very close to the examiner's ear, almost right at the end of the stethoscope. Bronchial sounds may be louder than normal, but not always.

Bronchial breathing is not normally heard over the lungs. However, a similar

sound, called tracheal breathing, can be heard by listening over the trachea just below the larynx. Like bronchial breathing, tracheal breathing has a relatively prominent expiratory phase, but it is louder, harsher, and even more hollow than bronchial breathing. These tracheal sounds have no pathologic significance. Bronchial sounds, on the other hand, always indicate an abnormality. They result from any condition in which the lung tissue is compressed, such as pleural effusion or consolidation, as in pneumonia. Either compression or consolidation causes a denser area, which results in greater transmission of sound from the bronchial tree than through the sound dampening air sacs.

Bronchovesicular Breath Sounds. Bronchovesicular breath sounds have been described as an intermediate between vesicular and bronchial breath sounds. As stated previously, bronchovesicular sounds are normally heard in the upper midthorax. In other areas, if there is both aerated lung and a small degree of pulmonary consolidation or compression, transmission of sounds from the bronchial tree is enhanced to some degree, and abnormal bronchovesicular breath sounds result. If the degree of compression or consolidation is very mild, this sound may be described as vesicobronchiolar; as compression becomes more severe, the breath sounds become truly bronchial.

Asthmatic breath sounds. Asthmatic breath sounds, like bronchial breathing, have a short inspiratory phase and a prolonged expiratory phase, usually even longer than bronchial breathing. However, there is no hollow or tubular quality to the breath sound. Instead, inspiration is often short and gasping, and expiration has a much higher pitch and is accompanied by wheezing and rhonchi. This type of sound indicates that there is airway narrowing, caused by edema and spasm (as with asthma), presence of foreign bodies or mucus in the airways, or stenosis of the airway. The bronchi still increase in diameter during inspiration, but during expiration the decrease in size is exaggerated and narrowing results.

Decreased or Absent Breath Sounds. Breath sounds are absent in an area when complete occlusion of the bronchus occurs, although the lung tissue distal to the obstruction may be healthy. Diminished breath sounds not representing a pathologic condition in the lung may be due to exaggerated thickness of the chest wall, as in obesity or in those with large thick muscles or large breasts. However, breath sounds may also be diminished in intensity with a variety of alterations. Any cause of generalized shallow breathing, such as the pain of pleurisy or generalized muscle weakness, may result in diminished breath sounds. The dilated air sacs of emphysema cause diminished velocity of air movement and also greater damping of sound transmission, and thus breath sounds are decreased. Any other alteration interfering with the transmission of sound, such as air or fluid in the pleural space, thickened, fibrosed pleura, or tumor, will cause decreased intensity of breath sounds on auscultation. Many of these alterations also diminish ventilation in that area of the lung and consequently diminish breath sounds.

Amphoric Breath Sounds. Amphoric breath sounds (from *amphora,* the Greek word for jar) resemble the sound heard when blowing over the mouth of an empty bottle. The sound has a harsh quality and a fairly high pitch. Expiration is prolonged, as in bronchial breathing, but expiration, unlike that of bronchial breathing, has a lower pitch than inspiration. This sound is heard infrequently, but may be heard over an open pneumothorax or a large, thin-walled cavity that has a communication with a bronchus.

Cavernous Breath Sounds. These sounds are much like the amphoric sound, but are relatively low in pitch and hollow. They are like the sound produced by blowing *very softly* over the mouth of an empty bottle.

Cog-wheel Respirations. Cog-wheel respirations are like vesicular breath sounds, except that the inspiratory phase is discontinuous and jerky. These interruptions are caused by nonsimultaneous and unequal inflation of the alveoli, such as occurs with pleurisy or muscle weakness.

Voice Sounds   Voice sounds heard on auscultation, called *vocal resonance,* have the same origin as the vibrations perceived as vocal or tactile fremitus. The sound produced in the larynx travels down the bronchial tree and is heard less distinctively as one auscultates toward the periphery of the lung.

When a person speaks in a normal manner, the sound heard on auscultation is soft and muffled as compared with the sound heard directly. The words themselves are not distinct, and one cannot understand what has been said. Often, the client may be asked to speak in a whisper, since the spoken voice may be too loud for the examiner to detect alterations in the sound transmitted.

Abnormal Voice Sounds

There are several abnormal voice sounds; these furnish clues to pathologic conditions in the chest.

Bronchophony. Bronchophony is used to indicate decreased clarity and loudness of words, heard as if they were close to the ear. However, the syllables are still somewhat distorted. The word *bronchophony* literally means the sound normally heard when listening directly over a large bronchus. This sound is heard over other parts of the thorax when pulmonary consolidation or compression of lung tissue is present. With those alterations the alveoli lose some of their sound-damping quality, and this causes the increased clarity and loudness of sounds heard on auscultation. Bronchophony is usually associated with increased tactile fremitus, bronchial breath sounds, and dullness on percussion.

Whispered Pectoriloquy. Whispered pectoriloquy describes the transmission of whispered speech to the chest wall in distinct and recognizable syllables. Whispered speech is often more effective than spoken words in detecting abnormalities. Normally, whispered speech is faint and almost inaudible except over the trachea and main bronchi, where it is heard more clearly but still indistinctly. With even small amounts of consolidation, the whispered speech may still be faint, but it is clear, with definite recognition of words. The words may sound as if they were whispered into the end of the stethoscope. This change occurs before bronchophony and bronchial breathing develop and consequently aids in early diagnosis of pneumonia.

Egophony. Egophony is another type of auscultated voice sound which may represent consolidation or compression of lung tissue. Normally, when the client pronounces a long "e" softly, the examiner hears the long "e" sound. Consolidation or compression of lung tissue alters the character of this auscultated sound, so that the examiner hears a long "a" with the stethoscope. This change from a spoken "e" to an auscultated "a" indicates egophony.

Adventitious Sounds   Adventitious sounds are not normally heard over the chest and, when present, are always abnormal. They are not modifications of breath or voice sounds, but are heard in addition to breath sounds, which, in themselves, may be either normal or abnormal. The most common adventitious sounds are the various types of rales or rhonchi and the pleural friction rub (Table 9-2).

Table 9-2.
Adventitious Sounds

Type	Description	Origin of Sound	Possible Cause
Rales			
Fine	Discontinuous crackling sounds; soft, high-pitched; end of inspiration	Thin secretions in alveoli due to inflammation or pulmonary vessel congestion	Pneumonia Pulmonary edema
Medium	Medium pitch, crackling or popping; mid-inspiration	Mucus in bronchioles	Bronchitis Pulmonary congestion
Coarse	Loud, low-pitched, bubbling or gurgling; early inspiration	Mucus in trachea, bronchi	Resolution of acute inflammation Severe pulmonary edema Moribund client
Rhonchi			
Sibilant	High-pitched, wheezing, prolonged continuous sound	Edema of bronchi, bronchioles; stenosis or tumor	Asthma Emphysema
Sonorous	Low-pitched, snoring	Thick secretions	Bronchitis
Pleural friction rub	Coarse, crackling, grating sounds close to ear	Roughened pleural surfaces moving over each other	Pleurisy Pulmonary embolus

Rales and Rhonchi

Rales are sounds produced during one or both phases of respiration where there is excess fluid of any sort in the alveoli or in any portion of the tracheobronchial tree. This fluid or exudate may be from inflammation, infection, edema, or retained secretions. Rales of one type or another are the most commonly heard adventitious sounds. Unfortunately, some of the terms used to describe variations of rales have evolved with several meanings and hence are most confusing. An attempt will be made here to identify the most common meaning of the various terms used and to identify other terms that may be used in describing the same sound.

Rales are subdivided into (1) continuous coarse sounds, called rhonchi, and (2) discontinuous crackling sounds, also called rales, the same as the parent term. Rhonchi usually imply the presence of exudate in the larger bronchi, while most medium or fine rales indicate bronchiolar and alveolar disease. Rhonchi may also be caused by events that narrow the bronchial lumen. Rales are heard mainly or only during inspiration, whereas rhonchi are heard during inspiration and expiration and may be more prominent during the latter.

Rales are often further divided and described as fine, medium, or coarse (Fig. 9-18). Fine, or crepitant, rales have a high-pitched, interrupted sound, which may be simulated by holding a lock of hair near the ear and rubbing it between the fingers. This sound can also be mimicked by moistening the thumb and forefinger with saliva and separating them slowly near the ear. Medium or crackling rales are both louder and lower pitched and resemble the "fizz" of a freshly opened carbonated drink or the crackling of rolling a dry cigar between the fingers. Coarse, bubbling, or gurgling rales are lower pitched

Figure 9-18. Schematic representation of rales. Note that rales consist of a number of discrete sounds, and that as they progress from fine to coarse, they occur earlier in inspiration. (Adapted from J. A. Prior and J. S. Silberstein. *Physical Diagnosis: The History and Examination of the Patient* (4th ed.). St. Louis: Mosby, 1973.)

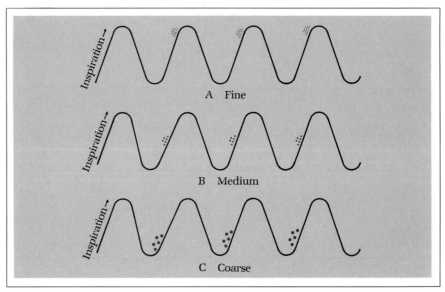

and loud. They are at times referred to as the "death rattle." They often are relieved by vigorous cough or mechanical aspiration.

Fine rales imply alveolar inflammation, exudate, and congestion, conditions found in clients with diseases such as pneumonia, congestive heart failure, and pulmonary edema. Fine rales are produced by the passage of air through secretions and also by the reinflation of alveoli whose walls have adhered together as a result of moisture and secretions. These rales often occur in "showers" at the end of inspiration as the alveoli distend. The fine rales of both pulmonary congestion and impaired pulmonary ventilation may disappear after a few deep breaths or coughs, but congestive rales reappear shortly thereafter.

Occasionally, fine rales are heard only after a cough and are then called *latent, or posttussive, rales.* To demonstrate these rales, have the client exhale completely and then cough without first taking a breath. You should hear a shower of medium rales on inspiration following the cough. You will probably have to demonstrate this maneuver to him. These rales, elicited only by coughing, are often present with a tuberculous lesion.

Atelectatic, or marginal, rales are crepitant-type rales that may be heard with initial deep breaths in the periphery of the lungs or the dependent portions. The lungs are never fully expanded during normal respiration, and secretions and moisture tend to accumulate in the unaerated portions, especially in dependent ones. These rales are heard only in the periphery with the first few deep breaths and then disappear after a few breaths as that portion of the lung becomes aerated. They have no pathologic significance.

Medium rales represent a gradation between fine and coarse rales and are thought to originate with the passage of air through mucus in the bronchioles or separation of the bronchiolar walls that have adhered because of exudate. These rales are most commonly heard in bronchitis and pulmonary congestion.

Coarse rales have their origin in the trachea and main and smaller bronchi. These bubbling, gurgling rales are often heard with the resolution of acute inflammation, when large amounts of thick exudate are present in the airway. They may diminish or disappear with a vigorous cough that clears the exudate. However, they may also be heard in the acutely ill, moribund client who has a depression of the cough reflex and accumulation of thick secretion. Coarse rales are also heard with severe pulmonary edema.

A *rhonchus* is a prolonged, continuous rale that has a musical note like that of a reed instrument or the violin. It is present in both phases of respiration, although there may be distinct differences in pitch, intensity, quality, and duration in one phase as compared with the other. If high-pitched, these sounds are called *sibilant rhonchi* and are often wheezing or squeaking. If low-pitched, snoring, or moaning, they are called *sonorous rhonchi.* A dry, coarse rale is interchangeably called a rhonchus by many.

The sound of a rhonchus is caused by an obstruction or narrowing of the

Figure 9-19.
Causes of rhonchi. *A.*
Narrowing of entire
circumference of lumen,
which may be caused by
inflammation with edema,
stenosis, or tumor. *B.*
Strands of thick secretions,
which vibrate with the
passage of air. *C.* Unilateral
narrowing of lumen,
caused by presence of a
tumor or resulting from
extrinsic compression by
enlarged lymph nodes or
tumor. (Adapted from J. A.
Prior and J. S. Silberstein.
*Physical Diagnosis: The
History and Examination
of the Patient* (4th ed.).
St. Louis: Mosby, 1973.)

tracheobronchial tree (Fig. 9-19). The change may be due to fluid or solid tissue within the lumen (for example, thick wet mucus), in which case the bronchial lumen becomes smaller during expiration and the rhonchi higher-pitched. If this is the case, the rhonchi can sometimes be cleared by several coughs. Narrowing of the bronchial lumen may also result from extrinsic compression on the bronchus, as with enlarged lymph nodes or a mediastinal tumor, or intrinsic narrowing from an endobronchial tumor. Edema of the mucosa and bronchial spasm also cause intrinsic narrowing and may themselves cause rhonchi or exaggerate rhonchal sounds caused by exudate within the lumen. In clients with asthma or emphysema, conditions in which rhonchi are expected, they can sometimes be heard only by having the person exhale as completely as possible as one listens below the clavicle.

Friction Sounds

The pleural friction rub results when inflammation of the pleura causes loss of lubricating fluid so that the opposing roughened surfaces produce a creaking or grating sound when they rub together, rather than sliding silently over each other. This is caused most commonly by pleurisy, often from an inflammation of the lung tissue that has spread to the pleura. It may also be caused by a pulmonary embolus, peripheral pneumonia, or trauma to the chest wall that causes change in the parietal layer. A friction rub may be imitated by placing the palm of one hand over the ear and then stroking the back of that hand with the fingers of the other hand.

The friction rub characteristically sounds close to the ear. It is usually audible in both phases of respiration, although it may be heard only at the end of inspiration. Friction rubs are more commonly heard and are louder in the lower anterolateral chest, where there is greatest mobility of lung tissue. An existing friction rub generally becomes louder with a deep breath or when the stethoscope is held more firmly on the chest wall. A friction rub is almost always accompanied by discomfort.

It may sometimes be crucial to differentiate a rhonchus or coarse rales from a friction rub. A rhonchus frequently clears with coughing, unlike a friction rub, and is predominantly inspiratory, whereas a rub involves both phases of the respiratory cycle. Also, rubs are usually more localized, are felt or heard unilaterally, and have the characteristic of seeming very close to the surface. In

Table 9-3. Physical Findings in Common Respiratory Disease States

Disease	Thoracic Expansion	Vocal Fremitus	Percussion Note	Predominant Breath Sounds	Voice Sounds	Adventitious Sounds
Acute bronchitis	Normal	Decreased	Resonant	Decreased vesicular	Normal	Sonorous rhonchi, coarse rales
Chronic bronchitis	Decreased bilaterally	Decreased	Hyperresonant (esp. with emphysema)	Decreased or inaudible	Normal	Occasional rales at bases
Emphysema	Decreased bilaterally	Decreased	Hyperresonant	Distant	Decreased	Fine to coarse rales; sonorous rhonchi with associated bronchitis
Bronchial asthma	Diminished bilaterally	Normal	Normal	Vesicular	Normal	Sibilant rhonchi
Consolidation (pulmonary infections or pulmonary infarction)	Limited—splinting	Increased	Dull or flat	Bronchovesicular or bronchial	Increased; egophony; whispered pectoriloquy; bronchophony	Fine to coarse rales; occasional pleural friction rub
Localized bronchial infection with atelectasis (tumor, mucus plug, foreign body, stenosis due to inflammation)	Limited on affected side	Decreased or absent	Dull or flat	Decreased	Decreased or absent	Sibilant rhonchi; few rales if obstruction is incomplete
Pneumothorax	Limited on affected side	Decreased or absent	Normal or hyperresonant	Distant or absent	Decreased	
Pleural effusion	Limited on affected side	Decreased or absent	Flat	Absent over area of effusion	Decreased or absent	Possible friction rub
Compressed lung with patent bronchus	Decreased	Increased	Dull	Bronchovesicular or bronchial	Increased egophony; whispered pectoriloquy	
Pulmonary edema	Normal	Normal or diminished	Resonant	Often bronchovesicular	Normal	Fine, medium, or coarse rales; occas. sibilant rhonchi
Diffuse interstitial fibrosis	Diminished bilaterally	Decreased	Dull	Sometimes bronchovesicular	Usually increased	Fine and medium rales
Pneumonectomy	Absent on affected side	Absent	Dull	Absent	Reduced or absent	

addition, rhonchi do not become louder when one presses harder on the stethoscope. The physician should be notified of the possible presence of a friction rub.

Table 9-3 lists common respiratory diseases and the physical findings that most frequently accompany these diseases. These are included not because the nurse is expected to make a medical diagnosis, but to familiarize her with the features characteristic of certain diseases. In other words, the nurse should know that it is reasonable and expected for a person with chronic obstructive pulmonary disease (COPD) to have diminished chest expansion, wheeze, and other symptoms, but that it would be abnormal for that expansion to be significantly unequal—a finding that should immediately be reported to the physician.

If the nurse finds alterations during the respiratory system assessment, she should be able to use the data gained to counsel clients in the appropriate help-seeking behavior. It is not necessarily expected, however, that the nurse would use the complete examination at all times or in all situations. It is anticipated that she will be using parts of the examination intermittently to assist her in planning, validating, and evaluating nursing intervention. However, only by habitual and conscientious use of these physical assessment skills will they contribute to and enhance the nurse's practice.

RESPIRATORY SYSTEM-ASSESSMENT GUIDE

I. General Appearance
1. Posture—observe to see if client is leaning forward, propping clavicles
2. Skin color—look for cyanosis or ruddy cheeks
3. Neurologic status—observe for signs of air hunger, such as anxious facial expression, recent personality change, degree of alertness
4. Fingers—look for clubbing of fingernails, periodic flushing of nail bed
5. Cough and sputum production
   a. Ask client about frequency and forcefulness of cough, color, consistency, and amount of sputum
   b. Examine specimen

II. Nose and Paranasal Sinuses
A. Inspection
   1. Examine external nose for symmetry, nasal flare, adenoid facies; look for septal deviation and perforation (with pen light)
   2. Note color and size of turbinates; look for any ridges, spurs, polyps, or discharge in nasal cavity
B. Palpation
   1. Test each nostril for patency while occluding the other
   2. Palpate over paranasal sinus for tenderness

III. Oropharynx
A. Inspection
   1. Observe uvula for color and size
   2. As client says "ah" observe for midline uvular elevation and coordinated pharyngeal construction
   3. Look at palatine and lingual tonsils for their color and size; check for exudate or any other sign of inflammation and for presence of tonsillar tags
   4. Observe the anterior and posterior tonsillar pillars for their color and size

     5. Observe the posterior pharyngeal wall for color, edema, and presence of exudate

IV. Trachea

    1. Palpate for midline location

V. Thorax

  A. Inspection

    1. Observe the thorax for any scars or deformities

    2. Determine the width of the subcostal angle, the AP diameter, the amount of projection of the angle of Louis, the slope of the ribs

    3. Observe respirations for costal or diaphragmatic breathing, use of accessory muscles, refraction of interspaces, rales, depth and ease of respirations; ratio of length of inspiration to length of expiration

  B. Palpation

    1. Palpate over thorax for any tenderness or masses on chest wall

    2. Determine amount of thoracic excursion (expansion) of posterior thorax, anterior superior thorax, anterior inferior thorax; note both velocity and degree of movement

    3. Note degree of movement of costal margin

    4. Evaluate vocal fremitus for equal contralateral distribution; check for tussive, pleural friction or rhonchal fremitus

    5. Note the location and amount of any subcutaneous crepitation

  C. Percussion

    1. Percuss over the anterior, posterior, and lateral chest determining the location of the resonant note; also flat, dull, or tympanic notes

    2. Percuss to determine the amount of diaphragmatic excursion

  D. Auscultation

    1. Auscultate over the anterior, posterior, and lateral chest noting the location of bronchovesicular and bronchial breath sounds; note decrease or absence of breath sounds and any bronchial or asthmatic breath sounds

    2. Determine whether voice sounds are normal or whether bronchophony, whispered pectoriloquy or egophony is present

    3. Note any adventitious sounds, i.e., rales, rhonchi, or pleural friction rub

SUGGESTED READINGS

DeGowen, E. L., and DeGowen, R. L. *Bedside Diagnostic Examination* (3rd ed.). New York: Macmillan, 1976.

Forgacs, P. *Lung Sounds*. London: Bailliere Tendall (div. of Cassell and Collier Macmillan Publishers, Ltd.), 1978.

Judge, R. D., and Zuidema, G. D. (Eds.). *Methods of Clinical Examination: A Physiologic Approach* (3rd ed.). Boston: Little, Brown, 1974.

Delp, M. H. and Manning, R. T. *Major's Physical Diagnosis* (8th ed.). Philadelphia: Saunders, 1975.

Prior, J. A., and Silberstein, J. S. *Physical Diagnosis: The History and Examination of the Patient* (5th ed.). St. Louis: Mosby, 1977.

10. Physical Assessment of Circulatory Function

GLOSSARY   **aneurysm** Localized abnormal dilatation of the wall of a vessel, usually of an artery.

angina pectoris A paroxysmal, constricting substernal pain often radiating to the left shoulder and down to the hand.

apex of the heart Pointed portion of the heart, usually located near the left fifth intercostal space medial to the midclavicular line.

arrhythmia Any variation of rhythm from the normal (regular) rhythm of the heartbeat.

atrial fibrillation An arrhythmia which has rapid uncoordinated atrial activity associated with an irregular ventricular rhythm.

atrial flutter An arrhythmia in which atrial depolarization is extremely rapid (approximately 300/minute), regular, and uniform in its sawtooth appearance, and the ventricular rate and rhythm vary with the degree of atrioventricular block.

atrial tachycardia An arrhythmia originating in the atria, characterized by rapid, regular beating of the entire heart.

atrioventricular block (AV block) Slowing or interruption of impulse transmission from the atria to the ventricles. *Bundle branch block* occurs when there is impulse transmission alteration in the bundle of His and may be described as right or left bundle branch block, depending on the origin of the transmission alteration.

base (cardiac) Region of the aortic and pulmonic outflow tracts; usually the second or third intercostal spaces to the right and left of the sternum.

bradycardia Slow heartbeat (less than 60 beats per minute in adults).

bruit Extracardiac blowing sound auscultated over a vessel, usually an artery.

cor pulmonale Right-sided heart disease due to pulmonary disease.

cyanosis Bluish discoloration of the skin and mucous membrane due to oxygen desaturation, usually evident when circulating reduced hemoglobin exceeds 5 mg per 100 m.

diastole Dilatation; period of "relaxation" during which the atria or ventricles fill; corresponding with the interval between the second and first heart sound.

edema Accumulation of excessive amounts of fluid in the interstitial space, tissue, or lungs.

embolism Sudden occlusion of a vessel by a clot or other obstruction carried to its place by the blood current.

gallop rhythm Characteristic cadence created by three heart sounds, in conjunction with a tachycardia.

hypertension Transient or persistent abnormal elevation of blood pressure.

infarct Localized ischemic necrosis of tissue due to interference with its circulation.

midclavicular line (MCL) Vertical line midway between the sternal line and the acromioclavicular joint.

murmur Any adventitious auscultatory sound produced by turbulent blood flow within or near the heart.

palpitation Unusually rapid, strong, or irregular heartbeat felt by the patient.

point of maximum impulse (PMI) Commonly synonymous with *apex impulse*, the point of maximal thrusting of the heart against the anterior chest wall during systole.

presystolic Period immediately preceding the first heart sound; pertaining to the latter one-third of diastole.

protodiastolic Period immediately following the second heart sound; pertaining to the initial one-third of diastole.

pulse Expansile wave palpated over an artery resulting from ventricular contraction, usually ten times the speed of the actual blood flow.

shock 1-Acute peripheral circulatory collapse marked by pallor, coolness and clamminess of skin, hypotension, weak, rapid pulse, and decreased respiratory depth. 2-Palpable, short, high-frequency vibration over a vessel or precordium.

syncope Temporary unconsciousness; fainting.

systole Contraction; period of contraction during which the atria or ventricles eject blood. *Ventricular* systole includes the interval inclusive of the first and second heart sound (used alone, systole generally refers only to ventricular activity).

tachycardia Rapid regular heartbeat (more than 100 beats per minute in adults).

thrill Sustained high-frequency vibration felt on palpation.

ventricular tachycardia Arrhythmia originating in the ventricles, characterized by rapid regular beating of the heart.

I N examining the circulatory system it is important to remember that a complete investigation demands not only an evaluation of the heart, but also a careful assessment of the peripheral circulation. Problems arising from alterations in the peripheral circulation, which can be detected easily on physical examination, may be overlooked by the nurse examiner because of overconcentration on the myocardium. In this chapter the complete evaluation of the circulatory system will be discussed in terms of techniques of examination and normal and abnormal findings that often present themselves in adult subjects.

In collecting data for assessment, we usually assume that the person is normal until the investigation demonstrates otherwise. Because cardiovascular phenomena are sometimes transient, this mode of thinking may not always be satisfactory and makes it too easy to miss something. To facilitate the examination, reverse this process and demand negation of alteration, rather than presuming normality. Questions should always be on your mind as you examine. Is the pulse irregular? Is the blood pressure elevated? Is there an extra heart sound?

Another key factor to be considered is organization. Although necessary for all areas of physical examination, it becomes especially important here because of a unique factor involved in circulation, namely, *timing*. For example, although pulsation is continuous, each individual heartbeat consists of heart sounds that are finite, necessitating simultaneous use of multiple observational skills to collect valid data. Again, questions should be kept in mind. What is it I see, feel, or hear? What is its duration? How can it be described? Planning must be done to ensure a complete and efficient examination. Use of techniques and the order of the overall examination should be by design, not accident. Start with the interview. In-depth data collection in this area should provide direction for the physical examination to follow. Inspection, palpation, and percussion then indicate what you should be listening for, and why, when you finally proceed to auscultation. The order for the overall examination should be as follows: extremities, neck, and precordium. In this way you move logically from the periphery toward the center, the heart. However, if circulatory assessment is included as part of a multisystem or complete physical assessment a cephalocaudal (head to foot) approach might be used. Whatever the approach, a preplanned organizational pattern is the essential factor, for a complete, efficient examination. As with all areas of assessment, complete assessment requires that subjective client information, interview data, be collected prior to physical examination. With respect to circulatory status, certain topics should be included as part of the complete interview or, if client status prohibits this, as part of the priority area assessment. These topics are past or present history of rheumatic fever, heart disease, hypertension, edema, chest pain, pain in extremities, hair loss on extremities, skin temperature changes, skin color changes, increased or decreased sensitivity to heat or cold, headache, epistaxis, dizziness, palpitations, night sweats, paroxysmal nocturnal dyspnea, or family history of heart disease, hypertension, or cerebrovascular accident. When collecting these data, keep in mind that if the client offers an affirmative response, follow-up is essential. Complete data should include information about where, when, character, duration, frequency, association, radiation, exacerbation, and relief of the problem (the what).

In physical assessment of the circulation, the four techniques—inspection, palpation, percussion, and auscultation—are used extensively. Because the quality of the data collected for assessment of the circulatory system depends on the nurse's ability to use these techniques with ease, they will be discussed first.

TECHNIQUES
Inspection and Palpation

As in any examination, the first concern should be to establish a general picture. Observation of body build, general color, character of respiration, obvious pulsations, and presence of emotional tension will give this overview (see Chaps. 5 and 6).

Extremities

Examination should include both the arms and legs. As you proceed, compare findings on opposing extremities. Symmetry, or the lack of it, may be significant. With the client in a sitting or supine position, start distally by inspecting the toenails (fingernails) for shape, color of plate and bed, thickness, ridging, and mobility. To evaluate mobility, stabilize the digit to be tested by placing the palmar surface of the distal joint of the third finger of the examining hand along the palmar surface of the distal joint of the digit to be examined. Next place the palmar surfaces of the distal joint of the thumb and index finger of the examining hand on either side of the nail plate being examined and attempt to rock the plate between the thumb and index finger. Then palpate for capillary refill by pressing the tip of the client's toenail (fingernail) to produce blanching; release and note the time taken for color to return (Fig. 10-1). Capillary pulsation, although not routinely tested, can be evaluated by using the same maneuver and observing for pulsation before releasing the pressure on the nail. Estimate the skin temperature along the extremities. Palpate with the dorsal surface of the middle phalanges, or with the plantar surface of the fin-

Figure 10-1.
Method for evaluating
capillary refill. *A.* baseline
presentation of fingernails.
B. Blanched third finger.
(Photo courtesy of Jon
Marino.)

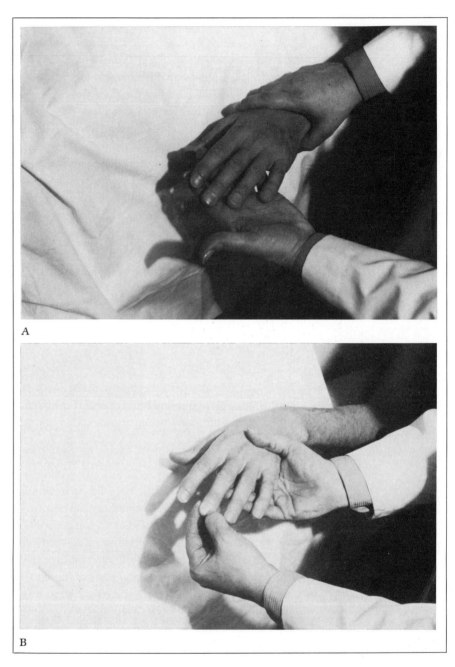

A

B

gertips, using a light rapid movement along the extremity (compare temperature gradations along opposing extremities simultaneously if possible). Skin color, hair distribution, and the presence or absence of any atrophy should then be observed.

Observe the pattern of venous circulation. Evaluate the degree of venous engorgement with the extremity in a dependent position and then gradually elevate the limb to heart level, noting the time and angle of dissipation of venous distention. Proceed by observing for the presence or absence of any swelling and then palpate for edema. The maneuver involves using the fingertip of one or two fingers to depress the skin surface over a bony area, removing the finger(s), and noting the appearance of the area immediately and the time taken for the depressed area to dissipate. Measure the limb circumference in centimeters wherever edema is suspected, and compare with the same area on the opposing limb. Note the location of the area measured in terms of centimeters proximal or distal to a bony landmark such as the malleolus or the tibial tuberosity. This notation helps to ensure that follow-up measurements are taken in the same place.

Before palpating the arterial pulses, observe for any obvious pulsations. Moving centrally, palpate the arterial pulses—dorsalis pedis, posterior tibialis, popliteal, femoral, radial, and brachial (Fig.10-2A–F). In palpating, use the three middle fingers, occlude the vessel completely, then lighten the pressure gradually. Determine the pulse rate, rhythm, force (amplitude), elasticity of the vessel wall, and quality. Elasticity of the vessel wall is established by occluding the vessel with the most proximally placed of the three examining fingers while lightly palpating the vessel with the two distally placed fingers. If two hands are used, occlude the vessel with one hand while palpating the vessel distal to the occlusion with the other. The quality of a pulse should be established after the examiner has lightened the initial pressure exerted over the vessel. The purpose of occluding or initially exerting a very firm pressure over a vessel is a technique to assist the examiner in identifying a pulse. The initial occluding or very firm pressure will dam some blood proximal to the pressure area. Thus, when the examiner lightens the pressure the first several pulsations palpated will feel more pronounced than subsequent ones. This technique in conjunction with the use of three fingers to palpate is especially helpful in identifying pulses that are weak or difficult to locate due to surrounding musculature. Quality of the peripheral pulses should be noted on a 4+ scale.

Palpation of the abdominal aorta should be done to ensure complete examination of the circulatory system. In addition to the data just mentioned, note any deviation of the abdominal aorta from the midline of the abdomen (see Chap. 11).

Finally, the lower extremities should be tested for calf tenderness and Homan's sign. Calf tenderness is evaluated by compressing the gastroenemius muscle anteriorly against the tibia and then pulling it away from the tibia. Homan's sign is elicited when the examiner sharply dorsiflexes the client's foot with the leg extended.

Neck

While the client is in a sitting position, observe for obvious pulsations and neck-vein distention. The carotid pulse can then be palpated in this position or after the client is placed in the supine position. Using the three-finger method, pal-

Figure 10-2.
Method for palpating
arterial pulses. (Note hand
placement for simultaneous
bilateral evaluation in A
and D). *A.* Dorsalis pedis,
B. Posterior tibialis, *C.*
Femoral, *D.* Radial, *E.*
Brachial, *F.* Abdominal.
(Photo courtesy of Jon
Marino.)

A

B

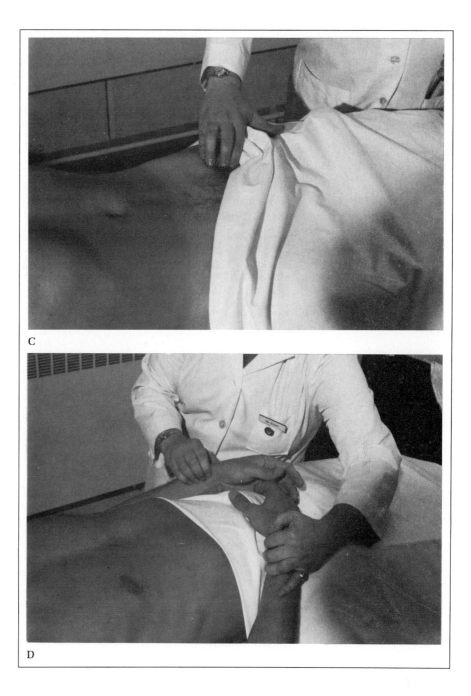

C

D

Figure 10-2.
Continued.

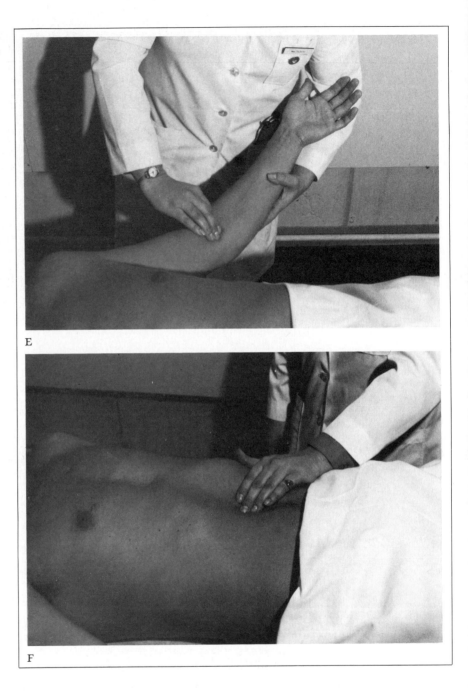

E

F

Figure 10-3.
Method for palpating the
carotid pulse. Note the
extension of the thumb on
the examining hand. (Photo
courtesy of Jon Marino.)

Figure 10-3.
Method for palpating the
carotid pulse. Note the
extension of the thumb on
the examining hand. (Photo
courtesy of Jon Marino.)

pate the carotid pulses by placing your fingers medial to the *sternocleido*mastoid muscle just below the jaw (Fig. 10-3). It should be noted that evaluation of pulsations of the neck should be done one side at a time to avoid possible occlusion of blood flow to the cerebrum. Collect data as delineated for the other arterial pulses.

Now, with the client in the supine position, observe for venous pulsations (Fig. 10-4). To be sure that you are observing the venous pulse, palpate a radial or carotid artery with one hand while gently palpating with the other what you consider to be the internal or external jugular vein. Note in the supine client the neck veins are distended and the venous pulse, undulating and diffuse in nature, differs from the arterial pulse, which is swift and localized. If difficulty is experienced, you can have the client inhale, hold his breath, and "bear down" briefly. This will cause the neck veins to distend further, as the change in pressure in the chest will diminish blood flow into the heart. Once the neck veins are located, perform the following maneuvers: (1) establish the character of the pulse; (2) observe the effect of respiration on pulsation; (3) observe the effect on pulsation of light pressure applied on the base of the neck; (4) observe the effect of a gradual elevation of the head of the bed to an upright position; and (5) time the pulsations. At present, use of the data on timing of venous pulsations is predominantly diagnostic in nature and falls primarily within the province of the physician. Details on the subject can be found in DeGowin and DeGowin [2], Judge and Zuidema [3], and Kampmeier [4].

Figure 10-4. Demonstration of jugular vein distention with the client in the supine position. (Photo courtesy of Jon Marino.)

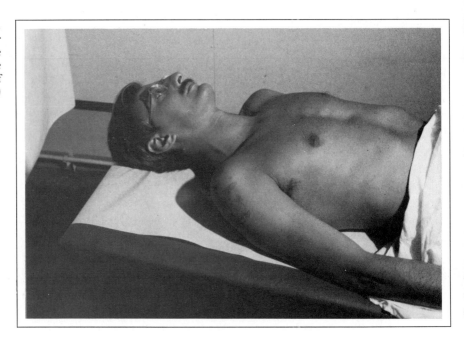

Precordium

Position yourself on the right side of the client with your right hip at the client's right hip and observe the anterior chest for any apparent pulsations in both the sitting and supine positions. Notation should be made of the character and location of the pulsations. Record the location of pulsations in respect to the intercostal space (ICS) and midclavicular line (MCL), or mid sternal line (MSL). To identify and number correctly the intercostal space, locate the angle of Louis, which is palpated as a prominence on the upper third of the sternum. Once the angle of Louis is located, move your fingers laterally, to identify the second intercostal space (see Fig. 9-8B and discussion on the landmarks of the chest). To facilitate demonstration of pulsations on the chest, have the client exhale and hold his breath. This maneuver reduces the lung volume between the chest wall and the great vessels, making the movement of the heart more obvious. If this technique is used, you should include in your instructions to the client that he hold his breath only as long as it is comfortable and that he should resume breathing at his discretion. In this way, you can concentrate on data collection and not be concerned about how long the client has been holding his breath. Placement of a tongue blade over the precordium and observation for the movement of the free edge also helps to amplify the pulsations (see Fig. 10-5). At the same time, note any bulging or prominence of one side of the chest as compared with the other. If the apical impulse is still not identified, try having the client turn to the left lateral position. This maneuver, like breath holding, moves the heart closer to the chest wall. If the PMI is located in this

Figure 10-5.
Method of amplifying the
apical impulse using a
tongue blade. *A.* Midpoint
of tongue blade resting over
apparent PMI. *B.* End point
of tongue blade held gently
over apparent PMI—useful
if curve of chest does not
permit midpoint technique.
(Photo courtesy of Jon
Marino.)

A

B

Figure 10-6. Palpation of the precordium. *A.* Correct palmar surface hand position in supine position. Note extension of the index finger to facilitate curve of palpating hand. *B.* Correct fingertip-hand position. *C.* Correct hand position when palpating chest with the client in left lateral position. *D.* Demonstration of correct position of the breast during precordial palpation of a female. (Photo courtesy of Jon Marino.)

A

B

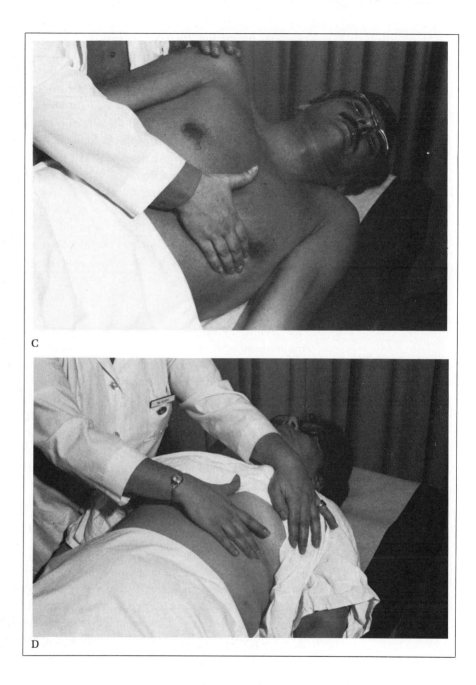

C

D

position, record that the PMI was located in the left lateral position. This notation is important as the heart moves laterally when the client is turned to the left. Next, palpate the precordium for pulsations, again noting their character and location. The main objective is to identify the apex impulse or point of maximal impulse (PMI).

In performing palpation, both the fingertip and palmar surface methods are acceptable. The application of the palmar surface of the first four phalanges, excluding the thumb, to the chest wall not only provides for the most comprehensive and accurate data, but also is easier to perform (Fig. 10-6). Shift your hand from place to place over the precordial area as you palpate. With female patients with large breasts, displace the breast upward with the palpating hand and hold it in this position with the other hand as necessary.

The four major areas of interest on the anterior chest are the apex or mitral area, the left sternal border or tricuspid area, the pulmonic area, and the aortic area (Fig. 10-7). Having the client exhale and hold his breath facilitates palpation, as the lungs will be retracted somewhat out of the heart's way, allowing for closer apposition of the heart to the chest wall and eliminating the distraction created by chest movement due to respiration. Again, if you use this technique, remember to instruct the client to hold his breath only as long as it is comfortable for him to do so. This technique is useful when examining a client with less prominent pulsations.

After palpating in the sitting and supine positions, have the client turn to his left side. This position makes it easier to locate the apex impulse if it has been difficult to do so with the client supine. It also assists in the identification of abnormal pulsations, as the heart is now angled more against the chest wall. The sitting position is useful when palpating the pulmonic and aortic areas of the heart. The technique of palpation is of great importance as it allows the identification of pulsations (including those of low frequency and intensity) that may be inaudible on auscultation.

Percussion   Of the four techniques used in the physical examination of the circulatory system, percussion offers the least information. It is not used in the examination of the extremities and neck. In the precordial examination percussion is used to appreciate the cardiac border. However, location of the border by percussion is affected by the client's respiratory movement and by any individual characteristic or event that causes elevation of the diaphragm. These factors, in addition to the fact that chest roentgenography more accurately demonstrates the size and contour of the heart, have led to the frequent omission of this portion of the examination. This author suggests that although x-ray examination may be more accurate, percussion gives the nurse examiner information that might not be readily available if x-ray equipment is not close at hand. In addition, percussion provides a way by which the nurse can easily note changes in the client's status.

Figure 10-7.
Demonstration of valve
areas on the chest. 1. Mitral
or apex area. 2. Tricuspid
area. 3. Pulmonic area. 4.
Aortic area.

Precordium

In examination of the heart, direct percussion (see Chap. 2 for discussion of direct and indirect percussion) can be most useful if guided by the following considerations:

1. Use a light tap rather than a slap (sound changes can be more easily identified with the lighter touch).
2. Place the fingers flat and tangentially along the anterior chest, as it is a convex surface.
3. The movement of your hand should follow the curve of the chest. In addition, when the patient has large breasts you will have a hand free to hold the breast out of the way

When using indirect percussion, the same guides apply, but examining the patient with large breasts is likely to be more difficult. In indirect percussion, the pleximeter (underlying) finger can be placed either parallel or at right angles to the heart. Either way is acceptable (Fig. 10-8). Stand to the right side of the supine client and percuss from the left axillary area to the midline in the seventh, sixth, fifth, fourth, and third intercostal spaces. Record the point of change in the percussion note in each space. This information gives you the left border of cardiac dullness (LBCD). Once the left cardiac border is estimated, attempt to locate the right cardiac border by percussing toward the sternum along the second, third, and fourth intercostal spaces on the right anterior

Figure 10-8.
Direct and indirect
percussion of cardiac
border. *A.* Correct and *B.*
Incorrect method of hand
placement for direct
percussion. *C.* Correct
placement for indirect
percussion. (Photo courtesy
of Jon Marino.)

A

B

C

chest. Usually, the right cardiac border is not percussable, as it lies below the sternum. Data are recorded again in respect to the ICS and the MCL, or MSL.

Auscultation   Auscultation, like percussion, is used predominantly in the examination of the heart with the notable exceptions of its use in measuring arterial blood pressure and in evaluation of the carotid artery and abdominal aorta for bruits. Before discussing auscultation of the precordium, some comment about arterial blood pressure is appropriate.

Extremities
In measuring arterial blood pressure, several points should be remembered. To ensure a true baseline measurement, the client should be in a stable position, sitting or supine, for at least five minutes before the arterial blood pressure is taken. The palpatory technique should be employed prior to auscultation to prevent excessive inflation of the cuff when auscultating. When palpating, inflate the cuff only until the palpable pulse disappears. Although an estimation of diastolic pressure is possible by noting the change from *bounding* pulsation to *normal,* the chief concern when palpating is to establish the systolic pressure by noting the first reappearance of the pulse. With the diaphragm endpiece of the stethoscope placed lightly over the brachial artery, cuff inflation should be only 20 to 30 mm Hg above the palpated systolic pressure. Release the cuff pressure 2 to 3 mm Hg at a time. The first sound to reappear, designated phase I Korotkoff, is the systolic pressure. Phase II, the bruit sound, and phase III, the

loud sharp sound, follow as the cuff pressure falls. Phase IV, the muffling or damping of the sound, is considered by the American Heart Association to be the most accurate measure of diastolic pressure. However, many sources still recommend the final disappearance of sound, phase V, as the best index of diastolic pressure. Recently, arterial blood pressure recording has included both the phases IV and V in addition to the systolic first phase (e.g., 130/86/70). Since the purpose of taking an arterial blood pressure is to determine a baseline for later comparative readings, it is more important for the health team to establish a consistent procedure than it is to debate the appropriateness of using phase IV or V, or IV and V, as any one of these is appropriate.

The final point to consider is cuff size. The rule of thumb is that the width of the inflatable bladder of the cuff should be 20 percent greater than the diameter of the extremity on which it is used [1]. The use of the wrong cuff size can lead to the collection of inaccurate data (usually, elevated results, as the cuff is too narrow). The question of cuff size becomes especially important when dealing with the obese client or when measuring the arterial blood pressure in the leg. When it is necessary to use the leg, the palpatory technique is usually satisfactory, as it generally is not essential to establish a diastolic pressure. When possible, the cuff should be applied to the calf and the posterior tibial artery palpated. The thigh usually demands a large cuff width that may not be readily available. To ensure complete data collection, the arterial blood pressure should be taken in both arms.

Several other extraneous factors can lead to error in measurement, for example:

1. Wrapping the cuff too loosely can give a false result, usually too high.
2. Emotional responses to the situation, the environment, or the examiner can also lead to elevated results. To overcome this, take the measurement at least twice during the examination with a minimum intervening time period of 10 minutes.
3. Presence of an "auscultatory gap" can lead to falsely low systolic values. This phenomenon occurs when sounds heard initially, as the cuff pressure is decreased from suprasystolic levels, disappear, only to reappear 10 to 15 mm Hg lower. Using correct palpatory technique before auscultation is the best defense against this possible error.
4. Presence of feeble Korotkoff's sounds can make auscultation difficult and thus unreliable. Having the client raise his arm prior to cuff inflation and then inflating the cuff in this position diminishes venous pressure. This may make sounds louder. Once the cuff is inflated, have the patient lower the cuffed arm and proceed as usual. If the sounds are still making measurement unreliable, you may have to accept the results of the palpatory measurement.

Neck

Auscultation of the neck, often omitted in the young adult, should be done on all clients. Using the diaphragm endpiece, the examiner should auscultate over each palpated carotid artery, checking for possible bruits. A firm pressure should be used with the diaphragm endpiece. At this time or when doing the abdominal examination, the abdominal aorta should also be auscultated.

Precordium

Auscultation of the heart, the most difficult of the techniques to master, is the most important of the four. Use of the stethoscope is the only means available to identify many valvular alterations, even with the development and use of cardiac catheterization. Trying to distinguish a sound, its quality, and its duration is not easy. Discussion and recordings are helpful, but expertise is attained only by extensive practice. The ability to hear sound depends not only on the characteristics of the sound, but also on the examiner's ability to perceive it. If the equipment is inappropriate, the difficulties involved increase dramatically (see Chap. 2).

Sound. Sound has three components: frequency, intensity, and quality. Frequency, commonly referred to as pitch, is the number of vibrations a sound creates per second (noted in cycles per second, or cps). Intensity is the magnitude of the vibration and determines loudness. Intensity is measured in decibels. When overtones are added to the basic frequency of a sound we have the third component, quality. This component allows the listener to recognize the source of a sound, e.g., whether the sound is produced by a violin or a trumpet. Both sounds may be of the same frequency and intensity, but because of the overtones, the quality is different, and the careful listener can make the distinction. The hearing ability of the examining nurse is another major consideration and influences the perception of any generated sound. Generally, the human ear can perceive frequencies ranging from about 20 to about 16,000 cps. Sounds below or above these frequencies are difficult or impossible to hear [3]. If a sound's magnitude of vibration (intensity) is too low, the sound may not be heard, even though the frequency is within the audible range. Therefore, the hearing of a sound is a function of both frequency and intensity.

The relationship of intensity and frequency to heart sounds is shown in Figure 10-9. Note that the majority of heart sounds are inaudible and those that are within audible range fall predominantly in the lower frequencies. Furthermore, an examiner's conception of sound can affect what she hears. If inexperienced, the nurse examiner may find the frequency of a sound coloring her perception of its intensity. For example, in loudness comparisons, a high-pitched sound is often described as louder than a low-pitched sound, even when its intensity is actually less than that of the low-pitched sound. This occurs because the listener believes high-pitched sounds are loud and low-

Figure 10-9.
Comparison of auditory
threshold with average
intensity of cardiac sound
at various frequencies. Note
that only sounds of 25 to
600 cps are in the audible
range. (Adapted from Judge
and Zuidema [3].)

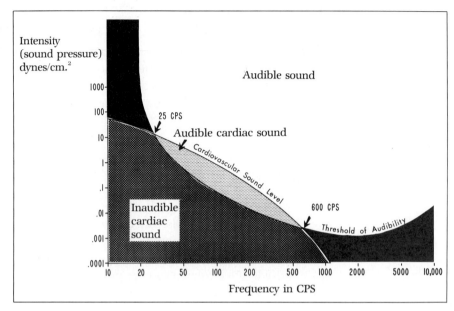

pitched sounds are soft. Thus it is important to note carefully what is heard, not only the overall impression of the sound, but also both of its individual components, pitch and loudness.

These factors, along with the masking phenomenon, are what make auscultation so difficult and palpation so important, for even though a sound may be inaudible, it may still be palpable. The *masking phenomenon* is the result of a defense mechanism of the ear, whereby it protects itself from loud (high-intensity) sounds by reducing its receptive ability. Masking comes into play when sounds following a loud one are faint. Because of reduced receptivity, these sounds may not be perceived by the listener.

Heart sounds may create this phenomenon, and so can extraneous room noise. The former must be accepted, but the nurse examiner must work constantly to overcome masking by consciously listening for the low-intensity sound which is so easily missed. Room noise can be minimized if not eliminated by preplanning, e.g., closing doors and curtains, turning off air conditioners.

Technique. A major difficulty for the inexperienced nurse is the identification of the first two heart sounds. Two maneuvers are helpful in making this discrimination. First, to identify S_1 correlate the sounds auscultated at the apex (PMI) or initial valve area with observation or palpation of the carotid pulse (Fig. 10-10). Because carotid pulsation is systolic in timing it is expected that the first heart sound (S_1) would just precede it, since it is produced, relatively speaking, by the closing of the mitral and tricuspid valves. In practice, you may perceive the sound to either immediately precede the carotid pulsation or occur simultaneously. In either case the sound isolated in this manner is S_1. The sec-

Figure 10-10.
Reference points for
localizing heart sounds.
Diagram demonstrates
actual valve locations and
the points to which their
sounds are usually referred.
(Adapted from Judge and
Zuidema [3].)

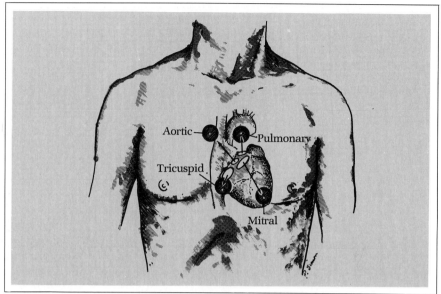

ond maneuver involves discrimination of the second heart sound (S_2). This is accomplished by listening at the aortic valve area of the chest (see Fig. 10-10). The second heart sound, produced by the aortic and pulmonary valves closing, is invariably loudest in this location. Once the loudest sound has been identified the examiner should move the stethoscope in a step fashion, on a diagonal line toward the apex (PMI), keeping this loudest sound as the focus. You will notice that with each step toward the apex (PMI) this loudest sound decreases in intensity. This changing sound is S_2. The former maneuver is also helpful in the timing of murmurs or extra sounds, especially when the heart rate is rapid or the quality of sounds is abnormal. Take time to develop skills in the use of these maneuvers. Effective auscultation of the heart requires confidence in your ability to distinguish S_1 from S_2.

Another problem auscultation often poses for the inexperienced examiner is the proper use of the bell endpiece. This endpiece is used to auscultate the precordium, as most heart sounds are of relatively low pitch and the bell provides for the best amplification of these sounds. If only the diaphragm endpiece were used in the examination, some sounds might be missed as it does not effectively transmit low frequency sounds. However, this feature of the diaphragm endpiece makes its use a helpful adjunct in the examination. Because it masks out low frequency sounds, its use enables the nurse examiner to concentrate more easily on the high pitch sound identified by the initial use of the bell endpiece. This is especially helpful when auscultating the base of the heart, where the relatively high pitch sounds tend to originate. However, when using the diaphragm endpiece the nurse examiner must keep its masking effect in

Figure 10-11. Correct method for holding bell endpiece of stethoscope, permitting use of variable pressure against the chest wall. (Photo courtesy of Jon Marino.)

mind. When using the diaphragm endpiece a *firm touch* provides the best results (for further discussion see Chap. 2).

To use the bell endpiece effectively a *light touch* is essential as too much pressure can destroy the transmission of low frequency sounds. To facilitate good control of the endpiece, consider the following maneuver. At the apex, place two or three fingers of your right hand (left, if you are left-handed) on the client's chest wall to allow for pressure variation against the chest wall while the other two or three fingers hold the bell endpiece in place (Fig. 10-11). While listening, start by pressing the bell firmly against the chest wall and then slowly lighten the pressure. The sounds should become louder and clearer, then eventually softer as you lift the bell endpiece off the chest. This maneuver helps one to develop the desired *light* touch.

Before beginning to listen, establish a routine. Determine what kinds of data you need to collect and how to proceed; doing this will help you to avoid omissions and facilitate efficiency. As for data collection, each time you place the stethoscope on the chest your routine should include:

1. *Notation of rate and rhythm.* Is the rate excessively fast or slow? Is the rhythm irregular in any way? How does the apical pulse correlate with the peripheral pulse?
2. *Identification of the first heart sound.* What is its intensity, pitch, and duration? Is it unusually loud, soft, or accentuated?
3. *Identification of the second heart sound.* What is its intensity, pitch, and duration? Is it unusually loud, soft, or accentuated?

4. *Relationship of the first and second heart sound.* What is the relationship of the first sound to the second in respect to intensity, pitch, and duration?
5. *Identification of extra sounds and murmurs.* Once the first and second sounds are described, concentrate on systole and diastole separately. Are there any extra sounds? If yes: When does it occur (systole-diastole)? What is its intensity, pitch, duration, and quality?

After listening over the entire precordium, note the location where any extra sounds you have identified were heard with maximum intensity. Finally, note the transmission of the murmur, if one was heard.

When developing your procedure, keep in mind that you should listen for one thing at a time in respect to your data collection routine (e.g., S_1 intensity). This suggestion may at first seem time-consuming, but in the long run it will actually reduce the time required for the examination.

Avoid "jumping" from valve area to valve area, or important data might be missed. Instead, move the endpiece in small increments across the chest from the apex toward the tricuspid area, up along the sternal border to the pulmonic area, across the sternum to the aortic area, and then diagonally back across the chest to the apex.

Changes in client position bring the heart closer to the chest wall, increasing the loudness of certain auscultatory sounds. The left lateral position usually provides for louder sounds at the apex, whereas the sitting position makes audible some murmurs otherwise inaudible at the left sternal border and base. Exercise can also assist in identifying extra sounds or murmurs; however, it is not usually considered part of the routine examination.

Alterations in respiration can affect the location and identification of sounds and murmurs, which is another reason listening over the four valve areas alone is not satisfactory. If breath sounds interfere with auscultation, having the client hold his breath at the end of expiration helps to intensify distant or weak heart sounds. Once again, if you use this technique remember to instruct the client to hold his breath only as long as it is comfortable for him to do so.

NORMAL AND ABNORMAL FINDINGS

To make proper interpretations of collected data, a thorough understanding of the physiologic interrelationships involved in the circulatory system is essential. While it is not the purpose to detail these interrelationships in this chapter, certain observations about them merit comment here.

The circulatory system is constantly adapting to changes in a person's internal and external environment. These adaptations, which maintain homeostasis, are expected to occur, and from them, the normal range of findings is established; for example, with exercise, an increase in pulse rate is expected. In addition to these variables, individual characteristics influence data interpretation. Thus, an acceptable blood pressure for a 72-year-old man may not be appropriate for a 21-year-old athlete or a 26-year-old pregnant woman. On examination, however, the findings in all three cases may still fall within the "normal" range, once their individual characteristics and the circumstances under which these data were collected are considered.

Proceeding from the extremities to the precordium, and from inspection to auscultation, the following should serve as guidelines to the detection of normal and abnormal findings.

Extremities   *Inspection and Palpation: Normal Findings*
Normally, the fingernails and toenails are convex in shape, the plates are transparent, the tips translucent white, the beds pink, the surface smooth or with some longitudinal ridges, and the mobility is negligible (Fig. 10-12). Capillary refill is immediate, and capillary pulsation is extremely difficult to demonstrate, if at all possible. Generally, skin temperature is warm over the entire extremity and symmetrical with the opposing extremity. Color and hair distribution are consistent with the rest of the body and are also symmetrical with the opposing limb. In the dependent position, superficial venous distention is apparent, and venous valves may be identified as nodular bulges. Collapse of the veins occurs when the extremity is elevated to heart level. The vessels themselves are easily movable, flexible, and without tortuosity. Swelling and atrophy are absent (see Fig. 10-12A and B).

Normal adaptation as a result of autonomic stimulation can create either vasodilatation or vasoconstriction. In either case, the responses observed in the extremities are symmetrical. Vasodilatation is demonstrated by warmth, rubor, capillary pulsation more apparent than usual, and throbbing of the digits. With vasoconstriction, the results are coldness of the extremities, pallor, and collapse of the superficial veins. A warm environment may cause vasodilatation. Vasoconstriction can be induced by smoking, anxiety, or a cold environment.

The normal resting pulse rate in the adult ranges from 60 to 100 beats per minute, with women tending to have higher rates than men. Rates greater than 100 beats per minute may be the result of anxiety and should be rechecked after the client has been at rest to ensure validity. Well-conditioned athletes can, and often do, have rates in the 50s without circulatory compromise. Generally, the rhythm is regular.

Two frequently demonstrated irregularities that are within normal limits are sinus arrhythmia and occasional premature beats. In *sinus arrhythmia,* the pulse rate increases with respiratory inspiration and decreases with expiration. This pattern is usually seen in children and young adults and occasionally in older people. The arrhythmia can also be created or exaggerated if the client takes several deep rapid inspirations in association with prolonged expiration or with irregular respiratory cycles. Anxiety over the examination can lead to such an alteration in respiration and to this arrhythmia. This can be evaluated by correlation of the pulse rhythm with respiration. If correlation between pulse rhythm and respiration is demonstrated, you should check the rhythm again later in the examination. If the arrhythmia is due to an altered respiratory cycle

Figure 10-12. Normal venous distention of the extremities. *A.* Upper extremity in dependent position; note apparent distention. *B.* Upper extremity at heart level; note absence of venous distention. (Photo courtesy of Jon Marino.)

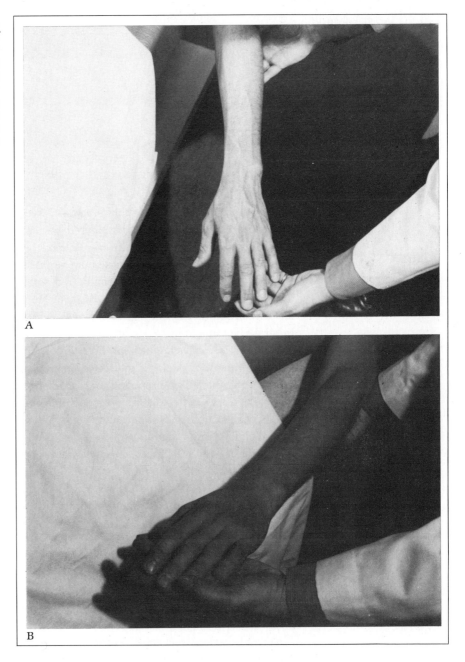

A

B

resulting from anxiety, it frequently dissipates as the client becomes more re-laxed during the examination. *Premature contractions* are usually the result of an early systole, with the pacemaker arising outside of the usual location, the sinoatrial (SA) node. They are common and generally present no problems except for a subjective effect they occasionally have on the people experiencing them, who often make the remark: "My heart skips beats once in a while"; or

Figure 10-13.
Diagramatic method of
recording peripheral pulse
quality. Rt (right), Lt (left),
B(brachial), R (radical), F
(femoral), AA (abdominal
aorta), p (popliteal), PT
(posterior tibialis), DP
(dorsalis pedis), Scale 0 to
4+ is used; 2+ is normal.
/ is used to indicate
absence of this portion of
the extremity.

	B	R	F	AA	P	PT	DP
Rt	2+	2+	2+		2+	2+	2+
Lt	2+	2+	2+		2+	2+	/

"Occasionally my heart stops for a second." Keep in mind it is the occasional premature contraction that is considered normal. Any degree of frequency of premature contractions noted in examination or from interviewing should be investigated more closely as disease may be present.

Force, or amplitude, is the reflection of the magnitude of the pulse pressure, the difference between systolic and diastolic pressure. As pulse pressure is related to stroke volume, any gross changes here will effect the force. Increases in stroke volume cause widened pulse pressures, thus creating an increased force. Exercise, ingesting alcohol, heat, and excitement all create an increased stroke volume. This factor is measured when pulse quality is evaluated.

Elasticity refers to the rebound and expansile action of the vessel wall. Normally, an artery is flexible, nontortuous, and nonpalpable after the blood has been forced out of it. *Quality* (character of the pulse wave) is a function of the rate of change and magnitude of the pulse pressure. It is best evaluated at the carotid artery (discussed in the section on the neck). Symmetry or lack of it is a key concern in evaluating the quality of the peripheral pulses. On a 4+ scale, normal, strong, localized pulses are recorded as 2+, absent pulses as 0, weak and thready pulses as 1+, bounding pulses as 3+, and water hammer pulses as 4+. Keep in mind that these numbers refer to the pulsation qualities, not how difficult the pulse was to identify. If a pulse is absent, such accompaniments as a cool to cold skin temperature and bluish skin color distal to the absent pulse usually are found. Figure 10-13 demonstrates an easy method of recording peripheral pulse quality.

Inspection and Palpation: Abnormal Findings
Abnormal findings reflecting cardiovascular disease and demonstrated by inspection and palpation of extremities are generally: clubbing, cyanosis, edema, varicosities, thrombosis, arterial occlusion, and aneurysm.

Clubbing. Clubbing of the fingers or toes in the early stages is demonstrated by a flattening of the angle of the base of the nail and increased mobility of the nail. Progressively the longitudinal curvature of the nail is increased, giving the finger a drumstick-like appearance (see Fig. 10-14). While the major cardio-

Figure 10-14.
Diagram of clubbing. Note
the drumstick or watch-
crystal-like appearance of
the nails.

vascular causes of clubbing are congenital cyanotic heart disease, cor pulmonale, and subacute bacterial endocarditis, there are many other causes of clubbing [3].

Cyanosis. Central or peripheral cyanosis is usually caused by congenital
heart disease with right to left shunting, pulmonary disease involving arteriovenous fistulas, or incomplete gas exchange. Clients with polycythemia frequently exhibit central cyanosis because of the changes in red blood cell production, even though their oxygen tension is relatively high. The bluish
discoloration is observed best in the inner side of the lips, tongue, and conjunctiva. Peripheral cyanosis occurs when there is a drastic decrease in systemic blood flow, usually as a result of a low cardiac output, as in congestive
heart failure or peripheral vascular obstruction. In this situation the restricted
arterial blood flow leads to an increased extraction of oxygen from the blood
in peripheral areas, thus increasing the amount of reduced hemoglobin. The
result is localized cyanosis, usually in conjunction with coldness and mottling
of the skin. This type of cyanosis is usually seen in the hands, feet, outer side of
the lips, and the earlobes. It is demonstrated by a light, one-finger pressure on
the bluish skin, producing a blanched imprint that dissipates slowly when the
testing finger is removed from the skin surface.

Edema. Cardiac edema is usually dependent (hands, feet, ankles), pitting,
and bilateral in nature. Pitting edema is graded from 1+ to 4+, with 1+
being a slight depression on the skin surface from finger pressure which disappears relatively quickly; 4+ is a deep depression which disappears very
slowly. As pitting edema is also graded on a 3+ scale, notation of the scale
used, in addition to the grade, promotes better understanding of the findings.
Although guidelines are available, the grading of edema is still subjective. Comparison of findings with associates and practice are the best ways to develop
confidence in one's judgments.

Edema can also be demonstrated unilaterally, in which case it is often the
result of some peripheral cause, e.g., occlusion of a deep vein or artery. This
edema may be nonpitting or "brawny" in nature. Differences in the circumference of the limb area from one extremity to the other is the key determination
to make here. Measurements (in cm) are made, using a bony prominence as a

landmark. Record the circumference measurements and the distal, or proximal, distance from the landmark used.

Varicose Veins. Varicosities, which are dilated and tortuous vessels, if present, are usually demonstrated in the superficial leg veins. Because of the vessel distention, blood flow through the affected area is decreased, while the pressure in the vessel is increased. Causation is either primary or secondary in nature. *Primary varicosities* are due to an inherent weakness in the vessel wall and the valves, and are often found to be familial. This alteration is often bilateral. *Secondary varicosities* are usually the result of obstruction.

Varicosities are demonstrated best by inspection of the extremities in the dependent position. In the early stages, vessel distention and tortuosity are the key signs. The client may complain of aching pain in the calf which is relieved by elevating the extremity. Night cramping may also be experienced. With further venous insufficiency, the appearance of edema, pruritus, paresthesia, skin ulceration, and dependent cyanosis becomes common. With prolonged venous insufficiency, a brown discoloration of the skin about the ankles (due to iron deposits) may be demonstrated.

Often, the varicosities are found in the greater or lesser saphenous veins, both of which lie superficially. The greater saphenous vein extends from the dorsum of the foot along the medial aspect of the calf and thigh, where it empties into the femoral vein in the groin. The lesser saphenous vein extends from the lateral malleolus along the posterior calf and empties into the deep popliteal vein at the popliteal space. Both veins also connect with the deep system by means of communicating, or perforating, veins. When the valves of these perforating veins are compromised, the saphenous varicosities may fill from the deep veins. Once superficial varicosities are identified, determination is made of the competency of the valves of the perforating veins and involvement of the deep veins (Fig.10-15).

The *Brodie-Trendelenburg test* [2, 3] is used to evaluate valve competency. With the patient in a supine position, elevate the extremity and drain the venous blood. Stroking the vessels toward the heart facilitates drainage. Once the vessels are empty, apply a tourniquet to the thigh to occlude the superficial veins. With the patient in the standing position, note the direction and time for venous filling, and then release the tourniquet. The tourniquet should not be left in place for more than 60 seconds. Normally, the veins fill from below in about 35 seconds, and once the tourniquet is released, there is no further vein distention. Valve incompetency is demonstrated by rapid filling of the superficial varicosities from above. Further distention of the veins after the tourniquet is released may also occur.

Deep vein involvement is evaluated by *Perthe's test* [2]. With the patient standing and the superficial veins distended, apply a tourniquet to the midthigh and have him walk for 5 minutes. As the patient walks, the superficial veins drain if the deep veins are patent. This is due to the pumping effect of the

Superficial circumflex iliac vein

Superficial epigastric vein

Saphenous opening

Femoral vein

Femoral artery

Pubic tubercle

Great saphenous vein

Lateral accessory vein

Superficial external pudendal vein

Great saphenous vein

Popliteal vein

Small saphenous vein

Perforating vein

Muscle

Superficial fascia

Skin

Saphenous vein

Venae comitantes

Deep fascia

"Venous pump"

Lateral malleolus

Medial malleolus

Dorsal venous arch

Figure 10-15.
Diagramatic presentation of the venous system in the lower extremities. (R. S. Snell. *Clinical Anatomy for Medical Students* (2nd ed.). Boston: Little, Brown, 1981. Reproduced with permission.)

muscles on the deep veins. If the superficial varicosities do not drain, incompetence of the saphenous and perforating veins is present. If the veins increase in prominence and the patient complains of pain, deep vein damage is indicated. The exact level of deep vein incompetence may be determined by the *Ochsner-Mahorner modification* [2] of Perthe's test. After demonstrating deep vein involvement, move the tourniquet distally along the extremity, each time repeating the walking after application until the veins collapse with activity.

The level at which the vessels collapse is the point above which deep-vein incompetence begins.

Venous Thrombosis. Venous thrombosis, an obstructive alteration of the veins, is usually the secondary result of some mechanical, thermal, or chemical injury. Inflammatory venous thrombosis, or thrombophlebitis, may be superficial or deep in nature. Superficial thrombophlebitis produces localized pain, tenderness, redness, induration, and swelling of the affected vein segment. The involved vein is usually thickened and cordlike when palpated. With deep thrombophlebitis there is warmth, tenderness, swelling of the involved extremity (rather than just of the vein segment), and the pain is frequently described as excruciating, piercing, or sharp. In the dependent position, there may be superficial vein distention in the extremity. Arteriospasm with resulting pallor and diminished or absent peripheral pulses may occur. A low-grade fever also may be present.

Asymptomatic venous thrombosis, or phlebothrombosis, frequently involves the deep femoral or pelvic veins. Because of this, it is important to be alert for possible thrombosis, especially in the bed-confined or pregnant patient. Signs suggestive of phlebothrombosis are:

1. Unilateral swelling detected by comparing circumference measurements of the extremities at thigh and calf.
2. Low-grade fever and tachycardia of unknown origin.
3. Minimal ankle edema.
4. Tenderness when the gastrocnemius muscle is compressed anteriorly against the tibia but not when the muscle is pulled away from the tibia.
5. A positive Homan's sign (calf pain on sharp dorsiflexion of the foot).

A positive result on points 4 and 5 must be distinguished from muscle or tendon pain. As you evaluate the venous circulation, it is essential to remember that pulmonary embolism is a major complication of thrombosis.

Arterial Occlusion. As with the venous system, the arterial circulation can be directly altered either by inflammatory or by degenerative processes in the vessel wall. Whatever the cause, arterial compromise (occlusion) presents signs that involve not only the vessels themselves, such as hardened tortuosity of the vessel in arteriosclerosis, but also of the surrounding tissue. As pointed out in Judge and Zuidema [3], in the investigation of the extremity with possible arterial compromise, the following may be noted:

1. Diminished or absent pulses. Audible systolic bruits extending into early diastole heard over major arteries—femoral or subclavian.
2. Reduced or absent hair peripherally—over the digits and dorsum of the hands or feet.
3. Atrophy of muscles and soft tissue.

4. Thin, shiny, taut skin.
5. Thickened nails with roughened transverse ridges and longitudinal curving.
6. Mild brawny edema.
7. Coolness on palpation.
8. Intense grayish pallor on elevation of the extremity. Dependency after a minute or two of elevation produces a dusky, plum-colored rubor which develops very gradually (in 30 seconds to 1 minute).
9. Flat, collapsed superficial veins.
10. Delayed venous filling time. Empty the superficial veins by elevating the extremity. Prompt filling (less than 10 seconds) occurs normally with dependent lowering.

With prolonged arterial insufficiency, four additional signs indicative of imminent gangrene may be apparent [3]:

1. Bluish-gray mottling of the skin unchanged by position.
2. Early ulceration between or on the tips of the digits.
3. Tenderness to touch.
4. Stocking anesthesia [3].

In the early stages of insufficiency no apparent signs may be noted, and exercise testing may be valuable in promoting the manifestation of signs of alteration. The changes demonstrated are usually diminished or absent arterial pulses, skin pallor of the distal portion of the extremity, and possible systolic bruits on auscultation over major arteries.

With chronic insufficiency at the bifurcation of the abdominal aorta, sexual impotence and intermittent claudication extending into the buttocks also can occur. Finally, in acute arterial occlusion the onset is usually noted by complaints of intense pain, pallor, cyanosis, and absent pulses; tenderness and stocking anesthesia may also be present distal to the occlusion.

Raynaud's disease is a vasoconstrictive alteration of the arteries and arterioles in the hands and feet, usually precipitated by exposure to cold or anxiety. In describing an episode, the client usually comments on pain, paresthesia, and color changes that occur. At onset the affected area becomes blue, due to partial occlusion, and progressively becomes white and then red as vasodilatation occurs. Skin ulceration and edema are not common. Because this disease is episodic in nature, it is important to be alert for cues when taking the history and to avoid discounting the client's complaints because they are not readily apparent at the time of examination.

Buerger's disease (thromboangiitis obliterans) combines arterial with venous compromise in addition to nerve involvement. The disease starts with an inflammatory process and develops into arterial occlusion with resultant pain, ulceration, and gangrene. It is seen more frequently in men than in women, in smokers than in nonsmokers, and most often in persons from 20 to 40 years of age. Considering the changing life styles of women and men, especially in western cultures, these incidence ratios between the sexes are probably changing. With more women and less men smoking, future studies of Buerger's disease can be expected to demonstrate a more equal incidence between men and women.

Aneurysm. Aneurysm most often involves the aorta and the popliteal artery. It is usually palpable as a pulsatile swelling along the involved arterial segment, and a systolic thrill may be felt over the area. If the thrill is continuous, an arteriovenous fistula may be present. Rupture of an abdominal aneurysm is commonly accompanied by complaints of persistent and intense back pain. Groin pain, either unilateral or bilateral, may also be present.

Auscultation: Normal Findings

Like height, weight, or eye color, arterial blood pressure varies greatly among individuals. Two constant influencing factors to be considered are age and sex. Part of the process of aging is progressive arteriosclerotic change. Although this process is slower in women than in men, the results are the same, namely, increased systolic pressure. While sources differ as to acceptable ranges of values for adults, systolic pressures of 95 to 140 mm Hg and diastolic pressures of 60 to 90 mm Hg are usually considered normal. The pulse pressure (difference between systolic and diastolic pressure) should be between 40 and 50 mm Hg. However, in the older adult (70 years and above) recent research indicates that a systolic pressure of up to 195 in men and 210 in women with an associated diastolic pressure of up to 105 in men and 110 in women can be considered acceptable if no associated symptoms are manifested.

A difference of 5 to 15 mm Hg in pressures in the left and the right arm is not uncommon. Comparisons made between pressures in the upper and lower extremities often show a 10 mm Hg difference in the systolic pressure, the higher pressure being found in the lower extremity. Relationships between lying and standing pressures should demonstrate a systolic drop of less than 15 mm Hg on standing, with a corresponding rise of less than 5 mm Hg diastolic pressure.

Bruits, the extracardiac blowing sounds auscultated over vessels, are normal in young adults. They may be heard over the abdominal aorta between the xyphoid process and the umbilicus, in the midline. However, they may indicate vascular disease.

Auscultation: Abnormal Findings

Abnormalities in arterial blood pressure fall into two general categories: hypertension and hypotension.

Hypertension. Hypertension is a persistent elevation of arterial blood pressure. Persistence is the key and in many cases is more helpful in making a determination of hypertension than the pressure itself. When the pressure is consistently above 140/90 mm Hg, it is usually considered significant, except in the older adult. Episodes of epistaxis, severe headache, and irritability may accompany the elevated pressure. In the presence of an elevated pressure, especially when no other alteration is noted, close questioning of the client as to family history is important, for essential hypertension has a strong familial tendency. Keep in mind that it is the elevated diastolic pressure more than the systolic pressure that causes increased stress on the cardiovascular and renal systems.

Hypotension. Hypotension occurs as a result of a decrease in cardiac output, peripheral resistance, or total blood volume. It is often associated with dizziness, blurring of vision, sweating, and occasional syncope. Pressures below 95/60 mm Hg are generally considered significant if the client's baseline "healthy" pressure was within "normal" limits. In the older adult obvious adjustments need to be made. For those persons who are hypertensive normally, hypotension may occur with much higher pressures. This example should serve to point out the need to establish norms for clients whenever possible before making decisions as to the significance of data.

Neck   *Inspection and Palpation: Normal Findings*

On examination, the carotid pulse presents the same information as the other arterial pulses. The additional information the carotid pulse offers is the basic quality of the pulse itself. The character of the pulse wave, or quality, is best evaluated in the carotid, as it is a function of the rate of change and magnitude of the pulse pressure, and these factors can be distorted as one moves to more peripheral pulses. Figure 10-16 shows a sphygmogram of a normal carotid artery in conjunction with a phonocardiogram of normal heart sounds and an electrocardiogram (ECG) of a normal cardiac cycle. Notice that the percussion wave is initiated after the mitral valve (S_1) has closed and systole has begun. This split-second delay represents the time needed to move the pulse wave to the neck. The percussion wave is separated from the dicrotic wave by the dicrotic notch, which is caused by the closing of the aortic valve. The upstroke of the percussion wave normally takes 0.10 second, and the rounding of the crest, 0.08 to 0.12 second. The actual timing of each segment of the wave is important, but it is the force (amplitude) of the wave and the relationship of the segments in respect to systole and diastole that is most significant. On examination, then, the pulse wave demonstrated by inspection and palpation should manifest as the relationship of the timing and force of the percussion wave to the dicrotic wave as seen in Figure 10-16. Distinctions between the waves are difficult to make, as differences in the timing and force are small.

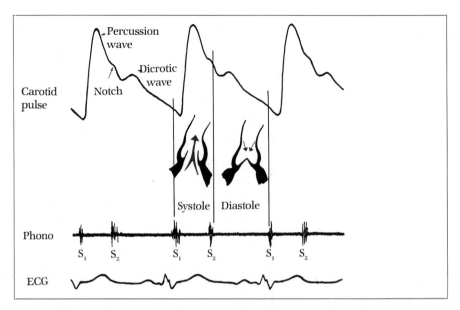

The normal carotid pulse is (1) localized and thrusting in character, (2) unchanged by respiration, (3) unaffected by light pressure on the root of the neck, and (4) unaffected when the client changes position.

The jugular veins of the normal person in the recumbent position are usually obviously distended, and pulsation is easily observed at the base of the neck. In the obese or "bull-necked" person this determination may be difficult to make.

The normal venous pulse is (1) diffuse and undulant in character; (2) decreases in rate with inspiration; (3) is obliterated by light pressure on the root of the neck; and (4) disappears when the client is elevated to a sitting position, usually by 45 degrees (Fig. 10-17A and B).

Inspection and Palpation: Abnormal Findings
Changes in quality of the arterial pulse when determined at the carotid artery provide information about various circulatory abnormalities:

1. *Anacrotic pulse* (see Fig.10-18A) is characterized by a delayed ascending limb of the wave (anacrotic notch) and a broadened summit. Although difficult to demonstrate, it can be appreciated on palpation as two beats during each systole, the ascending limb on the wave. This alteration is specific to aortic stenosis.

2. *Bounding pulse* is characterized by a widened pulse pressure in the presence of a normal or slightly lowered diastolic pressure. An increased stroke volume with a diminished peripheral resistance is also present. Common causes of this change in quality are complete heart block, anemia, hepatic failure, and fever.

3. *Water-hammer pulse* (see Fig. 10-18B) is an extremely bounding pulse with a low diastolic pressure. It is characterized by a steep ascending and descend-

Figure 10-17.
Jugular vein distention. *A.*
Venous distention in supine
position. *B.* Venous
collapse at 45-degree angle
of elevation. (Photo courtesy
of Jon Marino.)

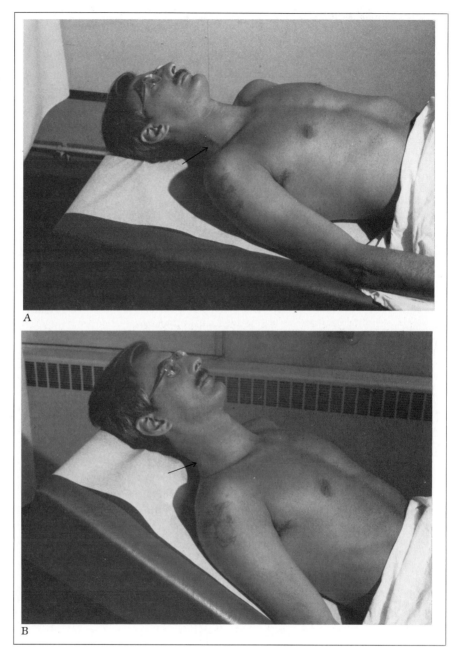

A

B

Figure 10-18.
Characteristic arterial pulse
wave sphygmograms with
simultaneously recorded
phonocardiogram and
electrocardiogram.
(Adapted from Judge and
Zuidema [3].)

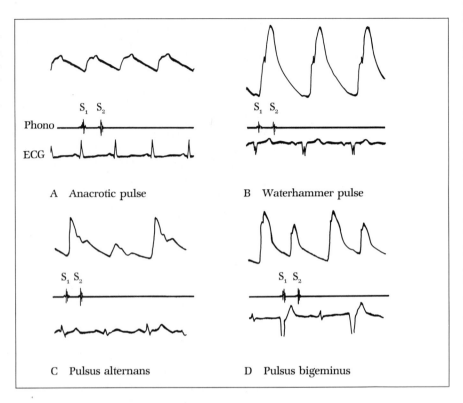

Figure 10-18. Characteristic arterial pulse wave sphygmograms with simultaneously recorded phonocardiogram and electrocardiogram. (Adapted from Judge and Zuidema [3].)

ing limb and a dicrotic notch that is absent or delayed downward. The pulse seems to tap or slap against the palpating hand. This collapsing, shock-like character is reinforced in the radial artery when it is palpated in the elevated extremity. This pulse is a classic sign of aortic insufficiency.

4. *Pulsus alternans* (see Fig.10-18C) is characterized by alternating large and small pulse wave amplitudes in regular rhythm. On palpation it is demonstrated as strong (high amplitude) and weak (small amplitude) pulsation. With a blood pressure cuff, the alternate systolic pressures may fluctuate as much as 25 mm Hg. This phenomenon is common in the presence of left ventricular failure.

5. *Pulsus bigeminus* (see Fig. 10-18D) is characterized by two beats coupled, followed by a pause (compensatory pause). The coupling usually is the result of alteration between a normal and premature beat. In addition, the second beat is weak, as the diastolic filling time is reduced. This can be seen with drug overdose (digitalis) or electrolyte imbalance.

6. *Pulsus paradoxus* is an exaggeration of the normal pulsation; that is, the pulse is perceptibly weaker on inspiration than on expiration, and vice versa. In normal persons, with inspiration there is an increase of the blood volume in the pulmonary system, which results in diminution of stroke volume and there-

fore of the volume in the peripheral system. With exhalation, the opposite occurs. These differences are slight and not usually demonstrated. Accentuation
of the differences occurs when there is an interference in the diastolic filling of
the ventricle. This is an important sign of possible cardiac tamponade, constrictive pericarditis, and sometimes of severe pulmonary emphysema.

Auscultation of the arterial blood pressure provides more objective data on
pulsus paradoxus. As pressure in the cuff is lowered, the first sounds are heard
only during expiration. With further reduction, the sounds are heard on both
expiration and inspiration. Differences of more than 10 mm Hg are usually
considered significant.

As indications of *localized alteration,* thrills and weakened or absent pulsation are the common carotid findings. Carotid thrill, which is common in aortic
stenosis, is also an indication of partial carotid occlusion. In the latter, a bruit
may be auscultated over the artery. Weakened or absent carotid pulses may be
the result of the aortic arch syndrome, a diffuse process involving the aortic
arch and its major branches. The syndrome can be caused by aortic aneurysm,
aortitis, or congenital anomalies.

Alterations that affect the jugular venous system are demonstrated by venous
distention or changes in the venous pulsation. *Jugular venous distention* is usually classified as mild, moderate, or severe. Venous engorgement (hypertension) is observed in right-sided congestive heart failure. However, any obstruction of blood flow to the heart can lead to venous hypertension. In long-
standing jugular venous hypertension, the veins are not only distended but tortuous in appearance. It is important to remember that distention must be present when the client is above a 45-degree angle from a supine position to be
considered abnormal. In addition, congestive failure can be demonstrated by a
positive hepato-jugular reflux (see Chap. 11).

Auscultation: Normal Findings
In the healthy adult no bruit is found over the carotid arteries. However, on
auscultation of the abdominal aorta, it is not uncommon to find a functional
bruit at or just above the umbilicus, as this is generally the location of bifurcation of the renal arteries. Typically it is heard as a systolic "blowing" or
"swishing" sound demonstrating the turbulence of blood flow at the bifurcation.

Auscultation: Abnormal Findings
A carotid bruit, demonstrated as a localized systolic "blowing" or "swishing"
sound, suggests a narrowing of the artery. This abnormality can be seen in
hypertension, especially in the older adult with arteriosclerotic changes, or as
a radiation of an aortic murmur.

An abnormal abdominal aortic bruit indicates partial obstruction. It can also
be a demonstration of turbulence resulting from an aneurysm.

Precordium   *Inspection and Palpation: Normal Findings*
What is seen and palpated over the anterior chest varies not only with the size and shape of the chest and amount of subcutaneous tissue, but also with position and phase of respiration. Normally, the chest is symmetrical and without bulges or retraction.

In the young asthenic (thin) person, the apex impulse is usually described as sharp, localized, and quick or prominent in nature. In the older person, it can be less prominent because of decreased elasticity of the chest wall. In the supine position it is generally visible and palpable at the fifth or sixth intercostal space, 1 to 3 centimeters medial to the midclavicular line (or 7 to 9 cm lateral to the midsternal line). It is 1 to 2 cm in diameter, occupying no more than one intercostal space with a duration of usually less than the first half of systole. In the short, deep-chested (hyperasthenic), or pregnant individual the apex impulse may be located at the fourth intercostal space, somewhat closer to or at the midclavicular line. The apex impulse may not be demonstrated either by inspection or palpation in the obese person.

Inspection and Palpation: Abnormal Findings
Abnormalities in precordial movement often represent hypertrophy of one of the ventricles. *Left ventricular hypertrophy*, commonly caused by aortic stenosis and hypertension, is demonstrated by an apex impulse that is displaced downward and laterally. The impulse is systolic and has a sustained, forceful, and thrusting nature described as a *heave* or *lift*. A palpable presystolic component or sound may occur, resulting in a double impulse (Fig. 10-19A). Use of the tongue blade technique shown in Figure 10-19B can facilitate its demonstration. With *left ventricular dilatation* a second impulse may occur, but it is protodiastolic (Fig. 10-20). *Right ventricular hypertrophy* presents a similar heaving impulse located over the precordium, just left of the sternum at the fourth or fifth intercostal space.

Impulses other than the apex or PMI can be identified. Pulsations that can be demonstrated in the second or third intercostal space are commonly found in pulmonary artery dilatation.

"Shocks," high frequency vibrations of short duration, are palpable heart sounds resulting from increased aortic or pulmonary pressure. "Thrills," high frequency vibrations that are well sustained, are palpable murmurs. It is important to note that although the presence of a thrill indicates a murmur, the absence of a thrill does not preclude the existence of a murmur.

Percussion: Normal Findings
Because of differences in body build and cardiac movement with respiration, specific measurements relating the normal left border of cardiac dullness can be misleading. Any individual characteristic or event (e.g., respiration) that causes elevation of the diaphragm moves the heart to a more horizontal posi-

Figure 10-19. *A.* Kinetocardiogram from patient with left ventricular hypertrophy. Note the presystolic extra sound, which correlates with presystolic component (a wave). *B.* Double apex impulse amplified by tongue-blade method. (From Judge and Zuidema [3].)

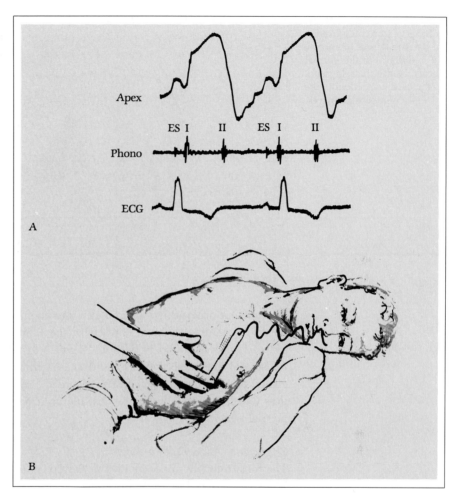

Figure 10-20. Double apex impulse with left ventricular dilatation. Sustained systolic component is followed by a smaller movement in early diastole. Notice the presence of a protodiastolic extra sound in this case. (From Judge and Zuidema [3].)

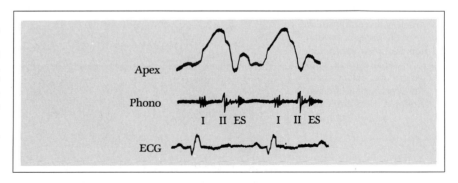

Figure 10-21. Characteristic configuration of the areas of cardiac dullness in the normal heart. Notice the relation of the cardiac borders to the intercostal spaces.

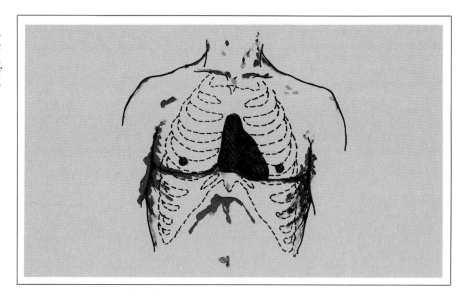

tion without necessarily indicating an alteration. In the asthenic client, the left border of cardiac dullness (LBCD) in the fifth, fourth, and third intercostal spaces is usually found to be 7 to 10 cm, 5 to 7 cm, and 2 to 4 cm from the midsternal line respectively (Fig. 10-21). Typically only the most laterally percussed point of cardiac dullness is recorded. The right border of cardiac dullness (RBCD) is usually not percussible as it lies beneath the sternum in the normal person.

Percussion: Abnormal Findings

The most frequent abnormalities in the precordium are related to cardiac enlargement. As Figure 10-22 illustrates, enlargement can be distinguished as to left or right ventricle by shape. In left ventricular enlargement, the displacement

Figure 10-22. Characteristic configuration of the areas of cardiac dullness in left ventricular enlargement, right ventricular enlargement, and pericardial effusion. (Adapted from Judge and Zuidema [3].)

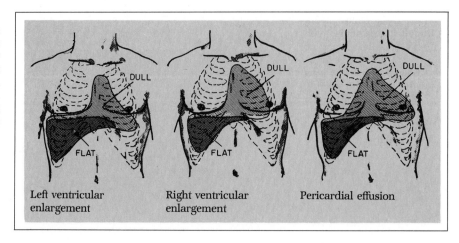

Left ventricular enlargement   Right ventricular enlargement   Pericardial effusion

is downward and lateral, usually about the fourth, fifth, and sixth intercostal spaces, creating a boot-shaped heart. With right ventricular enlargement the displacement is more lateral, showing changes in the third and fourth intercostal spaces. Pleural effusion, when considerable, is demonstrable and tends to create a triangle effect, with dullness to the left and the right of the sternum.

Auscultation: Normal Findings

The intensity (loudness), frequency (pitch), duration, and quality of the sounds heard are affected by such factors as location of the stethoscope in relation to the valves, client position, respiration, age, and body build. Sounds that are loud and clear in the young athlete may be almost inaudible or muffled in the older or obese person. Furthermore, listening at different locations on the same person can demonstrate differences in sound. Whereas individual characteristics form the basis for differences in the former situation, relative proximity of the valves to the anterior chest wall and the stethoscope in part determine the explanation in the latter.

Figure 10-23 illustrates the relationship between the cardiac cycle and the normal heart sounds in respect to their origin. The sounds of greatest importance are the first (S_1) and the second (S_2) sounds, since they divide the cardiac cycle into systole and diastole.

The physiologic third sound is a ventricular filling sound occurring in early diastole and is occasionally audible during periods of rapid filling. The physi-

Figure 10-23. Origin of heart sounds with correlation to the phonocardiogram and electrocardiogram. (From Judge and Zuidema [3].)

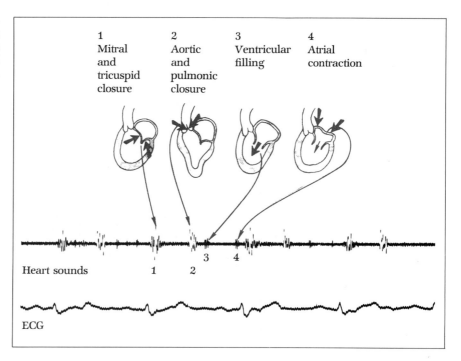

ologic fourth sound occurs late in diastole, just prior to the first sound. It is related to atrial contraction and is normally inaudible.

The illustrations in Figure 10-24 diagram the normal heart sounds at the valve areas, showing intensity (loudness) by height and the duration by width. The terms at the right of the diagrams are phonetic representations describing cadence.

The *first sound (S₁)* is louder, longer in duration, and lower in pitch than the second sound at the apex (see Fig. 10-24A). The mitral valve closes from 0.02 to 0.03 seconds before the tricuspid valve. Splitting of the first sound is therefore normally common, particularly in the tricuspid area (see Fig. 10-24B). Because the closing of the tricuspid valve usually is not heard well at the apex, a single-component first sound due entirely to the mitral valve is generally heard there.

The *second sound (S₂)* results from the combined closure of the aortic and pulmonic valves. This sound is almost always louder than the first sound at the base (see Fig. 10-24C). The aortic component is widely transmitted to the neck and over the precordium. As a rule, it is entirely responsible for S₂ at the apex. The pulmonary component is softer and is heard normally only at and near the second left intercostal space (pulmonic area). Splitting of the second sound is therefore best detected in this region.

Transient splitting of the second sound may be demonstrated in most normal persons at the end of inspiration (see Fig. 10-24D). Closure of the aortic and pulmonic valves during expiration is synchronous, or nearly so, because right and left ventricular systole are approximately equal in duration. With inspiration, venous blood moves into the thoracic cavity from the large systemic venous reservoirs. This increases venous return and prolongs right ventricular systole by temporarily increasing right ventricular stroke volume, thereby delaying closure of the pulmonic valve. At the same time, venous return to the left side of the heart diminishes, owing to the increased pulmonary capacity during inspiration. This in turn shortens left ventricular systole and permits earlier closure of the aortic valve. These two factors combine to produce transient "physiologic splitting" of the second sound.

The *physiologic third sound* is a faint, inconstant, low-pitched sound audible at or near the apex (see Fig. 10-24E). It is heard best when the patient is lying on his left side and frequently disappears when he sits up. It varies in intensity with respiration, usually becoming louder with expiration. It is common in children and young adults, but is rarely heard in older individuals.

The *physiologic fourth sound* is a low-pitched, short sound heard best at the apex with the patient lying on his left side (see Fig. 10-24F). This sound is rarely heard in the normal person.

Murmurs are gentle blowing sounds produced by turbulent blood flow within or near the heart. The *functional, or innocent, murmur* is commonly heard in children and young adults. This murmur is systolic in timing and is

Figure 10-24.
Normal heart sounds in
respect to valve area with
phonetic representation
included. (Adapted from
Judge and Zuidema [3].)

Figure 10-24.
Normal heart sounds in respect to valve area with phonetic representation included. (Adapted from Judge and Zuidema [3].)

Figure 10-25.
Representation of a functional systolic murmur. (From Judge and Zuidema [3].)

characteristically soft, short in duration, and variable. It is usually heard best at the pulmonic area or at the left sternal border. These murmurs vary with position and respiration and are not associated with any demonstrable heart disease (see Fig. 10-25).

Auscultation: Abnormal Findings

Abnormal findings on auscultation consist of abnormal heart sounds, murmurs, and friction rub.

Abnormal Heart Sounds. Abnormal *first heart sounds* are either accentuated in nature, as in hyperkinetic disorders (e.g., fever or mitral stenosis), or they are diminished (e.g., low output failure or heart block). In either case, an irregular rhythm usually is present.

Changes in the *second sound* also involve accentuation or diminution. With accentuation, pulmonary or systemic hypertension may be present. A diminished or inaudible second sound is associated with aortic or pulmonary stenosis.

Delayed closure of the pulmonic valve, usually due to overfilling of the right ventricle causing prolongation of systolic ejection time, results in a persistent

Figure 10-26.
Abnormal heart sound.
Representation of revised
splitting of S_2. (From Judge
and Zuidema [3].)

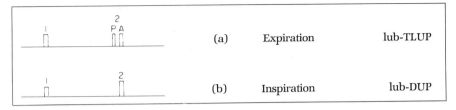

Figure 10-27.
Abnormal heart sound.
Representation of a
protodiastolic extra sound.
(From Judge and Zuidema
[3].)

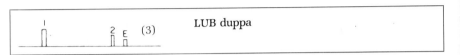

splitting of the second sound. This persistent splitting, splitting occurring throughout inspiration and expiration, may not vary with respiration (fixed splitting), or it may vary in the same manner as a physiologic split except that it widens more during inspiration. This is commonly associated with pulmonic valve stenosis and atrial ventricular septal defects. Right bundle branch block also may cause a persistent splitting.

Reversed or paradoxical splitting of the second sound results from delayed ventricular stimulation, as in left bundle branch block or prolonged left ventricular ejection time. In this situation the splitting occurs with *expiration* and disappears with inspiration as the normal mechanism of delayed pulmonic valve closure on inspiration compensates for the altered left ventricular activity (see Fig. 10-26).

Ventricular gallop is a pathologic appearance of the third heart sound, usually in the presence of an increased heart rate. Because it occurs early in diastole, it is also called a *protodiastolic sound.* It is heard best at the apex with the patient in the left lateral position. The sound occurs as a result of an overdistention of the ventricle in the rapid filling segment of diastole. Consequently, it is usually found in the presence of mitral insufficiency or ventricular failure. To facilitate distinction between normal and abnormal third sounds, remember that the normal third sound disappears when the patient is in the sitting position. With disease, the third sound persists (see Fig. 10-27).

Atrial gallop is the pathologic manifestation of the fourth sound. This sound, also called a *presystolic extra sound,* is dull and low-pitched and is heard best at the apex with the patient in the left lateral position. The sound occurs in the presence of forceful atrial contraction where there is resistance to ventricular filling late in diastole, such as in left ventricular hypertrophy. It is also seen with pulmonary stenosis (see Fig. 10-28).

Figure 10-28.
Abnormal heart sound.
Representation of a
presystolic extra sound.
(From Judge and Zuidema
[3].)

(4) E ⊓ | 2 ⊓   da-LUB dup

Murmurs. Except for the functional or innocent murmur previously mentioned, all murmurs should be considered abnormal. To make proper interpretations of information collected in respect to murmurs, the nurse examiner must understand the (1) production, (2) transmission, and (3) character of the murmur.

1. *Production.* Turbulence in blood flow can be produced by: (a) increasing the rate or velocity of the blood flow; (b) increasing or decreasing the diameter of a vessel or area through which the blood flows; (c) decreasing the viscosity of the blood; or (d) altering the normally smooth inner surface of the vessel wall. Blood flow velocity is a key determinant of intensity (loudness) and frequency (pitch) of the murmur. Increase the velocity of the flow (e.g., as in exercise), and the murmur becomes louder and higher in pitch.

2. *Transmission.* Murmurs, like all sounds, are loudest at their point of origin, and the closer the site of origin to the anterior chest wall, the louder the sound on auscultation. Frequency (pitch) is also affected by the amount of interposed tissue the sound must pass through before reaching the chest wall. Another factor affecting the frequency of a murmur is related to the transmission of the sound within the cardiovascular system itself. As a sound moves against the stream, as in regurgitation, high frequencies tend to be preserved while low frequencies are damped out. When moving downstream with the flow, the opposite is true. Consequently, many murmurs sound very different when auscultated from different locations on the chest.

3. *Character.* Description of a murmur should take into account and include in the record the following six categories: timing, location, intensity, frequency, duration, and quality.

a. *Timing* refers to the placement of the sound in relationship to the cardiac cycle—systolic, diastolic, continuous.
b. *Location* is the point of maximal intensity of the murmur, using the valve areas and the intercostal spaces for accuracy of reference points.
c. *Loudness* is graded on a six-point scale, with grade I/VI being barely audible and increasing in loudness to VI/VI, which is audible without a stethoscope.
d. *Pitch* is noted as low, medium, or high.
e. *Duration* is noted as short, medium, or long in timing (see Fig. 10-29).
f. *Quality* refers to crescendo (increasing in intensity) or decrescendo (decreasing in intensity) and overall presentation, namely, blowing, harsh, rumbling, rasping, musical, ejection, regurgitant.

Murmurs are classified as systolic or diastolic and, within these two groups, are described as to quality.

Figure 10-29.
Duration of heart murmurs.
(From Judge and Zuidema
[3].)

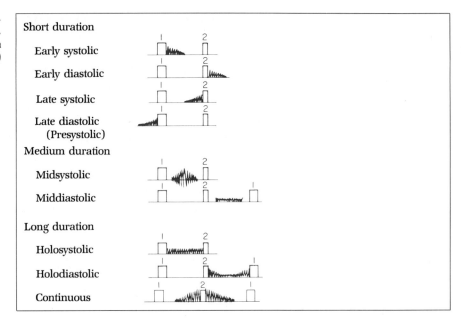

Figure 10-29. Duration of heart murmurs. (From Judge and Zuidema [3].)

1. *Systolic ejection murmurs* are produced by the forward movement of blood through the pulmonic and aortic valves. They begin after the first sound, swell and fade in a crescendo-decrescendo fashion, peaking in early or middle systole and terminating before the second heart sound. They tend to be of medium pitch and short in duration, and they do not override either the first or second sound. Examples of this type of murmur are the murmur of aortic and pulmonic stenosis and the functional or innocent murmur.

2. *Systolic regurgitant murmurs* are produced by the backflow of blood from the ventricles into the atria or through a septal defect. Because the blood moves from an area of high to low pressure, these murmurs tend to be high-pitched and longer in duration, usually holosystolic (pansystolic), that is, they extend through the entire systolic period. They tend to override the second and the first sounds. Their intensity tends to remain constant, occasionally increasing late in systole. In mitral regurgitation, the murmur is usually blowing in quality and loudest at the apex. With tricuspid regurgitation, the murmur tends to increase in intensity on inspiration. Septal defect murmurs are usually coarse in quality.

3. *Diastolic regurgitant murmurs,* as in systole, are high-pitched, long, usually holodiastolic (pandiastolic), and transmitted in the direction of regurgitant blood flow. Examples are the murmurs of aortic and pulmonic regurgitation.

4. *Diastolic filling murmurs* are low-pitched, localized, and rumbling. They tend to be middiastolic. In mitral stenosis, an opening snap of the mitral valve is often heard, and the murmur has a decrescendo quality. With tricuspid stenosis, the timing and quality are similar; however, the murmur tends to be high in pitch.

Pericardial Friction Rub. Pericardial friction rub is a grating-like sound resembling the rubbing together of two pieces of sandpaper. It has also been described as a "leathery" sound, suggestive of the squeaking of a shoe. Its appearance is a sign of pericardial inflammation. Friction rub may be heard over any part of the precordium, but is usually demonstrated at the left sternal border. Occasionally it is loud and continuous throughout systole and diastole; however, it is more commonly muffled, high-pitched, and transient in nature. The quality of the sound can be created by moving the stethoscope endpiece lightly over a "hairy" skin surface while auscultating.

CIRCULATORY SYSTEM-ASSESSMENT GUIDE

I. Interview
   A. Past or Present History of: rheumatic fever, heart disease, hypertension, edema, chest pain, pain in extremities, hair loss on extremities, skin temperature changes, skin color changes, increased or decreased sensitivity to heat or cold, headache, epistaxis, dizziness, palpitations, night sweats, paroxysmal nocturnal dyspnea
   B. Family History of: heart disease, hypertension, or cerebral vascular accident
II. Physical
   A. Extremities
     1. Inspection and Palpation
       a. Fingernails and toenails
         1. Shape, plate color and texture, bed color
         2. Mobility, presence of thickening
         3. Capillary refill
         4. Capillary pulsation
       b. Skin color
       c. Skin integrity
       d. Hair distribution
       e. Venous pattern
       f. Edema
       g. Atrophy
       h. Obvious pulsation
       i. Arterial pulses—brachial, radial, abdominal aorta, femoral, popliteal, posterior tibialis, dorsalis pedis, rate, rhythm, elasticity, quality
     2. Auscultation
       a. Arterial—blood pressure
   B. Neck
     1. Inspection and Palpation
       a. Obvious pulsations (supine and upright)
       b. Carotid pulses—rate, rhythm, elasticity, and quality
       c. Jugular pulses—supine position: distention, rhythm angle of collapse
     2. Auscultation
       a. Carotid bruits
       b. Abdominal aorta—bruits
   C. Precordium
     1. Inspection and Palpation
       a. Identification of PMI
       b. Obvious pulsations—heaves or lifts

      c. Thrills

      d. Shocks

  2. Percussion—left border of cardiac dullness (LBCD)

  3. Auscultation

      a. Rate and rhythm

      b. Identify S_1—intensity, pitch, duration

      c. Identify S_2—intensity, pitch, duration

      d. Compare S_1 with S_2 re: intensity, pitch, duration

      e. Identify extra sounds—timing (systolic or diastolic), intensity, pitch, duration, quality, location(s) heard (radiation) and where heard best

REFERENCES

1. Burch, G. E., and DePasquale, N. P. *Primer of Clinical Measurement of Blood Pressure.* St. Louis: Mosby, 1962.
2. DeGowin, E. L., and DeGowin, R. L. *Bedside Diagnostic Examination* (3rd ed.). New York: Macmillan, 1976.
3. Judge, R. D., and Zuidema, G. D. (Eds.). *Methods of Clinical Examination: A Physiologic Approach* (3rd ed.). Boston: Little, Brown, 1974.
4. Kampmeier, R. *Physical Examination in Health and Disease* (3rd ed.). Philadelphia: Davis, 1964.

SUGGESTED READINGS

Ask-Upmark, E. *Bedside Medicine Selected Topics* (2nd ed.). Stockholm: Almquist & Wessell, 1969.

Caird, F. I., Dall, J. L., and Kennedy, R. D. *Cardiology in Old Age.* New York: Plenum, 1976.

Delp, M. H., and Manning, R. T. *Major's Physical Diagnosis* (8th ed.). Philadelphia: Saunders, 1975.

Feinstein, A. R. *Clinical Judgment.* Baltimore: Williams & Wilkins, 1967.

Hochstein, E., and Rubin, A. *Physical Diagnosis: A Textbook and Workbook in Methods of Clinical Examination.* New York: McGraw-Hill, 1964.

Hopkins, H. *Leopold's Principles and Methods of Physical Diagnosis* (3rd ed.). Philadelphia: Saunders, 1965.

Kampmeier, R., and Blake, T. M. *Physical Examination in Health and Disease* (4th ed.). Philadelphia: Davis, 1970.

Pearson, L. J., and Kotthoff, M. E. *Geriatric Clinical Protocols.* Philadelphia: Lippincott, 1979.

Prior, J. A., and Silberstein, J. S. *Physical Diagnosis: The History and Examination of the Patient* (5th ed.). St. Louis: Mosby, 1977.

Candace M. Burns

11. Physical Assessment of the Abdomen and the Male Genitourinary System

anuria Total suppression of urinary secretion.

ascites Free fluid in the abdominal cavity.

ballottement Palpation technique to detect a floating enlarged organ when accompanied by ascites.

borborygmus Sounds produced during hyperperistalsis.

burning Urethral irritation with sensation similar to voiding hot water.

dyschezia Difficult or painful defecation.

dysphagia Difficulty in swallowing.

enuresis Voiding involuntarily or during sleep.

fluid wave Transmission of an impulse through fluid in the abdomen.

frequency Felt need to void often.

guarding Tension of the abdominal musculature over an area of tenderness.

hematuria Blood in the urine.

linea alba A vertical, tendinous line between the rectus muscles, extends from the xyphoid to the symphysis pubis.

megacolon Enlarged or dilated colon.

nocturia Excessive urination during the night.

oliguria Deficient secretion of urine.

paradoxical (overflow) incontinence Loss of urine due to chronic urinary retention or secondary to a flaccid bladder causing constant dribbling.

pneumaturia Gas or air in urine.

polyuria Excess in amount of urine voided.

pyuria Pus in the urine.

rushes Accentuation of normal bowel sounds but longer and higher-pitched.

strangury Difficult, painful passage of urine accompanied by spasm.

stress incontinence Involuntary urinary discharge resulting from an intravesicular pressure increase as in sneezing, coughing, or straining.

succussion splash Sound created by moving air and fluid in a hollow organ.

tinkles Very high-pitched bowel sounds, musical in quality.

urgency Sudden strong desire to urinate.

THIS chapter presents various aspects of the physical examination currently not generally performed by most nurses. At present only a few female nurses are carrying out complete genitourinary examination of male patients, and these nurses usually are functioning in some specialized clinician role. However, with little controversy, male nurses in a wide variety of clinical settings have employed and continue to employ successfully the various techniques of physical examination. As these techniques are learned and utilized by more nurses and as more liberalized views and expectations as to the role of the female nurse emerge, this situation will change rapidly.

EXAMINATION OF THE ABDOMEN

Physical examination of the abdomen differs from examination of other body areas in several features. Auscultation is generally less important in examination of the abdomen than in the thorax. Palpation of the abdomen provides less exact and useful information because the abdominal contents are separated from the examiner's hands by a thick muscular wall.

Order of the Examination

Although the same four basic techniques (i.e., inspection, palpation, percussion, and auscultation) of examination are employed by the nurse examining the abdomen, auscultation should in this instance be performed before palpation and percussion, since the latter two may alter bowel sounds that might normally be heard, creating a false impression. For example, a "normal" abdomen may suddenly present hyperactive bowel sounds after stimuli from palpation, or percussion, or both.

Positioning and Draping the Patient

Correct positioning of the patient is important for proper examination. The optimal position is to have the patient supine, with his hands at his sides. Do not allow the patient to put his hands behind his head; this causes contraction of the abdominal musculature, making it difficult to palpate the abdomen. Relaxation of the abdominal musculature is essential for successful palpation. The following techniques may be employed to assist the patient to relax.

The head should lie flat, preferably on a small pillow, and the knees kept slightly flexed to help prevent tensing of the abdominal musculature. The nurse examiner should stand at the right side of the patient, regardless of whether she is right- or left-handed. When examining for the presence of a hernia, bulges of the abdominal wall, or psoas sign, it is most desirable to have the patient standing. Abdominal organs drop in the upright person owing to gravity, thus increasing pressure on the mass and causing its descent and easier detection. The patient should be draped to provide for his modesty and comfort and ease of examination. The equipment needed for examination of the abdomen is: (1) stethoscope, (2) tape measure (preferably cloth or plastic that will not stretch), and (3) skin marking pen.

Landmarks

Certain specific landmarks are generally used to describe findings. These landmarks are identified in Figure 11-1. The examiner should be familiar with them as they will assist her in describing findings in a clear, concise manner and will support uniform interpretation. In descriptions of physical assessment findings, the abdomen is frequently divided into sections. Two methods are seen most often. The first method divides the abdomen into quadrants by drawing a line from the tip of the sternum to the pubic bone through the umbilicus. These four sections are namely; right upper quadrant, left upper quadrant, right lower quadrant, left lower quadrant. First a line should be drawn from the tip of the sternum through the umbilicus to the pubic bone. Then another

Figure 11-1.
Anatomical landmarks. 1.
Tip of sternum-epigastric
hollow. 2. Costal margin. 3.
Midline extending from
sternum to pubic bone (os
pubis). 4. Umbilicus. 5.
Anterosuperior iliac crest.
6. Superior margin of os
pubis. 7. Symphysis.

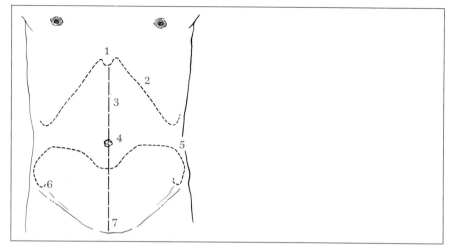

line is drawn at a right angle to the first line through the umbilicus. The abdominal structures located in each quadrant are as follows:

Right Upper Quadrant
Liver
Gallbladder
Duodenum
Pylorus
Portion of right kidney
Right adrenal gland
Hepatic flexure of colon
Portions of ascending and transverse
  colon

Left Upper Quadrant
Left lobe of liver
Stomach
Spleen
Body of pancreas
Portion of left kidney
Left adrenal gland
Splenic flexure of colon
Portions of transverse and descending
  colon

Right Lower Quadrant
Lower pole of right kidney
Cecum
Appendix
Portion of ascending colon
Right spermatic cord
Right ureter

Left Lower Quadrant
Lower pole of left kidney
Sigmoid colon
Portion of descending colon
Ovary and salpinx
Left spermatic cord
Left ureter

Figure 11-2 shows the quadrants and the abdominal organs usually located in each and should serve as a guide for the physical assessment. The second method of division, used less often than the quadrant method, sections the abdomen into nine areas.

Inspection   Inspection is an important part of the physical assessment and is too often rushed or entirely omitted. A single source of light is used in inspection of the abdomen. The light should be directed at a right angle to the long axis of the patient. With the patient properly positioned, the nurse notes the presence or absence of distention, symmetry, and midline protuberances. These are best seen by the nurse first standing and then sitting to one side and looking across

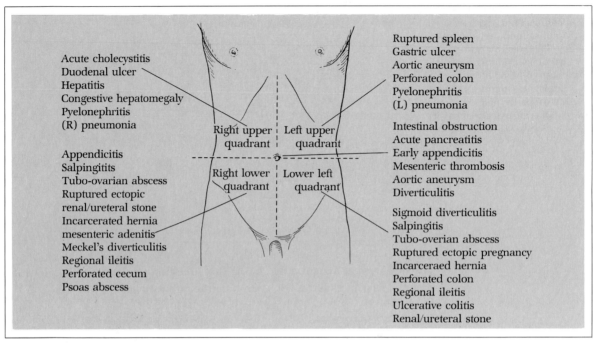

Acute cholecystitis
Duodenal ulcer
Hepatitis
Congestive hepatomegaly
Pyelonephritis
(R) pneumonia

Appendicitis
Salpingitits
Tubo-ovarian abscess
Ruptured ectopic
renal/ureteral stone
Incarcerated hernia
mesenteric adenitis
Meckel's diverticulitis
Regional ileitis
Perforated cecum
Psoas abscess

Right upper quadrant | Left upper quadrant

Right lower quadrant | Lower left quadrant

Ruptured spleen
Gastric ulcer
Aortic aneurysm
Perforated colon
Pyelonephritis
(L) pneumonia

Intestinal obstruction
Acute pancreatitis
Early appendicitis
Mesenteric thrombosis
Aortic aneurysm
Diverticulitis

Sigmoid diverticulitis
Salpingitis
Tubo-overian abscess
Ruptured ectopic pregnancy
Incarceraed hernia
Perforated colon
Regional ileitis
Ulcerative colitis
Renal/ureteral stone

Figure 11-2.
Topographic anatomy of the abdomen. (Modified from R. D. Judge and G. D. Zuidema (Eds.). *Methods of Clinical Examination: A Physiologic Approach* (3rd ed.). Boston: Little, Brown, 1974.)

the surface of the patient's abdomen. The resultant shadow should be high so that even small changes in contour will be evident. Standing may help the nurse to detect unusual abdominal shadows and movement; the sitting position provides a plane horizontal to the eye. Asking the patient to take a deep inspiration helps to accentuate an enlarged liver, spleen, or distended gallbladder, making detection easier.

Inspection of the abdominal skin for scars, dehydration, malnutrition, venous patterns, and discolorations can provide an abundance of information about the patient's general state of health (Fig. 11-3).

Venous Patterns

Normally, the venous pattern is faint with blood flow centrifugal from the umbilicus. The venous pattern becomes more prominent with thin skin and with decreased elasticity of the skin, as in aging. Irregular patches of faint pigmentation on the abdomen, flank, and back may be indicative of von Recklinghausen's disease.

Because of obstruction in large intra-abdominal or intrathoracic venous channels, a collateral circulation may develop in the veins of the abdominal wall. To determine the direction of flow, the nurse should compress and "strip" the veins and observe their refill. In obstruction of the superior vena cava, the blood from above finds its way to the heart via the inferior vena cava; thus the blood flow is downward. In portal obstruction, the flow is commonly upward

Figure 11-3.
Inspection of the abdominal
area may yield pertinent
clues about previous
trauma or surgery and may
signal the possibility of
adhesions or bowel
obstruction. (Reproduced
with permission from R. D.
Judge, G. D. Zuidema, and
F. Fitzgerald (Eds.).
*Methods of Clinical
Examination* (4th ed.).
Boston: Little, Brown,
1982.)

to anastomose with part of the veins in the attachment of the diaphragm. When describing venous patterning, it is important to record the flow pattern in a diagram.

Umbilicus

The position and shape of the umbilicus is important to note. Normally, it is a flat sphere with a long vertical axis and is positioned midway between the xyphoid process and the pubis. Intra-abdominal hemorrhage may cause discoloration of the umbilical area from the blood pigments reaching it via lymphatics in the medial umbilical ligament. This often is referred to as "Cullen's sign." Bluish, periumbilical patches frequently occur with pancreatitis. A yellow-tinged navel may be due to free bile in the peritoneal cavity. Reddish or purple mottling due to circulatory collapse also may develop. The mottling blanches with pressure, and the blanching lasts only a second or so.

Pelvic or lower abdominal masses may displace the umbilicus cephalad; masses of the upper abdomen may displace it caudad, as ascites also does. The umbilicus may protrude owing to an umbilical hernia. It may become dirty, infected, or lose mobility and become fixed as with malignancies, appearing as a hard, button-shaped mass. The umbilicus is a frequent site of fungal infection. When any abnormal findings are detected, prompt referral to a physician is indicated.

Hair Distribution

The nurse should observe and describe the distribution of the abdominal and pelvic hair. In the normal female the pubic hair is roughly triangular with the base above the symphysis. In the normal male pubic hair grows in the shape of a diamond, with hair frequently extending to the umbilicus. Disturbances of hormonal balance may alter the distribution of pubic hair to patterns characteristic of the opposite sex (see Chap. 6). A female-type hair distribution found in a male may be an indication of cirrhosis and failure of the diseased liver to conjugate estrogenic substances. A typically masculine hair distribution in a female may suggest an adrenocortical or genital abnormality. Sparse or absent hair associated with thin, smooth skin may be due to pituitary insufficiency. When such observations are made, the patient should be referred to a physician for follow-up.

Respiratory Movement

The abdomen and the liver, spleen, and gallbladder typically follow thoracic respiratory movement because of the pull of the diaphragm. In general, females usually breathe with costal movements only, whereas males (breathing quietly) breathe abdominally. Decreased respiratory movement occurs with increased rigidity of the abdominal muscles or undue distention. An ulcer perforated into the peritoneal cavity usually results in little or no respiratory movement of the abdomen. Frequently, appendicitis with local peritonitis causes immobility of the hypogastric region. Retraction of the abdominal wall upon inspiration is known as Czerny's sign and is generally associated with some central nervous system disease. Findings indicative of any abnormality should be referred to a physician.

Abdominal Contours

A flat abdominal contour is seen when the anterior wall extends in a horizontal plane from the level of the costal margins to the pubic bone. This is often seen in the young, athletic, well-nourished person or in the spare elderly person. A round abdomen is convex to the horizontal plane as the body is observed from the side. In the supine patient the height of the convexity is in the area of the umbilicus, whereas in the erect patient, gravity causes a shifting of this point to a lower position between the umbilicus and pubis. The round abdomen, characteristic of young children (see Chap. 15), is seen more commonly in the female than in the male and is due to excess subcutaneous fat or to lack of activity, or of muscle tone, or both. The aged frequently have this abdominal contour, owing to these factors mentioned, as well as to kyphosis of the dorsal segments of the spine. The scaphoid abdominal contour, when viewed laterally, is seen as a concavity to the horizontal plane and may be seen in patients of all ages. Asymmetry of abdominal contour may be an important indication of disease. The examiner should inspect the patient from above as well as from the sides in order to detect asymmetry.

Abdominal Distention. Abdominal distention is an abnormal state that requires further assessment. Distention may be localized or generalized, often resulting from gas in the intestines, fluid in the abdominal cavity, or tumor. Generalized distention is abdominal protuberance. If distention is caused by gas, the flanks do not bulge, and the lateral walls slope toward the midline as toward a rigid pole. The percussion note is resonant, bowel sounds are usually increased, and the patient may be nauseated and vomit. When the distention is due to fluid, the weight of the fluid causes the flanks to bulge (unless the abdominal musculature has *excellent* tone), resulting in a more flattened anterior abdominal area than is seen in the abdomen distended with gas. If the patient is relaxed and is asked to roll from side to side, a protuberance is seen on the dependent side of the abdomen as the fluid shifts from side to side. There is no change in the area of maximum distention if the abdomen contains gas. This maneuver is known as *shifting dullness.* The air-filled bowel floats on the fluid so that the difference between the dullness of fluid and the tympany of air is readily detected by percussion.

To elicit a *fluid wave,* one hand is placed on the lateral aspect of the abdomen while the other hand taps the opposite side of the abdomen gently but sharply. If fluid is present, a wave is seen as the fluid transmits the impulse through the abdomen (Fig. 11-4).

The *puddle sign* indicates the presence of small amounts of intra-abdominal fluid. To test for this sign, request the standing patient to assume a hand-knee position for several minutes. This will encourage any fluid present to "puddle"

Figure 11-4.
Eliciting a fluid wave to demonstrate the presence of intraabdominal fluid. (Modified from R. D. Judge and G. D. Zuidema (Eds.). *Methods of Clinical Examination: A Physiologic Approach* (3rd ed.). Boston: Little, Brown, 1974.)

around the umbilicus. Then the examiner should percuss around the umbilicus to detect small (several hundred milliliters) amounts of fluids. Ascites occurs for a variety of reasons, and its causes will not be detailed here. Whenever fluid is detected, the patient needs referral to a physician for further evaluation.

An extremely large amount of feces in the colon may cause abdominal distention, as in megacolon.

Localized distention may be caused by an enlarged organ, a tumor, localized fluid, or distended loops of bowel. A bulging is evident in one specific area of the abdomen and not in other areas. For example, an enlarged spleen may cause the left side of the abdomen to be distended, whereas hepatomegaly (enlarged liver) may cause right-sided distention. An ovarian cyst may cause asymmetric fullness in one or the other lower quadrants. Large hypernephromas or polycystic kidney may fill one or both sides of the abdomen.

Bowel contours should also be noted. Peristaltic waves may be visible through the abdominal wall(e.g., in mechanical obstruction). The bowel is frequently distended with gas, and this distention is obvious in the peristaltic waves observable.

An enlarged abdomen due to obesity cannot truly be classified as distended. Yet it is important to note that this is a common cause of abdominal enlargement. Folds or aprons of fat are usually deposited in the suprapubic or flank areas, and the umbilicus is usually deeply inverted. When obesity is caused by hypopituitarism, the body fat is centrally rather than peripherally distributed. Results elicited may be similar for abdominal fat as for fluid. Doubt as to the cause of abdominal distention may require that paracentesis be performed by a physician.

It is important that the patient be observed while straining, since this may yield information concerning the abdominal wall. When the patient rises from a supine to a sitting position without using his hands, diastasis recti (separation of the rectus abdominalis in the midline) may be noted, indicating weakness of supporting tissue between the longitudinal rectus muscles.

Hernias. Hernias result from weakness of the abdominal wall or structure or undue stress on the wall or region. A hernia is a protrusion of bowel or other tissue through an abdominal hiatus, enclosed in the peritoneal sac. An epigastric hernia occurs in the midline, penetrating the linea alba above the umbilicus, and frequently contains omentum rather than intestine. An umbilical hernia occurs through a weakness at the site of former (fetal) umbilical vessels. A femoral hernia occurs in the femoral canal at the midpoint of Poupart's (inguinal) ligament and is most common in women. Inguinal hernias occur more often in men. A direct inguinal hernia penetrates the abdominal wall at the internal ring and appears as a variable-sized tumor medial to the site of the deep epigastric artery. An indirect hernia enters the internal ring and later moves down the canal to protrude through the external ring into the scrotum (Fig. 11-5).

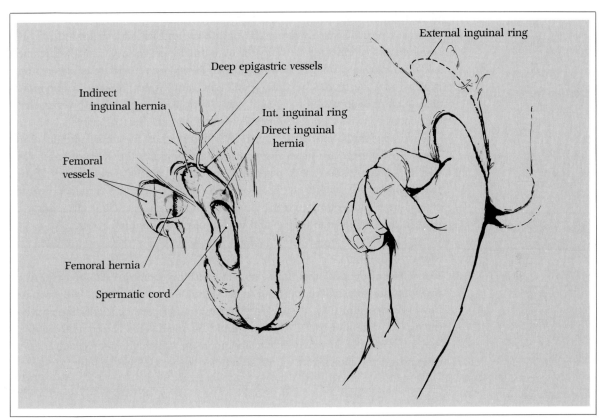

External inguinal ring

Deep epigastric vessels

Indirect
inguinal hernia

Int. inguinal ring

Direct inguinal
hernia

Femoral
vessels

Femoral hernia

Spermatic cord

Figure 11-5.
Inguinal hernias.
(Reproduced with
permission from R. D.
Judge and G. D. Zuidema
(Eds.). *Methods of Clinical
Examination: A Physiologic
Approach* (3rd ed.).
Boston: Little, Brown,
1974.)

Abdominal Pulsations

An abdominal pulsation may be readily evident. Pulsation of the abdominal aorta may be observed in the midline, cephalad to the umbilicus, and is systolic in timing. Pulsations from the normal aorta may be transmitted to the abdominal wall and may be difficult to separate from the expansile pulsation of an abdominal aneurysm (a local enlargement with a pulsation). One method of determining whether the pulsation is expansile or transmitted is to hold two matchsticks lightly over the pulsating mass. If their motion is in a vertical direction only, it is probably a pulsation transmitted from the aorta. Horizontal movement of the matchsticks indicates that the pulsation is possibly expansile. Although this simple test is by no means precise, it may be informative during an initial assessment. Findings indicative of any abnormality should be immediately reported to a physician.

Pigmentation

The skin of the abdomen is frequently protected from exposure to sunlight, thus facilitating the detection and differentiation of pigmentation changes caused by exposure to sunlight from changes caused by an increase in pigment. Unusual pigmentation, such as jaundice, may also be observed. The linea alba, usually seen as a narrow furrow above the umbilicus and invisible below it, may become notably pigmented, or hairy, or both during pregnancy. Lineal albicantes, which are striae produced by stretching of the skin and rupture of elastic fibers of skin, may be seen. They may result from any rapid increase in abdominal size, such as that caused by weight gain, fluid, and pregnancy. However, striae that occur as a result of Cushing's syndrome remain pink to purple.

Cutaneous angiomas (spider nevi) may be noted on the upper abdomen and chest. Spider nevi are generally found in association with liver disease. They may be distinguished from petechiae and other lesions because they blanch when pressure is placed on the nevus and/or when pressure is placed over the central arteriole feeding into the clump of dilated vessels. Tight glistening skin is often associated with ascites and edema of the abdominal wall.

Scars

Inspection of the abdomen for scars can yield important information regarding previous surgery or trauma and may signal the possibility of adhesions or bowel obstruction (Fig. 11-6). Deep irregular scars are generally indicative of burns. The size and shape of scars should be noted. This is frequently done by making a simple drawing of the abdomen on which the four quadrants are drawn and the dimensions of the scar noted in centimeters as follows:

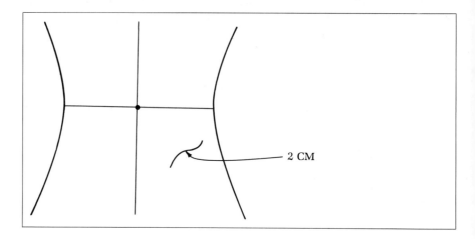

If the cause of the scar(s) was not determined in the history, the patient should be asked what type of operation or injury he had for each scar.

Pain

The patient's description of pain experienced may be helpful and should be carefully elicited. Facial expression, posture, restlessness, or immobility observed prior to and during the examination may yield useful data. The nurse

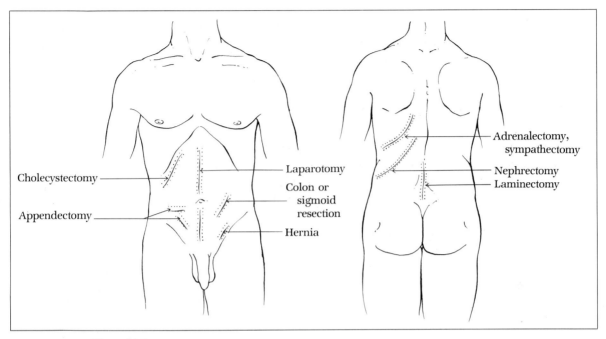

Figure 11-6.
Common surgical scars.
(Reproduced with
permission from R. D.
Judge, G. D. Zuidema, and
F. Fitzgerald (Eds.).
*Methods of Clinical
Examination* (4th ed.).
Boston: Little, Brown,
1982.)

must determine such facts as where the pain is, where it started, and where it radiates. Often, the manner in which the patient points to painful areas is helpful in identifying the source of the pain. For example, pain with peptic ulcer is usually localized, and the patient uses one finger to point to the specific area. Functional distress is more diffuse, and the patient moves his hand across the abdomen, unable to localize it in any one site. Figure 11-7 shows the common causes of abdominal pain.

Generally there are two major categories of abdominal pain: (1) visceral pain

Figure 11-7.
Some causes of acute
abdominal pain. (Modified
from R. D. Judge, G. D.
Zuidema, and F. Fitzgerald
(Eds.). *Methods of Clinical
Examination* (4th ed.).
Boston: Little, Brown,
1982.)

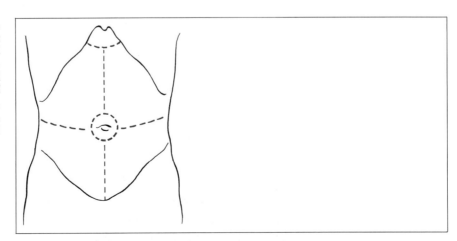

and (2) peritoneal pain. Visceral pain is caused by intra-abdominal disease affecting pain fibers located in an abdominal organ. Peritoneal pain occurs when pain fibers in the mesothelial tissue layer that surrounds the abdominal organs and lines the abdominal wall are affected. Visceral pain is usually felt in various areas of the abdomen (i.e., poorly localized, dull, and difficult for the patient to describe). Peritoneal pain is usually sharp and easily localized. If the type of pain does not become evident during the history-taking, the nurse should determine whether the abdominal pain is associated with any other symptoms such as vomiting, melena, bloating, diarrhea, and/or constipation.

The character of the abdominal pain may be described as sharp/knife-like, burning/firey, colicky/stabs of pain that gradually increase and then decrease in intensity, crampy, and/or radicular/shooting pain that starts in the back and radiates to the front.

An accurate description of the pain can be most helpful in determining its source. Patients reporting abdominal pain should be referred to a physician for a follow-up.

Palpation

General Guides

Palpation is used to confirm and amplify findings from inspection. The nurse should position herself at the right side of the patient and palpate with uniform pressure. Her hands should be warm, since cold hands are uncomfortable for the patient and may cause abdominal tensing. Fingers are to be held together; nails should be trimmed and smooth. To make accurate measurements, centimeters rather than fingerbreadths are used, since finger size varies greatly among examiners. During palpation it is important to determine whether a detected mass is in the abdominal wall or intra-abdominal. This can be accomplished by asking the patient to flex and tense his abdominal muscles. Masses in the abdominal wall continue to be palpable, whereas those in the abdominal cavity become more difficult to detect or completely nonpalpable.

Light palpation—just indenting the skin—should be used initially to detect tenderness. Soft organs may be detected in this manner, and distended hollow visceral organs may be missed if only deep palpation is used.

In moderate palpation, used to detect enlarged organs or masses, the side of the hand is used rather than the fingers to prevent digging the fingertips into the patient and producing involuntary guarding. Organs that move with respiration (e.g., liver, spleen) are first palpated with normal respiratory effort and then with deep inspiration. An organ undetected with normal respiration may be felt on deep inspiration.

Deep palpation is used to detect tenderness and organs not found with light or moderate palpation. Retroperitoneal masses such as the kidneys may be felt in this manner.

Various methods of bimanual palpation are used. Using both hands placed on separate parts of the abdomen enables the nurse to delineate the extent of an organ or mass and to measure the dimensions with the fingertips. This technique is useful in detecting a pulsatile mass. Pulsations felt in the fingertips of both hands indicates that the organ itself is pulsating rather than that the pulsation is being transmitted from the aorta. Placing one hand anterior and one posterior to the organ or mass serves to "trap" the organ and is a very useful technique to determine size, consistency, and texture of the organ. For example, in palpating kidneys, the right hand presses down from the anterior and the left hand presses up from the posterior. In attempting to detect minimal descent of an organ (e.g., liver, spleen), the nurse may find it useful to place one hand next to the other for palpating.

Palpation to detect *rebound tenderness* is an important maneuver when examining the abdomen. To elicit this sign, one hand is pressed slowly into the abdomen and then quickly withdrawn. Discomfort is elicited when the hand is suddenly withdrawn rather than with the downward pressure.

General Survey

A general survey of the entire abdomen should be done with light palpation, using the distal phalanges of the fingers of the examining hand (the right hand of a right-handed person). Systematically explore the abdomen with light pressure to detect an increase in abdominal muscle tone, enlarged solid organs (liver, spleen, kidneys, uterus), or hollow organs (bowel, stomach, bladder, aorta). Deliberate, firm, but gentle pressure is used to avoid tickling or sudden jabbing thrusts. It is best to examine areas of suspected or known discomfort last. Determine the area of greatest tenderness and location of possible resistance. In general, the degree of resistance (rigidity) is proportional to the degree of peritoneal irritation. An exception to this is the rigidity with peritonitis, which is initially very intense and then decreases or even ceases within a short period. Note the size and shape of the resistance, the character of its limits, its relation to the surrounding area, and whether it is in connection with an organ or corresponds to an enlargement of an organ. The relationship of resistance to respiratory movements should also be noted in terms of directions and limits of movement. The nature of the resistance should be described, e.g., soft, elastic, compact, cartilaginous, glandulous, tumorous, or fluctuating. Muscular resistance may also be due to increased tone of the abdominal musculature or reflex action spasm. Resistance should also be palpated from the vagina or rectum.

Guarding

Guarding may be voluntary or involuntary. Voluntary guarding is a conscious response by the patient on palpation over a painful abdomen; involuntary guarding is a reflex contraction of abdominal muscles and is not responsive to conscious effort on the part of the patient. Involuntary guarding often indicates the presence of a more serious pathologic condition. Rigidity is an extreme form of guarding and may be seen in conjunction with absent bowel sounds.

Organ Survey

Deep palpation is utilized to determine abnormality of organs when tenderness indicates underlying disease (e.g., tender liver edge, spleen, gallbladder). If an abnormality is felt, note its size, movement with respiration, tenderness, position, consistency, and attachment to underlying tissue, viscera, or both. Examination should also include palpation of the left supraclavicular space, since this may reveal an enlarged lymph node, an important sign of possible intraabdominal malignancy. A systematic survey of the following is made by deep palpation.

Abdominal aorta. Deep palpation of the epigastric area may reveal the aortic pulsation. The examiner's fingers will feel the thrust of the systolic pulse against the rigid spine. Tenderness is frequently elicited from pressure on this structure. Aneurysms may form in the abdominal aorta as saclike enlargements of the vessel. They are generally felt as pulsatile masses in the mid portion of the abdomen and may be accompanied by complaints of abdominal pain.

Colon. In the older person, or one with lax abdominal muscles, the examiner may be able to outline the transverse colon across the abdomen just above the umbilicus. It is soft and moveable. The sigmoid colon forms a ropelike structure in the left lower quadrant almost parallel to Poupart's ligament. Occasionally, the cecum and ascending colon can be palpated in the right lower quadrant.

Urinary bladder. Normally, the bladder, a pelvic organ, cannot be palpated unless distended well above the symphysis pubis.

Liver. The left hand should be placed under the patient's flank, fingers extended, palm side up, and lying parallel to the ribs. The hand is placed so that the patient's eleventh and twelfth ribs lie on the nurse's hand. Upward pressure with this hand pushes the liver toward the anterior abdominal wall. The right hand is placed flat on the abdomen, fingers in the long axis of the body and in the right upper quadrant, about midway between the costal border and the level of the umbilicus. The patient is then instructed to take a deep breath. The right hand should move with the abdominal wall as the patient inspires. With the descent of the diaphragm on deep inspiration, the liver moves downward. If it is to be palpated, one can feel it slip under the palpating fingers as they move with the abdominal wall (Fig. 11-8).

The edge of the normal liver is usually sharp, regular, and relatively straight in contour. To determine the size of the liver, measure in centimeters the distance it reaches below the costal margin and the total span by percussion of the thoracic cage with deep inspiration. The normal liver may be felt to descend to 1 to 2 cm below the costal margin. Normal liver size is about 10 to 12 cm.

Note whether the entire border is palpable (indicating diffuse enlargement). Also note any complaints of tenderness as the edge slips under the right hand, consistency, presence of nodes, and irregular or systolic pulsations or both.

Figure 11-8.
Techniques of palpating the liver. *A.* The anterior hand should parallel the rectus muscle. *B.* The hooking technique is occasionally preferable. (Reproduced with permission from R. D. Judge and G. D. Zuidema (Eds.). *Methods of Clinical Examination: A Physiologic Approach* (3rd ed.). Boston: Little, Brown, 1974.)

Nodules may be felt when the palm of the hand is placed over the liver surface as the patient takes a deep breath. Nodules on the liver wall can be felt as they move; whereas nodules on the abdominal wall cannot. When examining patients with severe, chronic emphysema, the liver may normally be displaced below the costal margin owing to displacement of the diaphragm by the over-expanded lung. (Percussion should reveal a low upper edge, thus revealing a liver of normal total size.) Cirrhosis may produce an enlarged liver with a firm nontender edge. An enlarged liver with a smooth tender edge may be indicative of inflammation or venous congestion. An enlarged liver that is firm or hard with an irregular edge is frequently associated with malignancies. The liver may or may not be tender. If any abnormalities are detected, the patient should be referred to a physician.

Ballottement is performed when ascites is present. The anterior wall is depressed with the fingertips over the suspected organ enlargement. Fluid is more readily displaced than a solid organ; therefore, when the fingers strike a floating organ, a distinct solid mass is felt.

Spleen. To palpate the spleen, the left hand reaches across the abdomen and is slipped under the flank. Fingers of the right hand are directed obliquely upward and laterally under the left costal margin. On deep inspiration, the right hand should move with the abdominal wall. The tip of the spleen may be felt as it is pushed downward by the descending diaphragm (Fig. 11-9). The spleen edge resembles a firm edge, similar to that of the liver. An alternate method for palpating the spleen is to stand on the patient's left side, facing his feet. The fingers of both hands are hooked over the costal margin, pressing upward and inward (Fig. 11-8B). Upon inspiration, the spleen may be felt by the fingertips. A normal spleen is rarely palpable, and its consistency is softer than that of the liver. Spleen size is more difficult to determine, but centimeters of descent below the costal margin should be recorded when possible.

Kidneys. Kidneys usually can be felt with bimanual palpation at the height of inspiration only in the young person, multiparous woman, or aged person with relaxed abdominal walls (Fig. 11-10). The right kidney lies slightly lower than the left and is the one most commonly palpated. The left hand should be placed under the flank, parallel to and just below the twelfth rib. The right hand is placed on the abdomen so that the fingertips are in the lower quadrant below the level of the umbilicus. The fingers must press deeply and move with the abdominal wall on deep inspiration. The kidney is felt as a solid, firm, but elastic mass.

To palpate the left kidney, the left hand reaches across the abdomen to be placed under the flank and similar technique is employed.

Figure 11-9. Palpation of the spleen. *A.* Positioning of examiner's hands. *B.* Patient's hand under his back. *C.* Patient rolled to right side. (Reproduced with permission from R. D. Judge, G. D. Zuidema, and F. Fitzgerald (Eds.). *Methods of Clinical Examination* (4th ed.). Boston: Little, Brown, 1982.)

A

B

C

Figure 11-10.
Palpation of the kidneys.
(Modified from R. D. Judge
and G. D. Zuidema (Eds.).
*Methods of Clinical
Examination: A Physiologic
Approach* (3rd ed.).
Boston: Little, Brown,
1974.)

The differences in palpation of an enlarged left kidney and the spleen are:

1. The splenic notch can be felt, whereas no kidney notch can, since blood vessels fill this space.
2. The spleen has a sharper outline than the kidney.
3. The spleen is usually enlarged anteriorly, whereas the kidney rarely is.

Inguinal rings. Palpation is especially important in detecting dilatations. The patient may be supine or, preferably, erect. The index finger is pressed upward through the scrotal wall along the spermatic cord into the external inguinal ring. Normally, the nurse should feel the sharp edge of the aponeurosis of the external oblique muscle (about the size of the tip of the index finger).

Gallbladder. Light palpation is best used in attempting to palpate this fluid-filled, hollow organ. The normal gallbladder is generally not palpable. A distended gallbladder may be felt below the liver margin at the lateral border of the rectus muscle. An enlarged and tender gallbladder may be indicative of cholecystitis; an enlarged but nontender gallbladder tends to be indicative of common bile duct disease.

Aorta. Normally, the aorta is palpable as a pulsatile, slightly tender epigastric structure less than 4 cm in diameter.

Stomach. The normal stomach cannot be palpated even after meals. Gastric carcinoma may cause a left upper quadrant mass when the distal half of the stomach is involved.

Pancreas. The pancreas cannot be detected by palpation due to its small size and retroperitoneal position. Even pancreatic masses are often undetected.

Percussion   *General Guides*

The purpose of percussion is to extend information gained by inspection and palpation or to substitute for palpation in certain circumstances. Using percussion, the nurse is able to outline air-containing or solid structures by the changing sounds. The normal percussion note over the abdomen is tympanic, except for dullness over the liver. Percussion is useful to delineate borders and contours of solid organs, i.e., liver, spleen. The technique employed is identical to that used in percussing the chest (see Chap. 9). Percussion should be light, so that small differences in densities may be perceived. A change in relative versus absolute dullness may be overlooked with too vigorous percussion.

General Survey

Just as with palpation, percussion should be systematic and orderly. First, percuss down the lower left thoracic border wall in the midaxillary line. Normally, this produces a resonant note over the lung. Below the level of the hemidiaphragm, there is normally a tympanic note, due to colon at the splenic flexure. Next, percuss down the right midaxillary line. The upper limit of liver dullness is usually detected at the seventh rib or interspace. Third, percuss to determine the lower limit of liver dullness by percussing down the right side of the chest in the midclavicular line. Normally, the lower limit of liver dullness is the costal margin. Last, percuss for the presence or absence of ascites. Percussion of a distended abdomen can assist the nurse in differentiating between fluid and gas. As described earlier, the percussion note changes to dull when percussing the dependent side or at the umbilicus (see shifting dullness and puddle sign, pp. 283 and 284). To detect distended loops of bowel filled with fluid or gas, the nurse can percuss with quick, repeated, slightly forceful taps at the left iliac fossa. Audible, one-wave "spash" sounds follow each tap rather than multiple waves, as with ascites.

Normally, when the spleen is percussed in the left axillary line and in the lowest intercostal space, the percussion note is resonant owing to the gastric air bubble. When the spleen is enlarged, the percussion note is dull because of stomach displacement. Free air from perforated air-filled viscera (duodenum) rises to the highest possible point, frequently between the liver and anterior ribs. This changes the percussion note from dullness to tympany when the liver is percussed.

Auscultation   *General Guides*

The diaphragm of the stethoscope is used rather than the bell, so that the usually faint peristaltic sounds are not missed. The stethoscope is placed lightly on the abdomen (Fig. 11-11), and each quadrant is auscultated for several min-

Figure 11-11.
Technique for auscultation
of the abdomen.
(Reproduced with
permission from R. D.
Judge, G. D. Zuidema, and
F. Fitzgerald (Eds.).
*Methods of Clinical
Examination* (4th ed.).
Boston: Little, Brown,
1982.)

utes. Interpretation of bowel sounds requires persistent practice and a fundamental knowledge of what causes the sounds. The nurse must auscultate the abdomen of many normal patients to establish a set of norms to serve as a basis for comparison. Any intestinal sound requires that both air and fluid are in interphase in the lumen of the intestine. Alone, neither produces a sound. A normal peristaltic wave produces audible sounds of air and fluid moving along a tube.

General Survey

The "auscultation center" is about 1 to 2 cm below and to the right of the umbilicus. At this point the active sounds of the bowels (especially the small intestines) are most audible. After examining this area first, proceed to auscultate the remainder of the abdomen. Under normal conditions, the best time to hear peristalsis is between meals or at night. Normal tones occur at intervals of about 3 to 5 seconds and are of short duration (about 0.5 second). They are low but distinct dry, rumbling sounds with only slight fluctuations of intensity. The sounds should not be bubbling, squelching, or dissonant in either tone or intensity. After a large meal, normal peristaltic sounds are multiplied, condensed, louder, and damped, and there is an increased rate of peristaltic movement. If abnormal bowel sounds are detected, the nurse should try to determine the point of greatest intensity.

Significant abnormal findings are usually at *two* extremes: (1) absent sounds when motility is inhibited, as in inflammation, gangrene, reflex ileus; and (2) a marked rush of persistent activity with waves of loud "gurgling" and "tinkling" sounds (borborygmi), as with gastroenteritis or diarrhea.

Esophageal bleeding frequently causes hyperperistalsis; intra-abdominal bleeding often results in a "silent" abdomen. Active bowel sounds are rare or absent for one to three days after abdominal surgery, but an abdomen silent for longer than three to four days may indicate a complication, and physician referral is necessary. Active peristaltic sounds may be decreased or entirely subdued by ascites, but a moderate amount of fluid intensifies the sounds of the intestines floating on the fluid. A peritoneal friction rub may be heard over the liver or spleen and usually indicates juxtaposition of two irritated or inflamed surfaces. It usually occurs over an abdominal organ, and the rubbing is associated with respiratory movement. The sound resembles two pieces of leather being rubbed together and is generally associated with carcinoma of the liver.

Rushes, tinkles, and succussion splash may occur with various types of bowel obstruction and should be brought to the attention of a physician. Systolic bruits are vascular sounds similar to a cardiac murmur and may indicate a dilated, tortuous, or constricted vessel. Loud bruits auscultated over the aorta may indicate the presence of an aneurysm. A venous hum may also be heard. It is generally heard over the upper portion of the abdomen or liver and is associated with increased collateral circulation between portal and systemic venous systems, as in hepatic cirrhosis.

EXAMINATION OF MALE GENITOURINARY SYSTEM
Penis and Scrotum

Examination of the male genitalia is based primarily on inspection and palpation (Fig. 11-12). The urethra is observed for discharge, inflammation, lesions, nodules, and swelling. The prepuce of the uncircumcised male should be retracted around the head of the penis. Normally, this should be accomplished with ease. A small amount of thick white secretion (smegma) is normally present between the prepuce and the glans. The shaft of the penis varies in size and is not considered abnormal unless very small and infantile in appearance. The urethra opens at the tip of the head of the penis. Ideally, the examiner should watch the patient urinate to observe the urinary stream. In adults, a poor urinary stream may indicate urethral stricture or prostatic obstruction.

Phimosis is an adhesion of the prepuce to the head of the penis, making it difficult or impossible to retract. *Paraphimosis* is an inflammation of the prepuce due to retraction that forms a tight ring around the penis, causing painful swelling of the glans. Edema of the penis is commonly seen with fluid retention due to dependent positioning. The penis should be examined from the tip to the base of the shaft for healed scars or any active lesions. An indurated, oval or round, painless ulcer is characteristic of syphilis. Carcinoma of the glans penis or prepuce is generally a dry, scaly, ulcerated, painless lesion. Condylo-

Figure 11-12.
Male genitalia. *A.* Cross
section. *B.* External.
(Reproduced with
permission from R. D.
Judge, G. D. Zuidema, and
F. Fitzgerald (Eds.).
*Methods of Clinical
Examination* (4th ed.).
Boston: Little, Brown,
1982.)

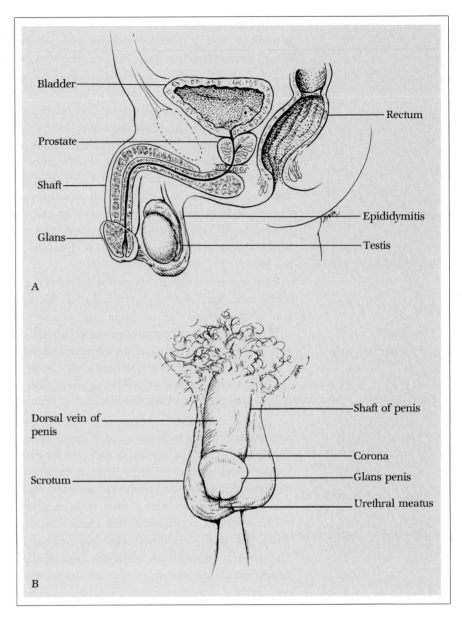

mata acuminata (venereal warts) are cauliflower-like lesions. They may be either dry or moist, appear singly or in multiple patches, and are caused by a viral infection. See Figure 11-13 for illustrations of these lesions.

The urethra should be examined for hypospadias, the abnormal positioning of the urinary meatus on the ventral surface of the shaft, or *epispadias,* an opening on the dorsal surface. Usually surgically corrected in childhood, these conditions are rarely seen in adults. The urethra should be observed for the

Figure 11-13. Some lesions of the penis. (Reproduced with permission from R. D. Judge, G. D. Zuidema, and F. Fitzgerald (Eds.). *Methods of Clinical Examination* (4th ed.). Boston: Little, Brown, 1982.)

Phimosis

Paraphimosis

Hypospachias

Syphilitic cancre

Herpes progenitalis

Condylomata acuminata

Epidermoid carcinoma

presence of any discharge. A thick, purulent discharge may be due to gonor-rhea and should be cultured. A thin, mucoid discharge may indicate urethritis.

The scrotum is examined and the testes palpated. An asymmetric position of the testes is normal, the left testes being slightly lower in the scrotum than the right. The normal size of the testes varies, but the largest should be about 2 centimeters in diameter and of firm consistency. Tenderness is normally present when anything but very light palpation pressure is used. Their size, shape, consistency, and tenderness should be noted. The epididymis surrounds the testes laterally and may be palpated with ease. The spermatic cord extends from the epididymis to the inguinal canal, where it is palpated between the thumb and forefinger as a thin cord. Testicular masses are frequently malignant. Atrophy may occur with other disease, e.g., mumps and liver disorders. Orchitis, or inflammation of the testes, is very painful, and pain is the patient's chief complaint.

Hydroceles, which are scrotal cysts filled with clear fluid, are rounded, non-tender masses and may be detected by transillumination. This is done in a very dark room, using a flashlight positioned under the scrotum. The entire cyst "lights up" as the light shines through the fluid. A *varicocele* is enlargement of the veins accompanying the epididymis and spermatic cord. A *spermatocele* is a cystic, localized enlargement of the spermatic cord or epididymis. Patients with any such abnormalities should be referred to a physician. Figure 11-14 illustrates these scrotal lesions.

Inguinal Region

Femoral pulses should be palpated first to detect evidence of aortic disease. Lymph nodes in the groin area are palpated and often felt as "shotty," firm, freely movable, half-centimeter masses.

The inguinal canal begins with the internal ring and extends in continuity with the scrotum. The external inguinal ring is the opening between the scrotum and the inguinal canal. The spermatic cord and accompanying vessels enter the inguinal canal at this point. To examine the inguinal ring for hernias, it is preferable that the patient be in a standing position. The index or little finger is directed upward from the distal aspect of the scrotum, turning the scrotal skin inward like the finger of a glove. The internal inguinal canal is a natural opening in the abdominal wall and is felt at the end of the canal as a fibrous circle of tissue with a soft center. If the patient is asked to "strain" as in defecating, the intra-abdominal pressure increases and accentuates any weakness of the internal ring or abdominal musculature. Straining is preferred to having the patient cough, since the intra-abdominal pressure is increased only momentarily with coughing and makes a thorough examination more difficult.

Other than increased or decreased femoral pulses or enlarged lymph nodes, the most frequently encountered abnormality in the inguinal region is a hernia (see Fig. 11-5). An *indirect inguinal hernia* is a herniation along the path of the spermatic cord. Both direct and indirect hernias may involve a variety of

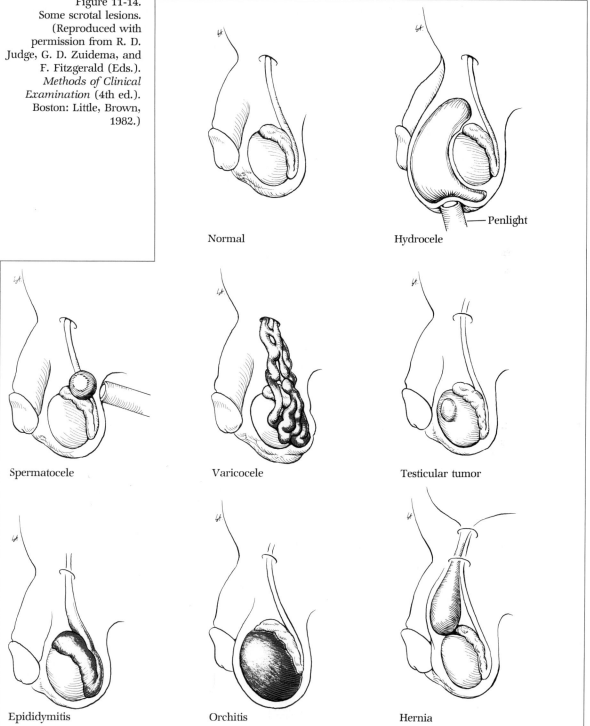

Figure 11-14.
Some scrotal lesions.
(Reproduced with
permission from R. D.
Judge, G. D. Zuidema, and
F. Fitzgerald (Eds.).
*Methods of Clinical
Examination* (4th ed.).
Boston: Little, Brown,
1982.)

Normal

Hydrocele

———Penlight

Spermatocele

Varicocele

Testicular tumor

Epididymitis

Orchitis

Hernia

Reducible	Can be returned into the abdominal cavity
Incarcerated	Nonreducible, entrapped
Strangulated	Blood flow to the bowel has been impaired

	Direct	Indirect
Description	Loop of intestine passes through posterior inguinal wall	Loop of intestine passes through abdominal ring and follows spermatic cord into inguinal canal
Cause	Increased intra-abdominal pressure against a weak posterior inguinal wall; congenital or acquired	Increased intra-abdominal pressure forces intestines into a congenital defect resulting from failure of the processus vaginalis to close
Incidence	Elderly, men	Infants and young persons and males 50 + years old

organs, including the mesentery, small bowel, colon, and urinary bladder. *Incipient hernias* are felt as a bulge at the internal inguinal ring when the patient strains downward while in a standing position. This small bulge may not be felt on the outside and may never progress to a true hernia. A small hernia produces a large bulge at the internal ring. It is felt by the examining hand placed externally over the area of the internal ring. Large hernias usually descend into the inguinal canal to variable distances and frequently enter the scrotum. A *strangulated hernia* is a medical emergency requiring prompt referral to a physician. Hernias may also be described as indicated in Tables 11-1 and 11-2.

A *direct inguinal hernia occurs* when the herniation is directly through a defect or weakness in the abdominal wall rather than along the inguinal canal. A small direct hernia differs from a small indirect one by invaginating into the scrotum. With the examining finger at the internal ring, the bulge can be felt pressing against the length of the finger rather than the fingertip. Direct hernias may produce scrotal masses and become incarcerated and strangulated.

Rectum and Prostate   The positioning of the patient for rectal examination varies. There are four possible positions:

1. Left decubitus position with the patient's knees drawn up to the abdomen.
2. Standing position with the elbows flexed and resting on the bed or table.
3. Supine position with the knees spread apart.
4. Knee-chest position with the patient's head turned to one side.

To inspect the external area, spread the patient's buttocks apart with both hands to expose the anal area for examination. Again the patient "bears down" to emphasize the anatomy and cause the normal anal sphincter to contract and demonstrate intact innervation.

To palpate internally, the examining hand should be gloved and well lubricated. Explain to the patient what is going to be done and the sensations he will feel (e.g., pressure), to help him stay more relaxed. Begin with gentle pressure of the ball of the index finger and gradually insert the tip of the finger as the sphincter relaxes. At this point, it may be helpful to tell the patient that he may feel the urge to have a bowel movement. Ask him to tighten his anal sphincter so that you can determine sphincter strength.

A bidigital examination may also be performed in the sphincter area. The thumb of the examining hand is pressed toward the index finger, and the tissue of the perianal area is palpated between the digits for masses or irregularities. Enlarged bulbourethral (Cowper's) glands can be detected in this manner.

The prostate gland is located anterior to the mucosa of the anterior rectal wall. The posterior aspect of the gland protrudes into the rectal ampulla, which allows this portion of the gland to be examined for abnormalities. The size of the normal prostate gland varies, but averages 4 cm in diameter (Fig. 11-15). It is divided into two lobes by a vertical median fissure. It should be of firm

Figure 11-15. Examination of the prostate gland. (Reproduced with permission from R. D. Judge and G. D. Zuidema (Eds.). *Methods of Clinical Examination: A Phyisologic Approach* (3rd ed.). Boston: Little, Brown, 1974.)

consistency and without "bogginess." The patient should not complain of tenderness when the normal gland is palpated; however, he may feel the urge to urinate. The seminal vesicles extend above the prostate gland and are normally not palpable.

The rectum normally can be palpated to a depth of 10 cm. The rectal valves normally are felt as protruding intrarectal masses. The lateral walls may be palpated by feeling the sides of the rectum. The examiner should be able to palpate the ischial spines and the sacrotuberous ligaments. The posterior wall of the rectum normally follows the curve of the sacrum and coccyx and feels very smooth.

External *hemorrhoids* can be identified by inspection of the anal area. Requesting the patient to "bear down" may make a visible hemorrhoid more prominent. Hypertrophied anal papillae resemble hemorrhoids, but there are no dilated veins. Perianal skin may be irritated or inflamed. Thickening of the surrounding skin may occur secondary to chronic scratching and pruritus ani. The pilonidal sinus is a tract into the skin overlying the tip of the coccyx. Normally, it contains hair. When it becomes obstructed and infected, a pilonidal cyst or abscess occurs.

Palpation of the anal sphincter may detect hypertonicity. This usually occurs due to tension or local irritation, as with anal fissure. Hypotonicity or a weak anal sphincter may be due to previous surgery or underlying neurologic disease. A perianal abscess may be found by bidigital palpation of the circumference of the anal sphincter.

Rectal masses are often malignant; approximately one-half of all carcinomas occur in the colon and rectum. A rectal shelf may be palpated as a stony hard mass above the prostate on the anterior rectal wall. This shelf usually occurs with metastatic carcinoma to the pelvic floor. Any abnormalities detected by the nurse require prompt referral of the patient for further evaluation by a physician.

Hesitancy and straining while voiding are early signs of prostatic obstruction. Loss of force and decrease of the caliber of the stream occur as urethral resistance increases, despite increased transvesical pressure. Terminal dribbling also increases with obstruction, and acute urinary retention may be seen in the patient who is unable to void. He has increasing suprapubic pain with urgency and is able to dribble only small amounts of urine. Chronic urinary retention involves little or no pain. There is a great deal of hesitancy in starting the stream and a marked decrease in its force and caliber. Constant dribbling (paradoxical incontinency) may also occur.

In benign prostatic hypertrophy the gland may be palpated as diffusely enlarged, without masses. Atrophy of the prostate occurs with loss of secondary sex characteristics. Tenderness on palpation is a common finding. Extreme tenderness may occur with urinary abnormalities. The gland may feel soft and "boggy" with prostatitis also.

Table 11-3.
Pain Characteristics of
Selected Genitourinary
Organs

Organ	Type	Duration	Location	Possible Causes
Kidney	Dull	Constant	Costovertebral angle, lateral; lateral to sacrospinalis muscle	Acute pyelonephritis with sudden edema Acute urethral obstruction with sudden renal back pressure
Urethra	Severe	Colicky	Back; may radiate from costovertebral angle to lower anterior quadrant of abdomen (radiates to vulva in females)	Acute obstruction (e.g., stone or blood clot) (Severity and colicky nature of pain is due to hyperperistalsis and spasm of smooth muscles in attempts to overcome the obstruction.)
Vesicle	Severe		Suprapubic; usually referred to distal urethra; related to urination	Overdistended bladder in acute urinary retention
Testicle	Severe Dull ache		Testicle Testicle	Trauma or infection Varicocele

Carcinoma of the prostate may be felt as a mass or node on the posterior lobe of the gland. Advanced tumors usually feel stony hard, are irregular, and not tender.

PAIN IN GENITOURINARY DISEASE

Pain is an important complaint of many patients with genitourinary alterations and may be localized or referred. Localized pain is felt in the region of the involved organ. Referred pain originates in a diseased organ, but is felt at some distance from the organ. It is also important for the nurse to remember that many genitourinary diseases are painless due to the slow progression of the disease (e.g., carcinoma, chronic pyelonephritis, and tuberculosis). Table 11-3 gives a brief description of types of pain that the nurse may encounter in patients.

ABDOMEN AND MALE GENITOURINARY SYSTEM-ASSESSMENT GUIDE

I. Abdomen
  A. Inspection
    1. Position—comfortable, hands at sides, relaxed
    2. Skin—venous patterns, scars, hydration, discolorations, pigmentation
    3. Umbilicus—direction, contour, lesions
    4. Hair—distribution, pattern
    5. Movements—pattern, pulsations

6. Contours—symmetry, normal age variations, distention due to air, fluid, tumor, hernia
7. Pain—visceral or peritoneal, character, localized or diffuse, accompanying symptoms, onset, duration

B. Auscultation
   1. Bowel sounds—absent, increased, gurgling/tinkling, borborygmi
   2. Circulatory sounds—bruits, venous hums, rubs

C. Palpation
   1. Light palpation—muscle tone and guarding, enlarged solid organs (liver, spleen, kidneys, uterus), enlarged hollow organs (bowel, stomach, bladder, aorta), tenderness, location, size, shape, consistency
   2. Deep palpation—note size, movement with respiration, tenderness, position, consistency, attachment to underlying tissue and/or viscera
      a. Aorta—pulsations, tenderness
      b. Colon—transverse: soft; movable sigmoid: ropelike
      c. Liver—contour, consistency, size, cm below costal margin, presence of nodules, pulsations
      d. Spleen—contour, consistency, size, cm below costal margin
      e. Kidneys—size, consistency

D. Percussion—delineate air, fluid and solid structures (dullness vs. tympany)
      a. Liver—dullness, size
      b. Spleen—resonancy, size
      c. Stomach—tympany
      d. Bladder—dullness when distended
      e. Masses—delineate borders and contours, size
      f. Fluid—shifting dullness, puddle sign, fluid wave

II. Male Genitourinary Examination: Rectum and Prostate
   A. Inspection
      1. Penis—distribution of pubic hair, parasites, size relative to age and general development, shape, skin color, lesions, edema, discharge, location of urethra
      2. Scrotum—symmetry, size, contour, skin color, lesions, edema, nodules
      3. Inguinal region—scars, lesions, enlarged lymph nodes
      4. Rectum—color, lesions, hemorrhoids, inflammation, pilonidal cyst
      5. Urinary stream—strength, force, urgency, dribbling, hesitancy
      6. Pain—localized or referred, type, onset, location, duration, accompanying symptoms
   B. Palpation
      1. Penis—retraction of prepuce, tenderness
      2. Scrotum
         a. Testes—size, location, consistency, tenderness, nodules
         b. Epididymis—location, size, tenderness, symmetry
         c. Spermatic cord—location, size, tenderness, symmetry
         d. Masses—size, location, consistency, tenderness, nodules, transilluminates
      3. Inguinal region
         a. Femoral pulses—strength, character, quality
         b. Lymph nodes—size, consistency, movability, tenderness
         c. Inguinal canal—indirect or direct inguinal hernia, reducible, strangulated
      4. Rectum—sphincter strength, rectal valves, perianal masses or enlarged glands, fissures, rectal masses: size, location, consistency, tenderness
      5. Prostate—size, consistency, nodules, tenderness

SUGGESTED READINGS

Boyce, H. W., Jr., and Palmer, E. D. *Techniques of Clinical Gastroenterology.* Springfield, Ill.: Thomas, 1975.

Buckingham, W. B., et al. *A Primer of Clinical Diagnosis* (2nd ed.). New York: Harper & Row, 1979.

Cope, Z. *The Early Diagnosis of the Acute Abdomen* (14th ed.). London: Oxford University Press, 1972.

DeGowin, E., and DeGowin, R. *Bedside Diagnostic Examination* (3rd ed.). New York: Macmillan, 1976.

Delp, M. H., and Manning, R. T. *Major's Physical Diagnosis* (8th ed.). Philadelphia: Saunders, 1975.

Sherman, J. L., and Fields, K. *Guide to Patient Evaluation*. Flushing, N.Y.: Medical Examination Publishing Co., 1974.

Smith, D. *General Urology*. Los Altos, Calif.: Lange, 1972.

12. Physical Assessment of the Female Reproductive System

adnexa The uterine appendages, the ovaries, uterine tubes, and ligaments of the uterus.

amenorrhea Absence of menses.

anteflexion of uterus The normal forward curvature of the uterus in which the upper part is bent forward.

atrophic vaginitis A nonspecific vaginal infection in which the epithelium may be spotted with small petechiae.

caruncle A small red eminence on the mucous membrane of the urinary meatus.

chronic cystic mastitis Inflammatory condition of the breast characterized by diffuse nodularity and cystic changes.

cul-de-sac A blind pouch posterior to the uterus.

cystocele Hernial protrusion of the urinary bladder through the anterior vaginal wall.

dysmenorrhea Painful menstruation.

dyspareunia Difficult or painful intercourse.

enterocele Hernial protrusion of part of the intestine through the posterior vaginal wall.

fibroma Fibroid tumor derived from connective tissue.

fornices The recesses formed between the vaginal walls and the vaginal part of the cervix. The areas are termed *anterior* or *posterior,* depending on their relation to the cervix.

greater vestibular (Bartholin's) glands Two small mucous glands on the inner aspect of the labia minora in front of the hymen.

gynecomastia Hypertrophy of breast tissue in the male, which causes resemblance to a female breast.

hypermenorrhea Abnormally increased volume of menstrual flow.

introitus The entrance into the vagina.

kraurosis vulvae Dryness, shriveling, and increasing fibrosis of the vulva and the vaginal vestibule, vulvovaginal stenosis. This condition frequently occurs in conjunction with leukoplakia.

leiomyoma Fibroid tumor of the uterus.

lesser vestibular glands Numerous minute mucous glands opening on the surface of the vestibule between the orifices of the vagina and the urethra.

leukoplakia The appearance of white, thickened patches on the vulvar surface. This condition frequently occurs in conjunction with kraurosis vulvae.

mastitis Inflammation of the breast, usually due to pyogenic infection.

menarche Beginning of the menstrual function.

menopause Termination of menses.

multipara Woman who has given birth to more than one child.

nabothian follicles Dilation of the mucus-secreting glands of the cervix caused by obstruction of their orifices and retention of the mucous secretions.

parametrium The loose connective tissue and smooth muscle lying beside the cervix and lower segment of the body of the uterus.

paraurethral (Skene's) glands Numerous mucous glands in the wall of the female urethra.

polymenorrhea Abnormally frequent menstrual flow.

polyp Protruding growth from any mucous membrane such as that of the cervix.

primigravida Woman pregnant for the first time.

primipara Woman who has given birth to one viable infant.

rectocele Hernial protrusion of part of the rectum through the posterior vaginal wall.

retraction Dimpling of the nipple or skin overlying the breast tissue.

retroversion of uterus Abnormal position of the uterus in which the entire uterus is tilted backward.

uterine prolapse Protrusion of the uterus through the vaginal orifice. *First-degree prolapse* The cervix lies between the level of the ischial spines and the vaginal introitus. *Second-degree prolapse* The cervix protrudes through the introitus. *Third-degree prolapse* Both the cervix and the body of the uterus have passed through the introitus, and the entire vaginal canal is inverted.

vestibule The area between the inner surfaces of the labia minora and below the clitoris which forms the entrance to the vagina.

INVESTIGATION and examination of the female reproductive system reveals considerable information on the status of the lower urinary tract and the lower abdomen, as well as the reproductive organs. The number of physiologic functions related to the genital area—micturition, defecation, menstruation, ovulation, copulation, impregnation, and parturition—makes a regular, thorough examination of this area exceedingly important. Examination of the female genitalia should, without question, be a part of every woman's annual physical examination.

The current sexual revolution and increasing frankness in relation to sexuality might lead one to anticipate only minimal reluctance from women in seeking or experiencing examinations of the reproductive system. However, it is important to remember that attitudes and behaviors developed over many years do not change quickly. Thus one must anticipate and respect a spectrum of reactions to and concerns about the history and the physical examination. Nurses have a vital role in educating women as to the importance of regular examinations and the necessity of early reporting of any alterations they themselves notice. It is hoped that the practice of having annual pelvic examinations will be conveyed from mothers to daughters, so that pelvic examinations will be a routine part of the health maintenance practices of each new generation of women.

HISTORY AND GENERAL ASSESSMENT

A thorough evaluation of the female reproductive system involves exploration of the woman's relevant history and observation of some general characteristics. The following should be included:

1. *General body stature.* Is the woman generally of a female body build?
2. *Secondary sex characteristics.*
   a. Distribution of facial and axillary hair.
   b. Pitch of voice.
   c. Breast development (see p. 311–314 for a thorough discussion).
3. *Family history.* Is there any history of cancer or other reproductive disorders, especially in the mother?
4. *Obstetric and surgical history.* Determine gravidity and parity. Has she had any abortions? If so, what type? What was the precipitating factor? Has she had previous gynecologic surgery, and if so, were there any complications?

5. *Menstrual pattern.*
   a. *Menarche.* At what age did she experience menarche? Were there any associated problems?
   b. *Menstrual periods.* Determine the interval between periods, the duration, and the amount of flow. What is the color of the menstrual discharge? Do clots occur? What is the date of her last menstrual period?
   c. Does dysmenorrhea or intermenstrual bleeding occur?
   d. *Menopause.* If she has experienced menopause, at what age did it occur? Was it natural, or was it artificially induced as by surgery or irradiation? Were there any associated problems? If she has not yet experienced menopause, what are her expectations regarding it? Does she have any questions as to what she may anticipate?
6. *Vaginal discharge.* Have her describe any vaginal discharge she has been having. Determine the amount (number of pads), character, color, odor, presence of tissue, and any precipitating factors.
7. *Sexual history.* How is her relationship with spouse or partner? How frequently does she engage in intercourse? Is it satisfying for her? Does she experience dyspareunia? This is a particularly important area to explore with the postmenopausal woman for whom menopausal dyspareunia is frequently a problem.
8. *Knowledge of own health care.*
   a. Has she had routine pelvic examinations and Papanicolaou smears? How often? When was her last one?
   b. Does she do monthly breast self-examinations?
   c. What method of contraception does she or partner use? Is it satisfactory to both? Does she need further contraceptive information?

BREAST EXAMINATION

A thorough, systematic examination of both breasts and surrounding lymphatic drainage sites is necessary because of the high incidence of disease in this organ. The breast is the most common site of cancer in the female [2].

The woman should disrobe to the waist so that both breasts can be exposed simultaneously for comparison (Fig. 12-1). Good lighting is important to ensure observation of areas of retraction. The woman is examined in both the sitting and the supine positions. Inspection is followed by palpation.

Inspection

Inspection of the breasts includes attention to symmetry, position and size, superficial appearance, nipples, and any skin retraction present.

With the woman in the sitting position, it is not uncommon to notice some asymmetry in the size and position of the two breasts. Generally, this is due to developmental differences, but it might indicate an abnormality such as a cyst, tumor, or inflammation.

In the thin, flat-chested woman, the nipple with its areola is approximately over the fourth intercostal space in the midclavicular line. With the accumula-

Figure 12-1.
Woman draped for breast
examination. (Reproduced
with permission from R. D.
Judge, G. D. Zuidema, and
F. Fitzgerald (Eds.).
*Methods of Clinical
Examination* (4th ed.).
Boston: Little, Brown,
1982.)

Figure 12-1.
Woman draped for breast examination. (Reproduced with permission from R. D. Judge, G. D. Zuidema, and F. Fitzgerald (Eds.). *Methods of Clinical Examination* (4th ed.). Boston: Little, Brown, 1982.)

tion of fat, there may be some dropping of the nipple below the fourth inter-costal space. In most women, the breasts extend in area from the third to the sixth ribs. However, with obesity, the loss of breast hypertrophy after lactation, or increasing age, the breasts sag and the nipples drop lower. The atrophy of breast tissue and muscular supports beginning at menopause results in the sagging, limp breasts of the aged female.

The skin overlying the breasts should be carefully observed. The examiner should look for local areas of erythema and signs of edema. The latter is man-ifested by hair follicles and follicular openings that are more pronounced or noticeable than usual, giving an orange-peel appearance.

The nipples should be carefully examined for bleeding, discharge, retraction, or ulceration. It is particularly important to note the color of any discharge, which may range from clear yellow to blue or green. Some asymmetry in the size and shape of the nipples is not necessarily abnormal. Inversion of the nipples may be present, but is significant only if it is of recent origin.

Careful inspection for skin retraction, or dimpling, is one of the most impor-tant aspects of the breast examination, and good lighting is essential for this purpose. Dimpling, which appears in different degrees, can be found on any part of the skin of the breast or nipple. It can occur with inflammation, but most often it denotes a malignancy.

To demonstrate best an early stage of retraction, the woman can perform a variety of movements to place pull on the suspensory ligaments (Fig. 12-2A). After she has been examined while sitting erect, ask her to raise her arms directly overhead (Fig. 12-2B). Also she can cause contraction of the pectoral

Figure 12-2. Demonstration of skin retraction. *A.* Diagram showing how shortening of Cooper's ligaments may produce skin retraction. *B.* Method of bringing out skin retraction by raising arms overhead. *C.* Method of bringing out skin retraction by pressing hands against hips. (Modified from R. D. Judge, G. D. Zuidema, and F. Fitzgerald (Eds.). *Methods of Clinical Examination* (4th ed.). Boston: Little, Brown, 1982.)

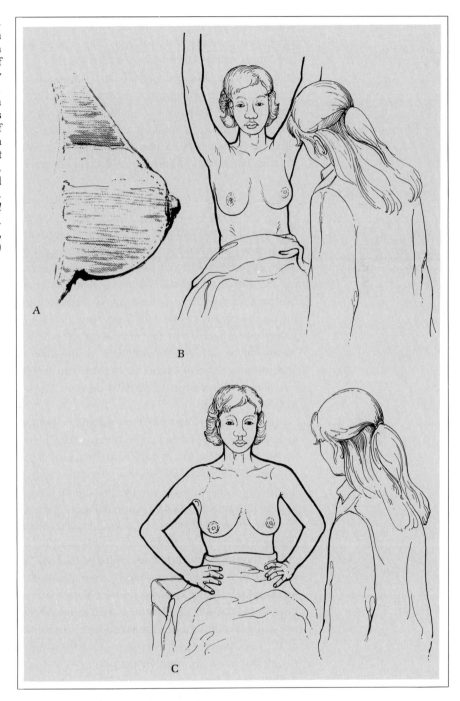

muscles by placing both hands together in front of her and pushing them against each other. A second way this can be accomplished is by her placing her hands on her hips and pushing forcibly against them (Fig. 12-2C). The latter two methods exaggerate any retraction that is present. The woman should continue one of these actions until all areas of both breasts have been inspected for retraction.

Observation of the axillary and supraclavicular regions is also important, to check for bulging, retraction, discoloration, or edema. These are the most important lymphatic drainage areas for the breasts.

Palpation   After the thorough inspection, the breasts, axillae, and supraclavicular regions should be systematically palpated. There is a wide variation in the consistency of normal breast tissue. Such factors as age, obesity, stage of the menstrual cycle, and pregnancy contribute to this variation. As the examiner becomes more experienced in the physical examination, she will gain an appreciation for the range of normal breast size and consistency. In young women, the breasts tend to be firm, somewhat elastic in consistency, and cone-shaped, with the border clearly delineated. The young breast may be particularly sensitive to palpation, especially at the time of its growth at puberty or just prior to the menstrual period. The breast tissue of the older woman is commonly stringy and nodular. The older breast develops an irregular consistency, with disappearance of the sharply delineated borders. Large breasts may become pendulous.

As palpation begins, the nurse should remember the monthly cyclic physiologic changes that occur in the breast. The breasts become engorged, lobular, and sensitive prior to the menses and decongest promptly thereafter. As a result of years of such cyclical changes, nodules may develop, giving the breast a granular consistency. During pregnancy, the breasts become firmer and larger, and the lobulations become more distinct. These well-defined lobules may easily be confused with tumor masses. Detailed recording and follow-up to ensure appropriate medical attention is mandatory.

For thorough examination, palpation of the breasts should be performed with the woman seated and then supine. In both positions, the breasts should be examined with the woman's arms at her side and then with her arms overhead (Fig. 12-3A and B). When examining the woman in the supine position, use a small pillow under the shoulder on each side as it is examined (Fig. 12-3C). This allows the breast to rest more symmetrically over the chest wall, permitting more accurate examination.

Palpation begins in the upper, lateral quadrant of each breast where most tumors occur. The examination must be systematic to ensure that the breasts are completely examined. The palpation can be done in a clockwise direction until the entire breast is examined, or palpation can proceed in and out, laterally to medially, forming a pattern like spokes of a wheel. If the woman com-

Figure 12-3.
Positions used for palpation
of the breast. *A.* Erect with
arms at sides. *B.* Erect with
arms raised overhead. *C.*
Supine. (Modified from
Judge and Zuidema [1].)

plains of tenderness or a lump in one breast, that area should be palpated last.

Palpation begins lightly and gently, using the palmar aspect of the fingertips, with a rotary to-and-fro motion. Following light palpation, each area is more deeply explored. It is important not to compress a portion of the breast tissue between the fingers of one or both hands, as this may give the erroneous impression that a lump is present. To avoid this, the breast tissue should be compressed gently but firmly against the chest wall (Fig. 12-3).

After examination of the breast tissue, attention is focused on the nipple. Any subareolar masses, induration, loss of elasticity, dry scaling, or excoriation should be noted. Gentle pressure or a stripping action should be used to see whether or not a discharge can be elicited.

The examiner should note the consistency and elasticity of the breast tissue and nipples, the texture of the skin, and any masses detected. If a mass is located, it should be characterized according to the following features:

1. *Location.* The. exact location of the mass must be designated. One method is to consider each breast as if it were the face of a clock with the nipple as the central point and the numbers of the clock placed clockwise in a 1 to 12 position. Thus a lesion can be stated to be along a specific axis, e.g., the 9 o'clock axis. Also, the mass should be located as to its distance from the nipple. It is often helpful to draw a circle and make a sketch of the mass, illustrating it on the proper axis.
2. *Size.* The size of the mass should be estimated as accurately as possible in three dimensions. It is particularly important to describe it in centimeters of length, width, and thickness for comparison with future progression or regression of the mass.
3. *Contour.* A description of the surface of the mass should be made. Is it regular and smooth or irregular and infiltrating?
4. *Consistency.* Determine the firmness or softness of the mass. It may be described as soft, cystic, moderately firm, firm, or stony hard.
5. *Tenderness.* Determine whether the lesion is tender and, if so, to what degree.
6. *Mobility.* Determine whether the lesion is freely movable, movable only in certain directions, or fixed. Is mobility of the mass limited by fixation to deep structures, to the skin, or to surrounding breast tissue?
7. *Discreteness.* Determine whether the boundaries of the mass are easily detected or difficult to differentiate.

After completion of the examination of the breast, the axilla should be carefully palpated. Thorough examination can be made with one hand while the examiner's opposite hand holds the ipsilateral arm of the woman, who may be either sitting or supine. The axilla should be thought of as having an apex and three walls. The lymph nodes are divided into three groups: anterior or pectoral group, central group, and posterior group. Cup the examining hand slightly and reach as high into the apex of the axilla as possible. Then pull the hand downward, exerting gentle pressure against the thorax with the fingertips (Fig. 12-4). Repeat several times so that each area is palpated with the woman's arm at her side and again while the arm is moved through a full range of motion. This is done to uncover any lesions hidden under muscle or fatty tissue. It is important not to abduct the arm too far, for this tenses the skin of the axilla, interfering with deep palpation and possibly causing the woman discomfort.

Figure 12-4.
Technique for examination
of the axilla. (Reproduced
with permission from R. D.
Judge, G. D. Zuidema, and
F. Fitzgerald (Eds.).
*Methods of Clinical
Examination* (4th ed.).
Boston: Little, Brown,
1982.)

Following examination of the breasts and axillae, both supraclavicular regions should be palpated. By deeper palpation check the deep jugular chain of nodes, as these are frequently routes of metastatic spread of breast cancer.

Significant Findings   As discussed earlier, there is a wide range of normal characteristics of the female breast. Experience in inspection and palpation of the breast best helps the nurse in developing skill in detecting abnormalities. Differentiating the nodules that occur with aging from tumor masses is one of the most difficult skills. Of course, where there is any question, the woman should be referred to a physician for biopsy of the lesion.

A thorough physical examination provides the following information:

1. Presence, location, and number of masses.
2. Consistency, size, tenderness, and mobility of mass(es).
3. Retraction or dimpling of skin over mass.
4. Displacement or retraction of nipple.
5. Palpable regional lymph nodes, if any.

These characteristics will be discussed here only in relation to the most common alterations.

Benign lesions, such as lipomas or adenofibromas, are most often soft and cystic, smooth-surfaced, with well-defined borders, and easily movable. In contrast, malignant lesions are generally firm with uneven surfaces, infiltrating, have irregular margins, and are often fixed to other structures as they become invasive. Tenderness is rarely found with a malignant lesion. An inflammatory

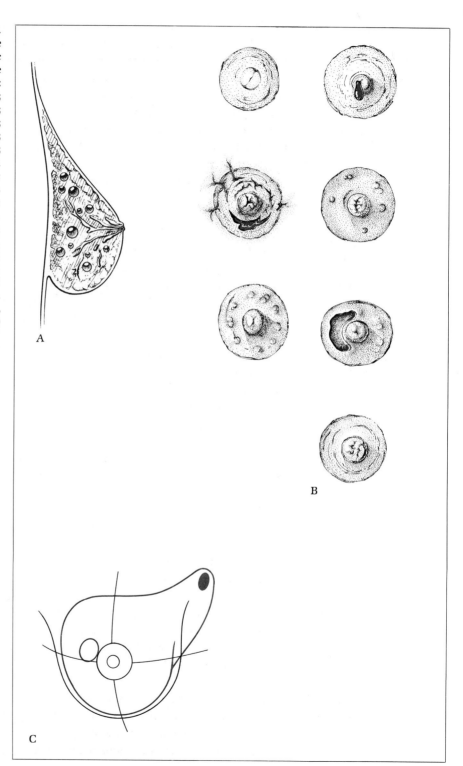

Figure 12-5. Lesions of the breast tissue and nipple. *A.* Chronic cystic mastitis. *B.* Some lesions of the nipple: (1) inversion; (2) discharge; (3) Paget's disease; (4) hyperpigmentation; (5) retention cysts; (6) ulceration; (7)inflammation. *C.* A sample sketch of a cystic left breast lesion, such as may be recorded in the written work-up. (Reproduced with permission from R. D. Judge, G. D. Zuidema, and F. Fitzgerald (Eds.). *Methods of Clinical Examination* (4th ed.). Boston: Little, Brown, 1982.)

process often demonstrates symptoms similar to those of a malignant lesion, having an irregular contour, a firm consistency, and being firmly or moderately firmly fixed to surrounding structures. One differing feature, however, is that inflammatory lesions are usually moderately to markedly tender.

Chronic cystic mastitis is an exceedingly common breast lesion characterized by multiple nodules diffusely located in both breasts. The breast tissue is usually thickened and may be tender to palpation. Occasionally, the process may be fairly localized. In either event, the woman should be referred for diagnostic biopsy (Fig. 12-5A).

Mastitis is a generalized inflammation of breast tissue, usually occurring during lactation. The involved breast tends to be red, edematous, and tender; chills and fever often accompany the inflammation. The usual cause is a pyogenic infection.

Any discharge from the nipple should always be considered significant and reported to a physician. Bloody or dark discharge can indicate intraductal papilloma or Paget's disease, a malignant disease of the nipple and areola (Fig. 12-5B). A sketch of the lesion will provide the best record of its size, its distance from the nipple, and its characteristics (Fig. 12-5C).

Male Breast   Examination of the breast in the male is just as important as it is in the female. Carcinoma of the breast does occur in males, though much less frequently than in females.

In examination of the male breast the same procedure is followed as in examination of the female breast. In the young, moderately thin man, the nipple and areola are found approximately in the fourth intercostal space, midclavicular line. With the accumulation of fat or with increasing age, this anatomic relationship is usually lost, with the nipple dropping below the level of the fourth intercostal space.

Carcinoma of the male breast usually occurs as an irregular, hard nodule underlying the areola, causing retraction of the nipple and fixation to the skin and deep tissues. The paucity of breast tissue accounts for the early metastasis to axillary lymph nodes.

Gynecomastia is usually unilateral and noninflammatory. In the young male, the breast has a glandular consistency and is conical in shape. With age, the nodularity increases, making differentiation from a neoplasm more difficult, and biopsy is necessary. Systemic disease, such as cirrhosis of the liver, may cause bilateral gynecomastia. In such cases the liver is no longer able to detoxify estrogens.

Self-examination of the Breast   Nurses play an exceedingly important role in instructing women in the technique of self-examination of the breast. The importance of regular examinations cannot be overestimated, and every woman should know and practice the technique. The method of examination is simple and easily learned. The nurse should stress that the exam can reveal the presence of disease while it is still in a curable state. Thus, it is a vital part of one's own health maintenance program. Additionally, mothers should begin teaching their daughters to do self-examination as soon as they begin to have significant breast development.

Ideally, the examination should be performed immediately following each menstrual period. Temporary changes preceding the menstrual cycle give the breasts a nodular consistency and increase their sensitiveness to palpation. Following menopause, breast self-examinations should continue on a regular basis. The woman should be taught to look for the following: any dimpling or puckering of the skin; retraction of either nipple; any thickening or change in consistency; or any alteration in symmetry, size, contour, or position. Also to be reported are pain, swelling, inflammation, or discharge. If she has some nodules that have been checked by a physician, they should be followed closely for any changes in characteristics.

After being given information as to what findings are important, women should be taught how to observe and how to palpate the breast.

Observation

The woman should place herself before a mirror with her arms at her sides. She should carefully examine her breasts in the mirror for symmetry, size, and shape, searching for any evidence of puckering, dimpling of the skin, or retraction of the nipple. She should then raise her arms above her head and again study her breasts in the mirror, looking for the same physical signs. She should also be alert for any evidence of fixation of the breast tissue to the chest wall. This may be displayed as she moves her arms and shoulders.

Palpation

Palpation should be performed in the reclining position. This position permits the breasts to spread over a greater area and thins the breast tissue, making accurate palpation easier. A small pillow or folded towel should be placed beneath the shoulder on the side of the breast to be examined. This raises that side of the body and distributes the weight of the breast tissue more evenly over the chest wall. The arm on the side to be first examined is placed at her side, and the breast is gently examined with the flat surface of the fingers of her opposite hand. The technique calls for gentle palpation of the breast tissue against the chest wall, usually beginning on the outer half of the breast and systematically covering the entire half of the breast, paying particular attention to the upper outer quadrant, where the axillary tail of breast tissue is thickest and where many tumors occur. She should then raise the arm above her head and thoroughly examine the inner half of the breast, beginning at the sternum (Fig. 12-6).

When the entire breast has been carefully palpated, the axilla should be examined carefully. With the arm on the side being examined again resting at

Figure 12-6. Self-examination of the breasts. *A.* The outer half of the breast is examined with the arm on the side being examined resting at the woman's side. *B.* The inner half of the breast, beginning at the sternum, is examined with the woman's arm raised above her head. (Reproduced with permission from R. D. Judge, G. D. Zuidema, and F. Fitzgerald (Eds.). *Methods of Clinical Examination* (4th ed.). Boston: Little, Brown, 1982.)

A

B

her side, she should cup her examining hand and reach as high into the apex of the axilla as possible. Exerting gentle pressure against the thorax she should pull her hand slowly downward. Repeating several times she should check in order the three lymph node groups: the anterior group, the central group, and the posterior group of lymph nodes. Each of these areas should be palpated again while the resting arm is taken through a full range of motion, to uncover any lesions that might have been hidden by fatty or muscle tissue. She should be reminded not to abduct the arm too far, for this interferes with deep palpation and may cause her some discomfort.

Following palpation of the one breast and axilla, the pillow is placed beneath the opposite shoulder, and the woman investigates the second breast and axilla in exactly the same manner.

Palpation of the breast and axilla should be thorough and unhurried. Every portion of the breast must be deliberately and carefully examined if small lesions are to be detected.

The woman should be instructed to place the greatest emphasis on the regions where most breast cancers develop, namely in the axillary tail of the breast and beneath the nipple. If the technique is to have any meaning she must establish a definite pattern and conduct a thorough examination at monthly intervals. The method will be effective only if used regularly [1].

PELVIC EXAMINATION

As discussed earlier, the pelvic examination should be a part of every woman's physical examination. Preparation for the examination includes both emotional and physical aspects. The degree of fear and embarrassment, of course, varies from person to person; but the nurse can expect nearly all women to experience some degree of apprehension. Cultural background and untoward experiences during previous examinations are often contributing factors. Thorough explanations of your actions and of what the woman can expect to feel will help her to relax sufficiently for satisfactory palpation with only minimal discomfort. Always be sure to meet the woman while she is sitting up and preferably clothed—at least the first time.

Certain basic items of equipment are needed for the routine pelvic examination. These are:

1. Examination table with stirrups
2. Instrument table and stool
3. Sink
4. Portable, easily adjustable light source
5. Assortment of bivalve vaginal specula of various sizes
6. Sponge forceps and cotton sponges
7. Lubricant
8. Rubber gloves
9. Cotton applicators or Ayres spatulas
10. Glass microscope slides
11. Specimen bottles and fixative solution or fixative spray

The woman should not have douched for at least 24 hours prior to the pelvic examination. Douching interferes with proper evaluation of vaginal discharge, cytologic studies, and cultures or stained smears for microorganism identification if necessary. She should void immediately prior to the examination, since an empty bladder makes palpation easier, eliminates possible distortion of the position of the pelvic organs caused by a full bladder, and obviates the danger and embarrassment of incontinence during examination. Since collection of a urine specimen is often indicated at this time, it should be routine. It is desirable that the rectum be empty, but it is not always mandatory. It may sometimes be necessary to have the woman return for examination after emptying the lower bowel by enema or laxative.

Positioning and Sequence

Proper positioning of the woman and good lighting are essential for an accurate examination. Avoiding unnecessary exposure and assuring privacy add to her comfort. The most satisfactory draping is a square sheet. For the common lithotomy position, she holds one corner over her xyphoid process, and the corners adjacent to this are placed over each knee. The fourth corner hangs between her legs and over her perineum. This fourth corner is turned back on her abdomen during actual examination of the perinium.

Pelvic examination may be performed with the patient in one of the following positions:

1. *The lithotomy position* is the most practical. With the woman lying on her back, the thighs are flexed and abducted, the legs are flexed, and the feet are supported in stirrups. Both legs are manipulated at the same time to prevent strain to the lower back.

2. *The left lateral prone (Sims) position* has the woman lying on her left side with her chest inclining toward the table. Her left arm is behind her, her right thigh is flexed about 90 degrees, and the left thigh is slightly flexed. This position is reserved primarily for women who have ankylosis of the hips or knees and those who are too weak for the lithotomy position. Also, it provides closer observation of the urethra and the anterior vaginal wall, especially if these areas are obstructed from view by uterine displacement when the lithotomy position is used. A single-blade retractor is placed in the vagina, retracting the posterior vaginal wall.

3. *The knee-chest position,* with the patient on her arms and knees and buttocks uppermost, may also be used for closer observation of the urethra and anterior vaginal wall. However, many women find this an uncomfortable position.

4. *The standing position* is used to evaluate hernias, uterine prolapse, relaxation of the vaginal walls or pelvic supports, and stress incontinence of urine.

For complete pelvic examination, the following sequence is suggested:

1. Examination of the abdomen
2. Inspection and palpation of vulva and perineum

3. Collection of specimens for cytologic examination
4. Inspection of the vaginal walls and cervix
5. Bimanual examination
6. Rectovaginal abdominal examination

Examination of the Abdomen

The pelvic examination begins with the examination of the abdomen, utilizing the usual four methods: inspection, palpation, percussion, and auscultation as is discussed in Chapter 11. Inspection may reveal enlargement or obvious tumors. Characteristics of such masses or areas of tenderness should be determined by palpation. Palpation of the inguinal lymph nodes should always be included.

Percussion aids in differentiating free fluid and encysted fluid within the abdomen. Usually, the tympanitic bowel floats on free fluid and is found in the midline or the most distensible part of the abdomen. In contrast, encysted fluid, whether it be that within a pregnant uterus, a distended bladder, or a large ovarian cyst, presents dullness in the midline and tympany in the lateral portion of the abdomen. Shifting dullness is characteristic of free fluid. A tense cyst may be differentiated from a solid tumor by demonstration of a fluid wave within it.

Auscultation of the abdomen provides detection and evaluation of bowel sounds, bruits, and fetal heart sounds.

Inspection and Palpation of Vulva and Perineum

The perineum is as tender and sensitive as any area examined during physical assessment. Anyone placed in the lithotomy position and then touched abruptly on the perineum experiences the anal sphincter reflex. The external anal sphincter and portions of the levator ani involuntarily contract, creating a barrier to comfortable examination. Thus the examiner's initial contact with the perineum should be at some distance from the labia and should be firm but gentle.

The pattern of pubic hair distribution should be that of a female, namely, an inverted triangle with its base anterior. The labia majora are usually plump and well formed in the normally developed adult female. They are free from erythema, edema, lesions, varicosities, hydroceles, tumor masses, or lacerations that may distort the normal configuration.

The labia minora are parted, with the examiner noting the clitoris, the vestibule, the urethral meatus, and the introitus. The size and development of the clitoris normally is variable, but true enlargement of the organ is obvious. The area of the vestibule between the inner surfaces of the labia minora and below the clitoris is the most common site of granulomatous and ulcerative venereal lesions in younger women and of malignant changes in the elderly. It should be checked carefully for erythema and ulcerations. The orifices of the lesser vestibular glands and the paraurethral (Skene's) glands are barely distinguishable unless infected. The external urethral meatus should be free from inflammation, tumor, and prolapse of the urethral mucous membrane. No discharge should be expressed from the urethra or the paraurethral glands when the examiner gently presses on the undersurface of the urethra and slowly withdraws her finger (Fig. 12-7).

In examining the introitus, the examiner notes its general appearance. In the nonparous individual, the labia minora lie together in the midline. If there is relaxation or laceration of the perineal muscles, the labia gape and fall to either side. The hymen or hymeneal remnants appear just inside the introitus. In the virgin, this structure is variable in thickness and in its restriction of the opening of the vagina. It normally admits one finger, sometimes two fingers, or may be impenetrable. The remnants of the ruptured hymen also normally vary in thickness and size in the nonvirgin (Fig. 12-8).

The ducts of the greater vestibular (Bartholin's) glands open into the margin

Figure 12-7.
External female genitalia. (Reproduced with permission from R. D. Judge, G. D. Zuidema, and F. Fitzgerald (Eds.). *Methods of Clinical Examination* (4th ed.). Boston: Little, Brown, 1982.)

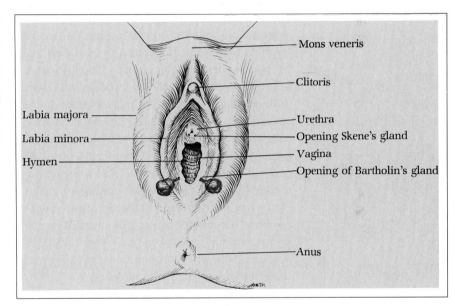

Figure 12-8.
Different appearances of hymen in *A.* virgin, *B.* woman who has had sexual intercourse, and *C.* multiparous woman. (Reproduced with permission from R. Snell *Clinical Anatomy For Medical Students* (1st ed.). Boston: Little, Brown, 1973.)

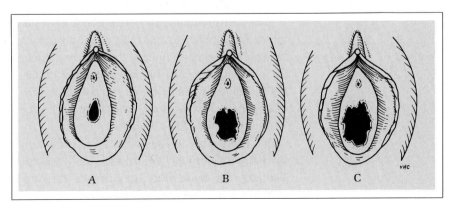

of the vaginal orifice just outside the hymen on either lateral side, slightly posterior to the horizontal midplane. They should be checked carefully for inflammation and swelling, but are normally not palpable. Nor are their orifices normally visible. If visible, an abnormality may exist. Palpation of enlargements on the surfaces of the labia and within the labia is accomplished by inserting the index finger into the vagina while exerting counterpressure with the thumb on the suspicious area.

Collection of Specimens for Cytologic Examination

Insertion of the bivalve Graves' speculum enables the examiner to obtain epithelium for cytologic examination, as well as inspect the vaginal walls and the cervix. The examiner must be adept at using the speculum to avoid unnecessary discomfort for the woman. The specula come in three different sizes, and the size of choice depends on the woman's size and parity. The posterior blade is fixed and the anterior blade movable. The two blades are held together by a thrumbscrew on the handle of the anterior blade. Loosening the thumbscrew allows the tips of the blades to come together. Depressing the anterior handle separates the blades, and tightening the screw holds the blades in position. Informing the woman of your actions and telling her what feelings to anticipate are particularly important during this phase of the examination. Instructing her to breathe deeply and slowly through her mouth helps her to relax.

To avoid interference with cytologic studies, the speculum should be lubricated only with warm water. For the right-handed examiner, the speculum is held in the right hand, and the labia are separated with the thumb and index finger of the left hand. With the first joint of the thumb against the underside of the thumb rest to hold the blades tightly together, the speculum handle is turned 45 to 60 degrees to the examiner's right (counterclockwise), so that the blades are held obliquely. The tip of the speculum is slowly inserted into the posterior part of the vaginal introitus that has been exposed, avoiding pressure on the external urethral meatus (Fig. 12-9A). If the flat surfaces of the blades are horizontal, the introitus may be stretched; if the blades are vertical, the suburethral area can be damaged.

As soon as the broad portions of the blades have passed the introitus, the speculum is rotated so that the blades are horizontal, and the handle is elevated so that the speculum is advancing at a 45-degree angle toward the examining table (Fig. 12-9B). Again, exert slight posterior pressure during this maneuver to avoid the sensitive area of the urethra. When the speculum is fully inserted, the blades are opened by pressing down on the thumbpiece to elevate the top blade, while the hand lifts on the handle to lower the fixed posterior blade. In this way the blades move away from each other, and the cervix and vaginal walls are exposed (Fig. 12-9C).

Another method of speculum insertion is to introduce one or two fingers of the left hand through the introitus and depress the perineal body backward. The posterior blade of the speculum is introduced into the vagina over the top of the fingers. This method also avoids pressure on the urethra.

Figure 12-9.
Insertion of the vaginal
speculum. *A.* Blades held
obliquely on entering the
vagina. *B.* Blades rotated to
the horizontal position as
they pass the introitus. *C.*
Blades separated by
depressing thumbpiece and
elevating handle. *D.*
Normal parous cervix.
(Reproduced with
permission from R. D.
Judge, G. D. Zuidema, and
F. Fitzgerald (Eds.).
*Methods of Clinical
Examination* (4th ed.).
Boston: Little, Brown,
1982.)

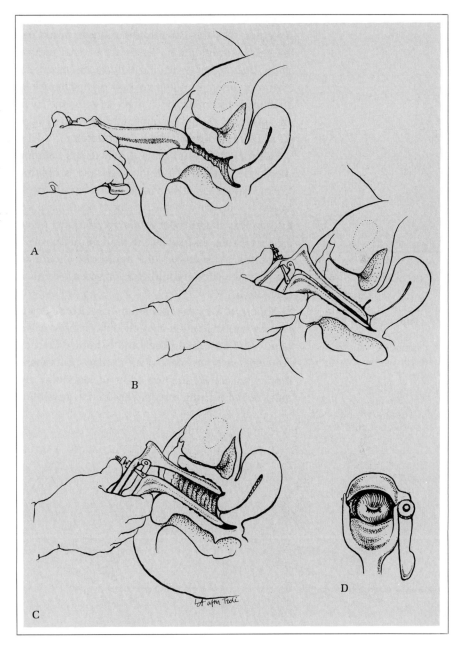

Because of its extreme value in the early detection of uterine cancer, a simple screening test, the Papanicolaou smear, must be considered a routine part of the pelvic examination. There are several methods for obtaining cells for the study, but only one method will be discussed here. Regardless of the method used, obtaining an adequate and representative sample of the endocervical epithelium is essential. Since this test is for the identification of epithelial lesions, the specimen should be obtained before the vagina and cervical face are wiped off or disturbed by bimanual examination.

The two slides and fixative, whether a solution of ether alcohol or a spray, should be readied before the specimen is obtained. With the speculum in position, exposing the cervix, use the handle of an Ayres spatula or a cotton-tipped applicator to collect a smear from the posterior fornix of the vagina. For the cervical smear, reverse the spatula and place the longer arm of the tip in the cervical os and rotate the blade a full circle. To avoid causing the woman unnecessary discomfort, the applicator should be inserted gently and not too far. The two slides should each be spread evenly and prepared with the fixative (Fig. 12-10).

Figure 12-10. Technique for obtaining the Pap smear. *A.* Cervical smear. *B.* Vaginal pool sampling. (Reproduced with permission from R. D. Judge, G. D. Zuidema, and F. Fitzgerald (Eds.). *Methods of Clinical Examination* (4th ed.). Boston: Little, Brown, 1982.)

Abnormal cervical epithelium can also be detected by Schiller's test, in which Lugol's iodine solution is applied to the cervix. Normal cervical epithelium contains considerable glycogen and is immediately stained dark brown. Abnormal epithelial cells are devoid of glycogen and therefore do not stain. Areas that remain unstained may be areas of glandular erosion, but the tissue certainly must be studied microscopically for the possibility of cancer.

Inspection of the Vaginal Walls and Cervix

After the specimens have been obtained, the cervix can be visually inspected with the speculum in position. The vaginal walls can be inspected as the speculum is withdrawn.

The normal cervix is 2.5 to 3 cm in diameter and extends into the upper vagina about the same distance. It is normally much smaller in the aged female, coinciding with uterine hypoplasia. The cervix is cylindrical in shape and points posteriorly, but if the uterus is displaced, as it is in about 20 percent of women, the cervix points anteriorly [2]. The cervix should be the normal pink epithelial color and should be free from lacerations, ulcerations, erythema, excavations, and new growths. It should be sponged vigorously and examined for any signs of bleeding. Ulcers or erosions usually present a beefy red color and have regular margins. Early carcinoma is difficult to differentiate visually from an erosion, though the margins are more likely to be irregular and the area may bleed easily. A cyanotic, bluish appearance of the cervix (Chadwick's sign) is an early indication of pregnancy.

Inspection of the cervical os includes the size, shape, and color of the os as well as observation of any discharge or polyps present. The normal os of the nulliparous adult female is small, closed, and usually in the horizontal plane. In the parous female, the os is more likely to be larger, with possibly some curvature and small, healed lacerations on it. There should be no discharge or polyps exuding from the cervical os. If there is a discharge, attention to its quantity, consistency, color, and odor are important. Chronic infection of the endocervical canal is accompanied by a thick mucous or mucopurulent discharge. In such a condition the cervix is enlarged and edematous in appearance, and nabothian follicles may be visible on the vaginal portion of the cervix. A cervical polyp generally appears as a dark, cherry-red mass, 1 to 3 cm in diameter, extending through the cervical os. It is smooth and uniform in contour and bleeds easily.

The lateral vaginal walls visible through the open speculum and the fornices should be inspected as to texture, color, support, and discharge. A more detailed inspection of the vagina may be made as the speculum is withdrawn. The normal vaginal epithelium of the adult appears thick and heavy and is obviously distensible because of its elasticity and its many folds. The color is normally pink and uniform. Any abnormal redness or blueness should be noted. If a discharge is present, again determine its characteristics and source—vaginal mucosa, cervical os, or both. Infection by Candida organisms, which are fungi, produces a thick, white, patchy, curdlike discharge that clings to the vaginal wall. Bacterial invasion of the vagina produces a thin, yellow, purulent material. In Trichomonas vaginitis the discharge is thin, yellow, often frothy, with a characteristic musty odor. Further, the vaginal wall may have a "strawberry" appearance, with small red spots seeming to show through the vaginal epithelium. A gonorrheal infection presents a situation similar to that seen with a Trichomonas infection, except that gonorrhea develops rapidly and typically produces a severe inflammation of the urethra and the greater vestibular (Bartholin's) glands, as well as of the vagina and cervix. The urethra and Bartholin's glands usually are not infected by Trichomonas organisms.

The anterior and posterior vaginal walls are inspected by rotating the speculum in the long axis of the vagina. The remainder of the vagina can be viewed as the blades are withdrawn. After the blades of the speculum clear the cervix, release the thumbscrew of the speculum and hold the speculum partially open by the thumb to allow the rest of the vagina to be viewed.

The integrity of uterine supports and the vaginal walls can be evaluated by asking the woman to bear down when the speculum has been withdrawn to the midpoint of the vagina. There should be no protrusion of the cervix nor bulging of the anterior or posterior vaginal walls. If the uterine supports are relaxed, varying degrees of uterine prolapse occur. The cervix protrudes into the open speculum and may follow it to the introitus. When there is relaxation of the anterior or posterior vaginal walls, a cystocele or rectocele bulges into the vaginal cavity. Vaginal palpation, as will be discussed, gives additional information on the presence of a cystocele, rectocele, or prolapse of the uterus.

Bimanual Pelvic Examination

The uterus and adnexa are palpated by the bimanual procedure, which involves placing two examining fingers in the vagina and a hand on the abdomen. The hand should move at least three-quarters of the way to the umbilicus to ensure that all the organs to be palpated are brought within reach of the intravaginal fingers. If the hand is too close to the symphysis pubis, the abdominal wall is pressed down in front of the uterus, and one is unable to feel the intrapelvic structures (Fig. 12-11A). Opinion is divided as to whether the intra-

Figure 12-11. Bimanual pelvic examination. The abdominal hand brings the pelvic contents to the intravaginal fingers for palpation of the uterus. (Reproduced with permission from R. D. Judge, G. D. Zuidema, and F. Fitzgerald (Eds.). *Methods of Clinical Examination* (4th ed.). Boston: Little, Brown, 1982.)

pelvic portion of the examination should be done with the right or left hand. This author believes the examiner should use the hand with which she feels she can best palpate the internal organs. Indeed, the examiner may find that to achieve a thorough examination, it may often be necessary to change the intra-pelvic hand, since the adnexal regions can often be felt best with the hand of the same side, for example, right hand for right adnexal region. Also, there are differences of opinion as to whether one or two fingers should be used intra-vaginally. It is advisable for the examiner to be skilled in the use of one-finger examination in order not to be handicapped in the examination of the virginal or elderly woman. However, whenever possible, the examiner is encouraged to use the two-finger technique because it permits a longer reach into the fornices and more thorough palpation of the internal genitalia. As with other skills, the examiner develops expertise in the bimanual examination only with consider-able experience in doing it.

Helping the woman to remain relaxed during the bimanual examination def-initely increases the likelihood of a thorough examination. Encourage her to breathe slowly through her mouth, relax her abdominal muscles and the ab-ductor muscles of the thighs, and to keep her knees as far apart as possible. The examiner begins with gentle pressure on the abdomen to prevent tighten-ing; deeper palpation follows as the woman becomes accustomed to the pal-pation. She should continue to be informed of the examiner's actions and of what she will be experiencing. She experiences some pressure, but unless ab-normalities exist, she should not experience pain if she is relaxed.

Before the lubricated fingers are introduced into the vagina, spread the labia apart with the other hand to avoid the discomfort of pulling pubic hair into the vagina. The examining hand is held with the palmar side superior, the thumb is hyperextended, the third and fourth fingers are completely flexed, and the first and second fingers are extended straight. With the fingers intravaginal, any firmness, tenderness, induration from scars, or adhesions can be felt if present. The amount of relaxation of the vaginal walls can be noted. Congenital abnormalities are quickly evident.

By maintaining slight pressure against the posterior portion of the vagina, the examiner avoids pressure on the bladder, which is normally sensitive. In-flammation of the bladder or bladder neck causes marked sensitivity on pal-pation. If the bladder is tender, there is frequently an associated reference of pain to the region of the umbilicus. The normally smooth bladder should be checked for tumor induration or stones. Though the anterior rectal wall and the rectovaginal septum may be examined at this time, a better evaluation can be made later by the rectovaginal examination.

The cervix is easily palpable. Note its size, shape, position, mobility, regular-ity, and consistency. In the normal adult, the length of the cervix is one-half the size of the uterine body. The external os of the cervix is normally small (3 to 5 mm) in diameter. The normal cervix feels like a firm, smooth, rounded button with a central depression. Invasion by carcinoma makes the cervix hard and gives it a granular feeling. Nabothian follicles are felt as small, firm nodules. Cervical polyps feel like soft, spongy masses. Lacerations, especially from childbirth, may be responsible for areas of deformity.

The position and direction in which the cervix may point are variable. As a general rule, the cervix points the opposite way from the fundus, so that in the normal position the cervix points posteriorly from the top of the anterior vaginal wall, and the fundus points anteriorly. If the cervix points anteriorly, the fundus usually is retroverted and found in the cul-de-sac, a condition occurring in 20 percent of adult women [2]. The normal cervix lies in the midplane of the pelvis with no displacement from the normal axis of the vagina, which is downward and backward. Changes in the axis and position of the cervix are usually caused by a tumor or an intrapelvic organ displacing the body of the uterus as well as the cervix. Normally, the cervix is freely movable for 2 to 3 cm in any direction. Motion of the cervix should not produce pain. Malignant infiltration or pelvic inflammatory disease may cause fixation of the cervix.

The position, size, shape, consistency, and mobility of the uterus should be determined. With the vaginal fingers placed in the posterior fornix, it should be possible to push the uterus forward and upward while the abdominal hand palpates for the fundus in the midline above the symphysis. A circular motion of the abdominal hand helps in penetrating the normal resistance of the abdominal wall. The normal, nonpregnant uterus is approximately 5 to 6 cm in length, with a smooth, firm surface. Softening of the lower uterine segment is an early indication of pregnancy (Hegar's sign). Irregular enlargement of the uterine body is suggestive of fibroid tumors. In either anteflexion or retroversion, the uterine body should be freely movable. The woman may experience some discomfort when attempts are made to move the retroverted uterus, but this should not occur with the anteflexed uterus (Fig. 12-11).

Palpation of the adnexa is the most difficult part of the pelvic examination, especially for the beginner and occasionally for the expert. The normal tube is usually not palpable, and in many instances, neither is the normal ovary. This is particularly true in obese women. The ovary is about 3 by 4 cm in size, soft in texture, and normally sensitive to pressure. It lies deep in the pelvis above the lateral fornix of the vagina and is best palpated by the vaginal fingers. To palpate the woman's right ovary, the abdominal hand is brought forward and inward just inside the anterior superior iliac spine while applying deep pressure in a direction slightly toward the midline. At the same time, the vaginal fingers in the lateral fornix should be directed slightly laterally and anteriorly to feel the ovary being pressed toward the palmar surface of the vaginal fingers by the abdominal hand. The same movements are employed in examining the left ovary on the other side. However, if the examiner is not satisfied with her examination of the left ovary, she may wish to change hands, using the left fingers intravaginally and the right hand on the abdomen. Any significant enlargement of the ovary, abnormal tenderness, masses, or indurations should be noted (Fig. 12-12A). When the normal tube is palpated medially to the ovary, it is approximately 4 mm in diameter, and has the consistency of a piece of rubber tubing. Marked tenderness of the adnexa is a characteristic finding in acute inflammatory changes caused by tuboovarian infections. In such instances, the tube and ovary usually cannot be differentiated by palpation but appear to be a single, tender, indurated area.

Figure 12-12. Bimanual pelvic examination. *A.* Palpation of the right ovary. *B.* Palpation of the right parametrial tissues. (From Judge and Zuidema [1].)

The parametrium (tissue beside the cervix and lower segment of the corpus of the uterus) is usually pliable, soft, and nontender. This tissue is palpable in the lateral and posterior fornices of the vagina. It contains the vascular supply and the lymphatics which drain the cervix; therefore it is indurated and tender if the cervix is inflamed (Fig. 12-12B).

Before removing the intravaginal fingers, the hand should be rotated and fingers pressed into the cul-de-sac to check for the presence of masses or any irregularities.

Rectovaginal Abdominal Examination

The pelvic examination is completed by rectovaginal abdominal palpation (Fig. 12-13). The well lubricated middle finger is gently inserted in the rectum and the index finger into the vagina. The rectovaginal septum can be palpated, and nodules, scarring, or induration noted. The vaginal posterior fornix and cul-de-sac can be better evaluated between rectal and vaginal fingers. With pressure from above, using the abdominal hand, the posterior wall of the uterus may be palpated with the rectal finger. By moving both fingers laterally, the adnexa and parametrial tissues may be palpated again.

For the young woman experiencing her first pelvic examination, the sensation she experiences on removal of the examiner's rectal finger may closely resemble the feeling of defecation. Telling her to anticipate this sensation will allay any fear that she, in fact, may have expelled some stool.

The First Pelvic Examination

Fortunately, the increased emphasis on health maintenance is increasing the individual's awareness of her body and her interest in its functions. The nurse can utilize a young person's first pelvic examination as an opportunity to increase her comfort with her total body and to educate her about her anatomy.

Figure 12-13. Rectovaginal abdominal examination. Note that one finger is inserted into the vagina and one into the rectum. (Reproduced with permission from R. D. Judge, G. D. Zuidema, and F. Fitzgerald (Eds.). *Methods of Clinical Examination* (4th ed.). Boston: Little, Brown, 1982.)

The discontinuance of draping is recommended as a way of establishing a better rapport between nurse and client and thus making the examination less impersonal. It also allows the examiner to detect the amount and duration of discomfort from the person's facial expressions. Adequate warmth is an important consideration during all examinations to increase client relaxation, but it becomes even more essential when the young woman is so exposed.

By raising the young woman to a semi-sitting position and with use of a mirror and good lighting, the nurse can point out both external and internal organs. These include the outer and inner labia, anus, urethra, clitoris, and vaginal orifice with hymenal ring. After speculum insertion, the vaginal walls and cervical os can also be viewed.

This anatomy lesson also provides the opportunity for health teaching such as wiping from anterior to posterior after voiding, the importance of voiding after intercourse, and various types of birth control measures [3].

THE POSTMENOPAUSAL WOMAN

The health professions are becoming increasingly aware of special problems experienced by the postmenopausal woman. This seems to be due both to the increasing number of women in this category and to a willingness to deal with conditions that previously were accepted as a normal part of aging for which treatment was believed to be of no benefit. In the gynecologic appraisal of the postmenopausal woman, the nurse should evaluate changes, both in the perineum and throughout the entire body, that may be resulting from the lowered estrogen level of menopause. These changes are the normal physiologic results of aging. In some cases, simple actions like using a lubricant during intercourse to decrease menopausal dyspareunia can offer some relief. In other situations, the knowledge that the changes one is experiencing are normal is sufficient to allay a woman's fears.

Systemic effects that the examiner should evaluate are related primarily to bone structure and the vascular system. A decreased serum estrogen level has been shown to increase the rate of osteoporosis, which may be responsible for the frequent complaint of back pain from the postmenopausal woman. Similarly, the changes in estrogen and follicle-stimulating hormone levels upset the balanced hormonal control of the vascular system, thus giving "hot flashes" a definite physiologic basis. Hypertension may also occur, as estrogen seems to have an inhibiting effect on the development of atherosclerosis.

Observing changes of appearance and structure, one sees atrophy and loss of fullness in breast tissue as well as in the genital area. The atrophy of breast tissue and muscular supports allows the breasts to sag and the nipples to drop far below the fourth intercostal space. The vulva loses its contour and becomes thin, due to reabsorption of fatty tissue. The vaginal mucosa becomes thinner and smoother, while the vagina decreases in length and width. With increased fibrotic tissue, much of its elasticity and ability to expand are lost. This loss of expansion may necessitate the use of only one finger intravaginally during a bimanual examination. In appearance the vaginal folds have disappeared, and the epithelium has a thin, velvety appearance. Examination of the uterus and adnexa reveals a smaller and firmer uterus and cervix, resulting from tissue hypoplasia. The ovaries and tubes atrophy also and become nonpalpable.

There are several alterations frequently seen in this age group. *Atrophic vaginitis* is a nonspecific vaginal infection in which the epithelium is frequently spotted with small petechiae. If this condition is exaggerated enough to result in shrinking and fibrosis, it is known as kraurosis vulvae. The white, slightly raised plaques of leukoplakia are also seen commonly in the postmenopausal group. Kraurosis vulvae and leukoplakia frequently occur together.

The postmenopausal woman may also develop a prolapsing or outpouching of the mucous membrane of the urethra. When the membrane is prolapsed to any extent, it frequently becomes infected, inflamed, and tender.

Weakening of the vaginal walls, as well as of the broad and round ligaments supporting the uterus, occurs to differing degrees in this age group, but many have some degree of uterine prolapse or development of a cystocele, rectocele, or enterocele.

The nurse may often find it worthwhile to explore with a woman her expectations or reactions to menopause. Numerous, inaccurate "old wives' tales" still exist about "the change." This time in one's life often involves many changes, but it need not be a depressing experience. Understanding why physiologic alterations are occurring should help one to accept them.

NURSING IMPLICATIONS

It seems obvious that the gynecologic assessment involves more than just the actual pelvic examination. It provides an excellent opportunity for health teaching, as well as for giving the woman a means of discussing concerns that may be related to the female-male relationship and interpersonal relationships within a family or with close associates. She should have the opportunity, if desired, to discuss her feelings or concerns about her sexuality, her role in society, her role as a wife, her role as a mother in helping adolescent daughters deal with their own evolving sexuality, and her reactions as she anticipates and experiences menopause and postmenopause.

Even though the general public is becoming increasingly knowledgeable about health matters, the nurse should not miss opportunities to emphasize important areas of health teaching. The opportunity given by the gynecologic examination enables her to stress the necessity for regular examinations of the breasts, which mothers should teach to daughters as soon as breast development begins; perineal cleanliness; and regular pelvic examinations and Papanicolaou smears. These practices should all be started by the mid-teens or certainly by the late adolescent years. The importance of the nurse's role in these areas of health teaching cannot be overemphasized.

FEMALE REPRODUCTIVE SYSTEM-ASSESSMENT GUIDE

I. Breast Examination (For Both Females and Males)—Seated and supine positions with arms at side and arms overhead; good lighting essential.
   A. Inspection
      1. Symmetry
      2. Position and size
      3. Superficial appearance—note erythema, orange peel appearance from edema
      4. Nipples—note bleeding, discharge, retraction, ulceration
      5. Skin retraction or dimpling present—demonstrated by raising arms overhead, pushing hands against each other, or by placing hands on hips and pushing forcibly
      6. Axillary and supraclavicular regions—note bulging, retraction, discoloration, edema
   B. Palpation
      1. Breast tissue
         a. Determine point of woman's monthly cycle
         b. Place small pillow under each shoulder as each side is examined
         c. Begin in upper outer quadrant
         d. Be systematic—palpate clockwise or laterally to medially over entire breast
         e. Palpate tender areas last
         f. Use gentle rotary to and fro motion followed by deeper palpation
         g. Note consistency and elasticity of tissue, texture of skin, and any masses
      2. Nipple—note subareolar masses, induration, loss of elasticity, dry scaling, excoriation, discharge
      3. Mass—for any noted, record: location, size, contour, consistency, tenderness, mobility, discreteness
      4. Axilla
         a. Examine with one hand while opposite hand holds woman's ipsilateral arm
         b. Begin at apex high in the axilla
         c. Pull hand downward with gentle pressure against thorax
         d. Repeat while arm is moved through range of motion
         e. Especially check axillary tail of breast
      5. Self-examination of the breast
         a. Do regularly after menstrual period
         b. Follows above outline and woman is taught to make same observations
   C. Record Findings
II. Pelvic Examination—Equipment needed: examination table with stirrups; instrument table and stool; sink; portable, easily adjustable light source; assortment of bivalve vaginal specula of various sizes; sponge forceps and cotton sponges; lubricant; rubber gloves; cotton applicators or Ayres spatulas; glass microscope slides; specimen bottles and fixative solution or fixative spray. Proper positioning of woman and good light are essential.
   A. Inspection, Palpation, Percussion, and Auscultation of Abdomen
   B. Inspection and Palpation of Vulva and Perineum
      1. Pubic hair distribution
      2. Labia majora and minor
      3. Clitoris, vestibule, urethral meatus, introitus—note erythema, ulcerations, and any noticeable glandular orifices
   C. Collection of Cytology Specimens
      1. Warm and lubricate speculum with warm water
      2. Insert slowly with slight posterior pressure
      3. Prepare slides and fixative for Papanicolaou smears
      4. Collect specimens from posterior fornix and cervical os and spread on slides
   D. Inspection of Cervix

      1. Leave speculum in position
      2. Sponge cervix vigorously and observe for bleeding
      3. Note size, shape, color of os, and any discharge or polyps
      4. If discharge present, note quantity, consistency, color, and odor

E. Inspection of Vaginal Walls
      1. Note texture, color, supports, and discharge as speculum withdrawn
      2. Describe discharge as above and check for its source
      3. Have woman bear down as speculum is removed to check integrity of walls

F. Bimanual Palpation of Uterus and Adnexa
      1. Facilitate woman's relaxation
      2. Spread labia apart with one hand and insert lubricated fingers of other hand into introitus
      3. Maintain slight pressure on posterior vagina
      4. Note firmness, tenderness, induration, or adhesions; bladder tenderness, induration, or stones
      5. Palpate cervix and uterus
        a. Use abdominal hand in circular motion to palpate fundus through abdominal wall
        b. Note size, shape, position, mobility, regularity, and consistency
      6. Palpate adnexa
        a. Normal tubes and ovaries may not be palpable
        b. Bring abdominal hand forward and inward while applying pressure, and direct vaginal fingers laterally and anteriorly
      7. Palpate parametrium and cul-de-sac before removing fingers

G. Rectovaginal Abdominal Examination
      1. Insert middle finger into rectum and index finger into vagina
      2. Check rectovaginal septum, vaginal posterior fornix, cul-de-sac
      3. With pressure above from abdominal hand, check posterior wall of uterus, adnexa, and parametrial tissues

H. Record Findings

REFERENCES

1. Judge, R. D., and Zuidema, G. D. (Eds.). *Methods of Clinical Examination: A Physiologic Approach* (3rd ed.). Boston: Little, Brown, 1974.
2. Prior, J. A., and Silberstein, J. *Physical Diagnosis: The History and Examination of the Patient* (5th ed.). St. Louis: Mosby, 1977.
3. Wells, G. M. Reducing the threat of a first pelvic exam. *Am. J. Mat. Child Nurs.* 2:304, 1977.

SUGGESTED READINGS

Cohen, S. Patient assessment: Examination of the female pelvis. Part I. *Am. J. Nurs.* 78:P. I. 1, 1978.

Cohen, S. Patient assessment: Examination of the female pelvis. Part II. *Am. J. Nurs.* 78:P.I. 1, 1978.

DeGowin, E., and DeGowin, R. *Bedside Diagnostic Examination* (3rd ed.). New York: Macmillan, 1976.

Liston, J., and Liston, E. H., Jr. The mirror pelvic examination: Assessment in a clinic setting. *J.O.G.N. NURS.* 7:47, 1978.

Magee, J. The pelvic examination: A view from the other end of the table. *Ann. Intern. Med.* 83:563, 1975.

Malasanos, L. *Health Assessment*. St. Louis: Mosby, 1977.

Margie J. Van Meter

13. Detection of Alterations in Neuromuscular Functioning

active range of motion Limits of motion through which a joint may be moved by those muscles that cross the joint.

ankylosis Complete loss of motion of a joint.

aphasia Loss of the power of expression by speech, writing, or signs (expressive aphasia), or of comprehending spoken or written language (receptive aphasia), due to injury or disease of the higher cerebral centers concerned with expression and comprehension.

arthritis Inflammation of a joint.

ataxia Failure of muscular coordination; irregularity of muscular action.

atrophy Wasting away of or diminution in the size of muscle.

bursa Potential space often filled with fluid found between tissue layers which move upon each other.

cavus foot Foot deformity in which a very high arch is present.

chorea Constant, rapid, and jerky but well-coordinated involuntary movements.

clonus Muscle spasm in which contraction and relaxation alternate in rapid succession.

consensual Similar reaction of both pupils to a stimulus applied to only one.

contractures Fibrosis of tissues supporting a joint, or disorders of the muscle fibers, limiting normal motion of the joint.

contralateral Pertaining to the opposite side.

crepitation Grating or crackling noise produced by rubbing together the ends of a fractured bone.

decerebrate posturing Hypertonic extension of the legs, internal rotation of the shoulders, arms extended at the elbows, and hyperpronated fingers hyperextended. Legs are extended at hip and knee, with plantar flexion of ankles and toes.

decorticate posturing Spontaneous spasms of rigidity consisting of flexion of the arm, wrist, and fingers, with adduction of the upper extremity and extension, internal rotation, and plantar flexion in the lower extremity.

dermatome The area of skin supplied with sensory nerve fibers by a single posterior spinal root.

dorsiflexion Backward flexion or bending.

dysarthria Imperfect articulation in speech.

dysphagia Difficulty in swallowing.

dysphasia Incomplete degree of aphasia.

eversion Position achieved by turning a part away from the midline of the body.

extinction Failure to perceive one of two identical bilateral simultaneous stimuli; if sensory perception is otherwise intact, extinction or suppression may indicate parietal cortex dysfunction.

fasciculation Visible spontaneous contraction of a number of muscle fibers supplied by a single motor nerve filament.

graphesthesia Sense by which figures or numbers written on the skin are recognized.

inversion Position achieved by turning a part toward the midline of the body.

ipsilateral Pertaining to the same side.

joint effusion Excessive fluid within a joint.

kyphosis Curvature of the spine, the convexity of which is posterior.

language Systematic means of communicating ideas or feelings by the use of conventionalized signs, gestures, marks, or especially articulated vocal sounds.

lower motor neuron Peripheral neurons whose cell bodies lie in the ventral gray columns of the spinal cord and whose terminations are in the skeletal muscles.

meniscus Fibrocartilaginous structure found between the articular surfaces of certain joints.

339

nystagmus Involuntary repetitive rapid movement of the eyeball.

paresis Weakness or partial paralysis. *hemiparesis* Muscle weakness affecting one side of body. *paraparesis* Muscle weakness of the legs and lower part of the body.

paresthesia Abnormal sensation such as burning or prickling.

passive range of motion Limits of motion through which a joint may be moved without use of the muscles which cross the joint.

plegia Complete paralysis. *hemiplegia* Paralysis of one side of the body and the limbs on that side. *paraplegia* Paralysis of the legs and lower part of the body, caused by disease or injury of the spinal cord. *quadriplegia* Paralysis of all four limbs.

pronation Position of the forearm achieved by turning the palm down; position of the foot achieved by turning the sole down.

proprioception Perception of movements and position of the body and joints.

sensory level Level below which there is a decrease or loss of sensation corresponding to the level of dysfunction of the spinal cord.

stereognosis Faculty of perceiving and understanding the form and nature of objects by the sense of touch.

supination Position of the forearm achieved by turning the palm up; position of the foot achieved by turning the sole up.

supine Position of lying on the back, face upward.

tic Spasmodic movement or twitching, as of the face.

tremor Involuntary trembling or quivering. *intention tremor* Associated with movement. *resting tremor* Occurring without movement.

upper motor neuron Neuron in the cerebral cortex which conducts impulses from the motor cortex to the motor nuclei of the cranial nerves or to the ventral gray columns of the spinal cord.

T HE intent of this chapter is to help the nurse practitioner determine abnormal from normal responses in the neuromuscular physical assessment of the patient, to monitor for progression or regression of symptoms of neuromuscular alterations, and to be able to describe the normal and the abnormal clearly. It is not intended to enable the nurse examiner to localize lesions. Additional knowledge is needed to correlate sensory changes, motor weaknesses, pathologic reflexes, and the patient's subjective symptoms, a correlation that is essential in localizing the site of the lesion in the nervous system.

To achieve the intent of the chapter the basic parameter will be identified and a detailed description of each manuever used for these tests will be given. This approach has been used for the following reasons: There are few nurses skilled in the neuromuscular examination to serve as preceptors, and so the nurse developing her skills needs textual references to help her analyze her particular problems in technique and to develop her skills with a minimum of direct supervision. The preceptor can then be used to validate the interpretation given to the patient's responses. The nurse can become confident in evaluating the responses elicited in testing because she has learned how to examine the patient carefully.

The patient who is a vague historian and with vague complaints then becomes less an enigma to the nurse who is skilled in obtaining and evaluating objective data. When a patient coming for evaluation of his hypertension regimen who has had a benign brain tumor removed complains of a headache and nonspecific left shoulder and left ankle symptoms, the nurse can systematically assess objective functioning and symptoms and be comfortable in referring or not referring him to the physician.

MENTAL STATUS The higher cerebral functions of orientation, mentation, and language are a beginning consideration in the neurologic examination. It is necessary to determine whether alterations in these functions have occurred, so that their effect on responses can be recognized and misinterpretation of the responses avoided.

Orientation and Memory Orientation and memory can be ascertained by the behavior and answers given during the history-taking interview. If the patient's general behavior is suggestive of confusion or forgetfulness, further investigations should be made in these areas. Tact is required when the mental incapacities of an alert person are being considered or exposed. The patient might be asked if he has noticed any difficulty with memory before being asked if he remembers your name, or what your role is, or what day, month, or year it is. It is helpful to begin with an explanatory statement to the alert patient indicating that you are aware of the simplicity of the questions you are going to ask, but for the sake of thoroughness, you want him to respond to them.

Recall ability is tested by asking the patient why and on what day he came to the health care facility, who visited him, or what he had for breakfast. The patient who cannot answer these questions may still be able to recall where he was born and other events of the distant past because remote memory may be intact.

Specific exercises can be utilized for testing recall and concentration. Give the patient an address, a color, and an object to remember. Have him repeat them immediately and instruct him to remember them. Later in the interview ask him to recall them.

A series of randomly selected digits may be given at the rate of one per second. A normal person can repeat a series of six to seven digits in order and a series of four digits in reverse order.

Direct testing can also include the serial 7 test. In this test the patient is asked to subtract 7 from 100, then 7 from the remainder (93), then 7 from 86, and so on.

Estimation of intellectual abilities can be made from the patient's vocabulary, the way he presents material having to do with his illness, his occupation and activities, and direct questioning. Included in the factors that influence testing results in this area are the ability to conceptualize, the level of education, life experiences, and social and cultural background. It is expected that a person can name several past presidents of the United States in order and name five large cities and five countries.

Interpretation of sayings such as "Cheaper by the dozen," or "A stitch in time saves nine" indicates the level of ability to understand and to make abstractions. Persons with impaired mentation make literal interpretations or are unable to do much more than rephrase the words. Cultural and social factors may influence the patient's interpretation of the saying. Educational level also can be an important factor in developing a person's ability to conceptualize.

Grammatical structure and vocabulary can be observed during the interview. There may be only simple words used. Sentence structure may consist only of essential words, e.g., subject and verb, or may be more complex, with many descriptive words and phrases included. Talking may consist only of a minimal response to questions asked or may be spontaneous, with additional information voluntarily supplied.

Language Function Assessing the ability of a person to communicate with others is necessary but complex. In order to determine the presence of language impairment, the patient's ability to communicate must first be determined.

The two main components of speech are the ability to receive incoming verbal or written symbols and the ability to communicate, or to send messages. Between these receptive and expressive components is the interpretation of the message. Language symbols are received by the eyes and ears and sent to the postcentral gyrus of the cortex. If the person is right-handed (and in some who are left-handed) the left cerebral hemisphere is more developed than the right and serves a major function in the interpretation of spoken and written language. The right cerebral hemisphere may be more developed in the left-handed person. Verbal expression is achieved by association tracts from the left postcentral gyrus to the motor strip or precentral gyrus. The words are then articulated by movements of the jaw musculature, vocal chords, and tongue and by coordinated respiratory movements.

A variety of tests may be used to evaluate a person's ability to receive and understand certain types of symbolic language such as letters and words. Before testing, it is important to know the patient's level of education and reading ability. Graduation from high school does not imply equivalent reading ability. How fluent is the person in the language in which he is being tested? The patient's visual acuity is assessed so that if corrective lenses are needed he is wearing them during the testing. Knowledge of the patient's hearing acuity is a significant factor because if he is hard of hearing and the examiner does not know it, it could be misinterpreted as an inability to comprehend.

Methods of Testing Language Function
The following are methods of testing the patient's basic language skills:

1. Point to common objects, such as pencil, clock, pillow, book, chair, and have the patient name each one. Use only single nouns and verbs.
2. Have the patient match printed and written words with pictures.
3. Have the patient read some simple words, both printed and written.

4. Write out some simple commands and ask the patient to read them and perform the activities, for example, "Tap right foot"; "Make a face."
5. Give simple verbal command for the patient to follow, such as, "Stand up"; "Bend your leg"; "Shake my hand."
6. Give a complex verbal command for patient to follow, such as, "Look at the ceiling and raise your arm"; "Left hand on right knee"; "Right hand on head."

It should be noted that when there is impairment of the cerebral centers for comprehension, the ability of a person to deal with abstractions is impaired. To facilitate testing of such patients, concrete objects associated with present circumstances should be used as much as possible.

Tests may be used to evaluate the ability of the patient to express himself verbally and in writing. For example he might be asked to write or verbally give a description of an object or a place. The nurse examiner already has some indication of the expressive abilities of the patient because, when testing for reception of communication, a verbal response is sometimes required.

In eliciting verbal responses it is necessary to avoid questions that are used so often in daily life that the answer is automatic; for example, "How are you?" "Fine." Some routine questions can be answered by patients who do not understand the words or are unable to express what they really want to say simply by timing of the question. For example, "Hello, how are you?" is usually said almost immediately on meeting a person, not in the leave-taking. Some persons who cannot express their thoughts because of brain impairment use what is called automatic speech, in which they can sing familiar songs, count, answer questions that are frequently asked, and give their name and address.

The character of the speech patterns should also be appraised. Does the patient initiate conversation and ask questions spontaneously? Does he speak in a monotone? Does the voice have a nasal quality? Does he use simple, single noun and verb sentences, or are his thoughts expressed in more complex sentences?

Responsiveness   Impairment of consciousness occurs on a continuum. The descending order of the continuum is from spontaneous verbal and motor activity and attentive cooperation to complete absence of any motor or reflex responses. Deterioration or improvement of consciousness occurs within the sequence [3]. With deterioration, the alert patient becomes less able to answer questions, slower and more difficult to arouse. First, there is a general uncooperativeness and then incapacity to cooperate.

Disorientation may follow or coincide with the loss of ability to cooperate. Disorientation is progressive and in a consistent pattern. First, the patient is disoriented in relation to time, to place, to person, from others, and then from self. The inability to follow simple commands, e.g., "Open your mouth," "Close your eyes," "Squeeze my fingers," usually occurs after disorientation to person.

Beyond this level of function it is necessary to use painful rather than verbal or auditory stimuli. Pain can be induced by applying pressure over the styloid process in the neck, on the supraorbital nerve, the root of the fingernail, or the periosteal surfaces of bone or by squeezing muscle bellies or tendons. The supraorbital nerve is located in the eyelid against the supraorbital bone, just above the globe of the eye. Pinching the biceps, Achilles tendon, or the pectoralis muscle of the upper chest may be sufficiently painful to elicit a response. At first, responses to pain are somewhat purposeful; there is resistance or withdrawal and grimacing. Purposeless responses of chewing or hyperventilating are indicative of extremely depressed levels of consciousness as are decerebrate and decorticate posturing. When motor responses to pain cannot be elicited, the corneal and cough reflexes may still be present.

When monitoring a patient for signs of improvement or deterioration of consciousness, it is important to be aware of where he is on the continuum and what direction the progression is. Some examiners record the progression on the continuum by dividing the continuum into stages or levels of consciousness such as lethargy, semicoma, and coma. These terms lead to ambiguity and the need for interpretation. It is better to describe the phenomenon observed or elicited from the patient and the type and amount of stimulation needed to elicit the response. This permits comparisons of the patient's responsiveness over time and between examiners and easier recognition of changes in the patient's responsiveness (Table 13-1).

Muscle strength, blood pressure, pulse, respiratory pattern, temperature, and pupillary light reflex are correlated with the level of responsiveness to recognize and evaluate increasing intracranial pressure. Changes in orientation, arous-

Table 13-1.
Mental Status

Area of Assessment	Assessment Method	Normal Response
Orientation	Assess time, person, place	Accurate
Memory and concentration	Ask to recall recent and past events	
	7 digits	Recall 6 to 7 digits
	3 items	Repeat and recall all 3 items
	Review historical events, personal data	Recall of chronologic sequence
Intellect	Vocabulary usage	Reflective of education, culture, etc.
	Interpretation of proverbs	Some degree of abstraction
Language		
Receptive	Commands to follow	Comprehends 2 or more step directions
Expressive	Name and label items	Accurate naming
Responsiveness	Progressive stimulation; verbal to tactile to painful	Requires only verbal stimulation
		Alert, oriented, follows directions

ability, and muscle strength are likely to be the first signs of increasing intracranial pressure in the patient who is on the alert, oriented, cooperative end of the continuum. A subtle hemiparesis can be first detected by testing for ulnar drift. This is done by instructing the patient to put his arms out in front with the elbows straight and the fingers spread and then to keep his eyes closed. He holds this position for approximately one minute, and the examiner observes for flexing and internal rotation of the elbow. Normally, a person can hold the position without flexing the elbows, but one with hemiparesis cannot do so. The patient with marked muscular weakness of an arm is not able to hold the

Figure 13-1.
Increasing intracranial
pressure signs.

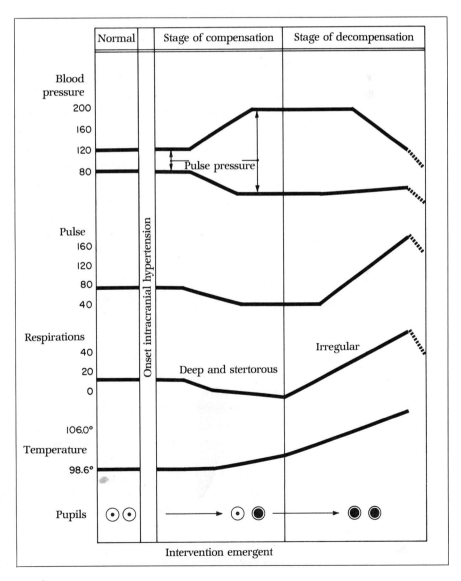

arm up at all, and the patient with hysterical or functional weakness lets the arm drop straight down with the elbow straight.

The effect of increasing intracranial pressure on the blood pressure, pulse, respirations, temperature, and pupillary light reflex is shown in Figure 13-1. Fixed, dilated pupils and cessation of respirations are the end states.

The patient should be roused to his fullest level of response each time he is evaluated. This is likely to be after activities are done with him or for him, or it may be achieved by a brisk massage around the mouth. The examiner should be careful to maintain the patient's dignity and be cognizant of the sequelae of the stimulation (i.e., bruising) and the need to clarify to family members the purpose of the vigorous stimulation.

If neurologic examination is needed to determine the presence of increasing intracranial pressure, it must be done thoroughly to establish a baseline for detection of deterioration or improvement and for the prescription of therapy. Delay in instituting therapy for increasing intracranial pressure may have dire consequences.

When examining an unresponsive patient, particularly in the primary care situation, one should always be looking for the cause of the altered consciousness. The breath odors, signs of trauma or of hemiparesis, previous illnesses, or drug use are clues to the possible cause.

CRANIAL NERVE FUNCTION EXAMINATION

The testing of the twelve pairs of cranial nerves is done in order of their numbers, so that none is omitted. A device for remembering the order of the cranial nerves is "*On old Olympus' towering top a Finn and German viewed some hops.*" The first letter of each of the 12 words is the same as the first letter of the names of the cranial nerves.

Olfactory Nerve (Cranial Nerve I)

Cranial nerve I subserves smell, and to test its function, the patient is instructed as follows: "Close your eyes and tell me when you first smell this, then try to identify the odor." One nostril is occluded by finger compression, and an odoriferous substance like tobacco, coffee, or peppermint is sniffed through the other nostril. The substance is first held away from the nose and gradually brought closer for the patient to identify. The other nostril is then occluded, and this time the substance is not presented. This assesses the patient's suggestibility and attention. In every sensory test such safeguards must be built in to ensure objective results. Finally a substance is presented to the untested nostril. Appreciation of an odor without precise identification of the substance is sufficient to rule out *anosmia* (loss of the sense of smell).

Anosmia may be caused by a number of factors. The common cold and allergic rhinitis are the most common causes; therefore, before testing the function of smell, possible obstructions of the nasal passages should be ruled out. The patient usually notices loss of taste rather than smell, since taste is influenced by smell.

The olfactory nerve need not be tested in routine examinations. It is pertinent in head trauma and tumors at the base of the frontal lobe, which may cause olfactory tract damage.

Optic, Oculomotor, Trochlear, and Abducens Nerves (Cranial Nerves II, III, IV, and VI)

Methods of assessing functions of these nerves and other assessment methods are detailed in Chapter 7, on vision. Evaluating visual acuity, visual fields, and motor function of the eye is an integral part of the neurologic examination.

Trigeminal Nerve (Cranial Nerve V)

The trigeminal nerve supplies sensation to the face and motor innervation to the muscles of mastication (Fig. 13-2). It consists of three peripheral branches from the gasserian ganglion outward: the ophthalmic branch (first division); the maxillary branch (second division); and the mandibular branch (third division). Sensations from the cornea and the forehead are transmitted via the ophthalmic branch. The maxillary branch is the sensory supply for the lateral aspect of the nose, the skin of the cheek, the upper teeth and jaw, and the mucosa of the uvula, hard palate, and nasopharynx. The mandibular branch is the only branch that has both motor and sensory fibers. It carries sensory stimuli from the ipsilateral side of the tongue, pinna of the ear, lower teeth, gums, jaw, floor of the mouth, and the buccal surfaces of the cheeks. The motor fibers innervate the temporal, pterygoid, and masseter muscles (the muscles of mastication).

The technique for testing sensations is as described in the section on sensory function examination. The patient is instructed to keep his eyes closed for facial testing to avoid responses based on visual rather than cutaneous clues. The skin of the forehead, cheek, and jaw should each be tested for pain, touch, and temperature and on both sides of the face, so that all three branches of both

Figure 13-2. Distribution of trigeminal nerve innervation to the face, and technique of eliciting corneal reflex. Note sparing of angle of the jaw.

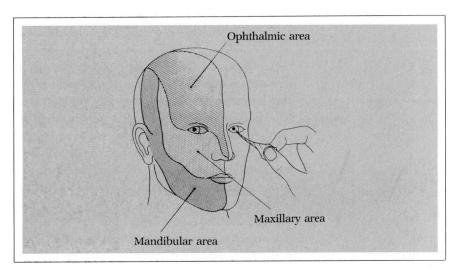

Ophthalmic area

Maxillary area

Mandibular area

the trigeminal nerves are evaluated. Start with a normal area, rather than a numb area, to establish that the patient understands the directions. Then alternate areas and sides randomly. Assess for decreased or increased sensitivity and equality of response of the two sides.

The afferent pathways of the corneal reflex are the trigeminal nerves; the efferent pathways are the facial nuclei. To test the right corneal reflex the patient looks to the left, and a cotton tip is introduced from the right, out of the patient's visual field in order to minimize visually stimulated blinking. The cornea is touched lightly with the cotton. The cornea, not just the sclera, must be touched. Care should be taken to stimulate but not scratch the cornea. The normal response is rapid closure of the eyelids, similar to that occurring when a foreign body enters the eye. It is common for both eyes to blink. If there is no ipsilateral blink, ask if the stimulus was felt and observe for a consensual blink. Each corneal afferent tract goes to both facial nerve (efferent) nuclei to close both eyes. If the facial nerve on the side tested is destroyed, the patient feels the stimulus, and there is a consensual blink, but no ipsilateral blink. On the opposite eye there is an ipsilateral blink, but no consensual blink.

The mastication muscles are tested by having the patient clench his teeth and palpating the muscles of the side of the face (masseter and temporal) for force of muscle contraction and bulk. Normally, they are firmly contracted, and attempts to open the jaw by downward pressure on the chin are resisted. The pterygoid muscle is tested by pressing laterally on the jaw while the patient's mouth is partly open. With one-sided pterygoid weakness, the jaw deviates toward the weak side. The deviation may be seen as the mouth is opened slowly. Look at the relative positions of the upper and lower teeth for jaw deviation when the mouth is opened.

Facial Nerve (Cranial Nerve VII) Motor innervation to muscles of facial expression, taste on the anterior two-thirds of the tongue, and general sensation to portions of the external ear are mediated by the facial nerves. Their function is determined by asking the patient to wrinkle his forehead by frowning and raising his eyebrows (frontalis muscle), closing his eyes tightly (orbicularis oculi muscle), pursing the lips by whistling (orbicularis oris muscle), retracting the angles of the mouth by smiling (lower facial muscles), and drawing his lower lips downward and laterally by vigorous effort to show teeth (platysma and triangularis muscles).

There should be equality of function and strength between the two sides of the face. Some degree of facial asymmetry is common, especially of the mouth with smiling and talking, and must be distinguished from muscle weakness. Gross weakness is apparent from marked asymmetry, but lesser degrees of weakness can be detected only when deliberately sought by testing the various muscles of facial expression.

Two types of facial nerve paralysis may be observed, depending on the site of the disruptive lesion. Lower motor neuron lesions in the facial nucleus of the facial nerve cause complete paralysis of one-half of the entire face. The muscles of that side of the face sag, and the normal lines around the lips, nose, and forehead are less pronounced. The mouth is drawn to the strong side with smiling; there is inability to close the eye; the patient may drool; and the cheek on the affected side may puff out with expiration. The central type of facial paralysis is due to a lesion above the facial nucleus, such as in the motor area of the cortex. The forehead function is intact because the primary motor neurons of the brainstem supplying the forehead muscles are innervated by both sides of the motor cortex. The lower facial muscles are paralyzed for voluntary movements, but an involuntary grin is still possible, with innervation from extrapyramidal circuits. There may be slight weakness of eyelid closing and palpebral fissure widening.

The muscles of facial expression are tested in the patient with a depressed level of consciousness by observing wincing in response to noxious stimulation, for example, applying pressure to the supraorbital nerve.

Taste on the anterior tongue is not routinely tested unless the examiner wishes to determine if the taste fibers of the facial nerve are also involved. The technique for testing taste is described in the section on the hypoglossal nerve.

Auditory Nerve (Cranial Nerve VIII)

Auditory nerve testing is discussed in Chapter 8.

Glossopharyngeal and Vagus Nerves (Cranial Nerves IX and X)

The glossopharyngeal and vagus nerves run close together, and because their functions are so similar they are tested together.

The glossopharyngeal is a mixed nerve. The motor portion produces elevation and construction of the pharynx. It is the sensory nerve to the posterior third of the tongue, soft palate, tonsillar pillars, and pharynx. The vagus is also a mixed nerve innervating the larynx. In addition, it has visceral innervation functions, with implications for the cardiovascular and gastrointestinal examinations.

The taste function of the glossopharyngeal nerve can be evaluated by having the patient first rinse his mouth with clear water to remove any existing substances that could affect taste. The tongue is then protruded. Sweet, sour, salt, and bitter substances are separately applied to the anterior two-thirds (innervated by the facial nerve) and posterior third (innervated by the glossopharyngeal nerve) of the tongue. The mouth is rinsed with water after the application of each substance. The patient is asked to identify each substance by pointing to or selecting a card on which is written the word describing the substance. Sugar crystals or glucose solution produces sweetness. Unsweetened lemon juice or vinegar gives a sour sensation; table salt gives a salty sensation; quinine elicits a bitter taste and should be used last. The substances in crystalline form can be applied directly with an applicator. Those in solution can be applied with a medicine dropper. Taste sensation is frequently diminished or absent in the aged and also following head injuries. If olfactory acuity is diminished, there is a direct effect on the gustatory sense, and taste may then be simultaneously decreased.

The lesions of the vagal system affect the patient's ability to swallow and can be determined by having him drink some water. This is best performed with the patient's head elevated. Nasal regurgitation or coughing indicates palatal weakness. Care should be taken to prevent aspiration of the liquid.

The gag reflex is stimulated by touching each side of the pharyngeal wall with a tongue blade. The glossopharyngeal nerve is the sensory component of the gag reflex and the vagus the motor component.

The presence of hoarseness or diminishing strength of coughing may indicate laryngeal weakness.

For good visualization of the back of the mouth, the tongue is depressed with a tongue blade and the oropharynx illuminated by a light directed from behind or to the side of the examiner. The pharyngeal walls and soft palate are observed for symmetry and their relationship to the midline position. As the patient says "Ah," the soft palate should elevate equally on both sides. The pharyngeal muscles contract during the "Ah," moving toward the midline. Weakness on one side produces deviation to the unaffected side and distorts the midline position. If there is weakness of the soft palate, the voice has a nasal quality.

The Spinal Assessory Nerve (Cranial Nerve XI)

The spinal accessory nerve innervates the sternocleidomastoid and trapezius muscles. The sternocleidomastoid muscle originates behind the ear and inserts into the clavicular area. When the head is turned to the side, this muscle can be observed as the longitudinal ridge which becomes prominent on the contralateral side of the neck. The sternocleidomastoid muscle is observed bilaterally for muscle mass, symmetry, and contour from the neck to the shoulders. Ordinarily its shape is readily identified, but atrophy of this muscle could make it difficult to observe. In athletes, the muscle contour is prominent but symmetrical. In the presence of abnormal head movements, the sternocleidomastoid muscle is likely to show more hypertrophy on one side.

Because of the origin and insertion of the sternocleidomastoid muscle, contraction of this muscle on one side causes a downward movement of the head, with rotation of the chin to the opposite side. The examiner tests muscle strength by placing one hand on the side of the patient's face and resisting movement as the patient turns his head forcibly in that direction. The examiner's other hand is placed on the firm longitudinal ridge that becomes prominent in the opposite side of the neck. The other sternocleidomastoid muscle is tested by reversing the process.

The trapezius muscles move the shoulders up and down. The patient in the upright position is observed both from the back and front to assess symmetry of the neck and shoulder junction. The shoulders should be at the same level. The scapulae should be at the same level, both with the arms down at the sides and when outstretched in front. If there is weakness in the trapezius muscle, one scapula may be lower and become more prominent than the other when the arms are extended in an anterior position.

Muscle strength can be assessed by having the patient shrug his shoulders and hold the position. The examiner places one hand on each shoulder and tries to push the shoulders down as the patient tries to maintain the shrug. Weakness is indicated by inability of the patient to maintain the position.

Hypoglossal Nerve (Cranial Nerve XII)

The hypoglossal nerve is a motor nerve, responsible for movements of the tongue. While at rest on the floor of the mouth, the tongue is observed for the amount of space it occupies, its contour, muscle mass, and the presence of any movements. The tongue should fill the entire space bordered by the lower teeth. No movements should be visible when the tongue is at rest. Normally, movements occur only when the tongue is under tension, e.g., in protrusion.

The strength of the tongue can be tested by having the patient push the tongue against the inner aspect of the cheek. As the examiner externally compresses the cheek at the point at which the tongue protrudes, the tongue should be able to maintain its position if no weakness is present. Both sides are tested.

The tongue is then extended out of the mouth. The tip of the tongue should be in a midline position between the two front teeth. If the tongue consistently deviates to one side, weakness of the nerve may be indicated. (The tongue deviates toward the side of the weakness because it is a thrusting muscle.) The tongue is again observed for symmetry and muscle mass. Any decrease in size or the presence of deep lengthwise ridges may be indicative of atrophy. The patient should be requested to make rapid, repetitive movements of the tongue into and out of the mouth. The movements should be quick and strong, improving during the testing. A table listing each cranial nerve, the appraisal methods, and the normal response is included to facilitate the examination of the cranial nerves. (See table 13-2.)

MOTOR FUNCTION EXAMINATION

For a thorough inspection of motor functioning it is important that the patient be undressed except for a loincloth. Women may also wear chest covering.

Muscle Bulk

Muscles are tested in pairs. The size, contour, and strength of the muscle on one side is immediately compared with the one on the opposite side. A general comparison of body contour is made with the average normal figure of like sex and age. A concept of normal muscle bulk is gained with experience.

The limbs are positioned symmetrically for comparison, and the muscle contours are inspected during contraction and rest. When there is suspicion of atrophy, measurements should be made of the circumferences of the limbs bilaterally at their maximum girth. Corresponding points should be accurately

Table 13-2.
Cranial Nerves

Nerve	Appraisal Method	Normal Response
I Olfactory	Identify odors with the alternate nostril occluded	Appreciation of the odor with or without precise identification of the substance
II Optic		
Visual acuity	Read Snellen chart or Jaeger chart with and without glasses	Less than 20/30 requires follow-up
Visual fields	Confrontation test	Movement perceived in all quadrants both eyes
	Cover one eye and identify movement in periphery while looking straight forward	
III Oculomotor	Tested together	
IV Trochlear		
VI Abducens		
Extraocular movements	Follow movement of finger in all directions of gaze	Able to look with each eye
Accomodation	Focus from a distant to a close object	Convergence, accomodation, and pupillary constriction
Pupillary light reflexes	Light shown in each eye separately	Direct and consensual pupillary constriction
Optic disc, vessels, and retina	Fundoscopic	Distinct smooth structures
V Trigeminal		
Facial sensation	Light touch with cotton to forehead, cheek, jaw bilaterally	Perception and accurate identification in all divisions. Equal bilaterally
Corneal reflex	Light touch with cotton to cornea bilaterally	Direct and consensual blinking
Jaw strength	Palpate muscles of the sides of the face while teeth are clenched	Symmetric Firmly contracted equal bulk and strength
	Attempt to open jaw	Jaw opens in midline
VII Facial		
Motor	Wrinkle forehead, raise eyebrows, frown, smile, purse lips, and keep eyes closed against resistance	Symmetry of function and strength
Taste	Sweet, sour, salt, bitter to anterior tongue bilaterally	Distinguish all four tastes May be diminished in the aged
VIII Acoustic		
Hearing	Ticking watch Whisper and spoken word	Able to hear barely audible whisper (15-25 db)
Weber	Tuning fork on midline of skull	Sound remains centralized
Rinne	Tuning fork on mastoid process then next to ear	Air conduction heard longer than bone

Table 13-2.
Continued.

Nerve	Appraisal Method	Normal Response
IX Glossopharyngeal		
X Vagus		
Gag reflex	Drink water	No cough, nasal regurgitation, etc.
	Touch each side of pharyngeal wall	Symmetric movement Immediate gagging
Taste	Posterior third of tongue bilaterally (See VII Facial)	
XI Accessory	Test strength of shoulder shrug and turning of head side to side	Symmetry of scapulae movements and strength of resistence
XII Hypoglossal	Protrude tongue Push tongue against tongue blade	Midline without tremor or atrophy Equal force bilaterally

marked for measuring above and below the patella, the elbow, and other appropriate bony prominences. The tension applied to the tape measure must be the same for both sides. The points at which the measurements are taken, as well as the circumferences, should be recorded for evaluation of the progression of the atrophy. Differences of less than 1 cm are not significant.

Asymmetric muscle wasting is not difficult to detect, but symmetric wasting is easily missed. Hypertrophied muscle is seen occasionally, but atrophy and weakness occur much more frequently. Wasting may be from lower motor neuron lesions, myopathy, or disuse from paralysis due to upper motor neuron lesion or joint pain, as in arthritis.

Muscle Tone

Muscle tone, or tonus, is the slight muscular resistance felt by the examiner when the relaxed limb is passively moved through its range of motion. It is the end result of all neural activity from many sources. The qualitative evaluation of tonus is difficult and largely a matter of personal experience.

The patient is instructed to relax and to let the limb being examined "hang loose." This is difficult to do, and to achieve the desired degree of relaxation it may be necessary to divert the patient's attention. Each limb in turn is palpated, passively shaken, and moved through flexion, extension, and rotation. The range of motion is done both rapidly and slowly while feeling the degree of resistance. Normal tone has a mild even resistance to movement through the entire range. It is a quality of resilience rather than complete flabbiness. The swing of extremities is determined by tonus. Swing can be tested by the examiner flipping the patient's arms out from the hips and allowing them to drop, and by raising the patient's legs and letting them drop while the patient sits on the side of the table. The duration, regularity, and pattern of the swing are observed. The normal limb swings freely with a regular motion like a pendulum, which decreases in a steady even manner.

Muscle tone may be increased (hypertonicity) or decreased (hypotonicity). The alteration may be general or focal, with tonus different in separate muscle groups. In hypertonicity the increased resistance may be predominantly in extensor muscles, in flexor muscles, or in both; there is increased flexion of joints, muscle bellies stand out more, and limbs at rest tend to remain in a fixed posture. Hypertonicity is associated with brisk reflexes and is characteristic of upper motor neuron lesions. Spasticity and rigidity are manifestations of hypertonicity. Sudden passive movements of the joints are initially met with considerable resistance, evidenced by spasms, but when overcome, the movement continues more easily. *Rigidity* is a steady contraction of flexors and extensors which causes increased resistance to passive movement throughout the full range of motion in any direction.

In hypotonicity the muscle feels soft and flabby, there is a looseness of extremities on shaking them, and the joint can be moved beyond the usual range of motion. The extremity tends to assume a position dictated by gravity. There is loss of the normal slight flexion of joints, and there is a flattened appearance of the muscle body instead of the rounded contour. Lower motor neuron lesions and muscle disease are causes of hypotonicity. The patient complains of such symptoms as slowness, dragging of the foot, and lack of arm swing in disturbances affecting muscle tone.

Muscle Strength   Ability and confidence in detecting muscular weakness, especially if minimal, can be attained only by testing a variety of patients with muscular weaknesses and normal strength. Practice is the only means of gaining a feel for what is normal range. When testing muscle strength, it is the muscle fibers and their innervation that are being tested. Knowledge of muscle innervation is essential in pinpointing neurologic lesions, and knowledge of the function of specific muscles is needed to understand abnormal gaits and muscular function deficits. The use of muscle and nerve anatomy charts can help one to determine and describe better which muscles, peripheral nerves, and spinal cord segments are involved.

Muscular strength can be tested and described with limited knowledge of specific muscles and nerves by the function performed in reference to a particular joint. The functions are flexion, extension, abduction (away from midline), adduction (toward midline), supination (face up, palm up), pronation (face down, palm down), and rotation. The muscle and joint functions are tested in a cephalocaudal (head to foot) order from the neck and shoulders down to the elbows, wrists, hands, hips, knees, ankles, and feet (Table 13-3).

For efficiency and assistance in localizing the lesion it is helpful to develop a scheme for examining muscle strength, tone, size, and reflexes that begins at the head and neck and moves downward to the arms and then the legs.

During the motor examination there should be unobstructed observation of the patient, so that the muscles and joints can be inspected, palpated, and tested for strength. The patient should be in the position that gives him the greatest body stability. In the routine examination, the patient should be seated. Symmetric muscle pairs are directly compared (i.e., one arm is tested, then the other) for relative strength. Proximal and distal muscle groups are tested. If the patient experiences muscular difficulty under certain conditions, such as cold or exertion, these conditions should be reproduced with cold water or repeated movements of the involved muscles. The examiner generally tries to match strength with the patient, using the principles of leverage and the fact that muscles are strongest when they act from their shortest (flexed) length.

Generally, the patient is instructed to hold a position of strength and to resist with maximal effort the pressure applied by the examiner and to continue to resist until instructed to stop. The opposing pressure is applied gradually and is continuously increased to the maximum or until the patient is overpowered. The comprehending, cooperative patient, with either strong or weak muscles, offers a smooth steady counterpressure, and the joint moves as the examiner varies the pressure applied.

The patient with a hysterical type of weakness is likely to have a jerky contraction, or sudden cessation of effort, or both. This abrupt giving way and lack of following through are major clues to functional (hysterical) weakness. Functional weakness of a leg may be detected by placing one's hands under the supine patient's heels while instructing him to lift the weak leg. Normally, with unilateral leg weakness, there should be pressure felt from the heel of the unaffected leg as it is used for leverage if full effort is put forth to move the contralateral leg. Much urging is required to get any muscle contraction in nonorganic weakness.

To make the patient's record meaningful for examiners and useful in determining changes in muscle strength a standardized scale is used for grading muscle power [3].

Value	Functional Level
5	Full range of motion against gravity with full resistance.
4	Full range of motion against gravity with some resistance.
3	Full range of motion against gravity.
2	Full range of motion with gravity eliminated.
1	Palpable increase in muscle tension. No joint movement.
0	No evidence of contraction.

This scale is intended for lower motor neuron lesions and is only useful in the fully cooperative person, for it is based on the ability of a person to contract a muscle group with his maximum effort against applied resistance.

Table 13-3.
Muscle Strength Testing

Muscle Function	Patient's Movement	Examiner's Resistant Motion
Neck		
Flexors	Chin on chest	Fingertips against forehead; palm of hand against occiput
Extensors	Head backward	
Fingers		
Flexors (C 8)	Squeezes examiner's fingers hard; makes fist	Compares grips and attempts to withdraw to straighten fingers
Extensors (C 7)	Fingers out straight	Attempts finger flexion
Adduction (C 8–T 1)	Holds paper between adjacent fingers	Pulls paper
Abduction (C 8–T 1)	Fingers straight out and spread apart	Squeezes adjacent fingers together
Wrist		
Flexors	Flexes wrists	Tries to extend wrist
Extensors	Pronates forearm and cocks up wrist	Presses dorsum of hand to push wrist down
Elbow		
Flexors (biceps, C 5–6)	Flexes elbow 90 degrees and attempts to bend more	Prevents flexion
Supinators (palm up) Pronators	Rotates wrist in one direction then the other	Resists efforts to rotate
Extensors (triceps, C 6–8)	Flexes elbow varying degrees and attempts to straighten	Prevents straightening
Shoulder		
Abduction (deltoid C 5–6)	Holds out upper arm horizontally	Attempts to depress elbow
Adduction	Holds upper arm close to chest	Attempts to raise elbow horizontally
Ankle		
Dorsiflexors (L 4–L 5)	Walks on heels; pulls foot and toes upward	Pulls downward on foot
Plantar flexors (S 1–S 2)	Walks on toes; push down	Pushes against bottom of foot
Knee		
Flexors (hamstring L 5–S 1)	Sitting: Holds knee bent at 90 degree angle. Prone: Partly flexes knee and tries to flex further	Resists above ankle
Extensor (quadriceps L 3–4)	Squats; arises; slight flexion of knee and resists bending	Attempts to flex knee
Hip		
Flexors (L 2–L 3)	In bed: Raises leg about 45 degrees and holds 15–20 seconds (wobbling or drifting downward indicates weakness). Sitting: Raises knee up	Downward pressure directly above knee

Table 13-3. Continued. Muscle Function	Patient's Movement	Examiner's Resistant Motion
Extensors (L 4–L 5)	Ascends step, rising from squatting position	
Abductors (L 4–L 5)	Holds knees apart	Tries to approximate knees
Adductors (L 2–L 3)	Holds knees together tightly	Tries to separate knees
Trunk		
Abdominal	Rises from lying to sitting	
Back	Side or prone: Elevates leg or head	

Contracture, pain, involuntary movements, spasticity, rigidity, ataxia, and deformity may all interfere significantly with evaluating muscle strength.

In the unconscious or demented patient, observations are made of his performance, noting, for example, whether there are spontaneous movements or withdrawal in response to noxious stimuli, the presence or absence of muscle tone when dropping the lifted limb of the unconscious, and equal bilateral body responses.

The motor examination begins the moment the examiner meets the patient, as she observes how the patient walks, stands, sits, and performs other spontaneous activities. In the routine physical examination, the strength of a few movements is always sampled. These include the cranial nerves, elbow, wrist, hip, knee, and ankle flexors and extensors. Depending on the patient's history and physical findings much more may be done.

The patient who has muscle weakness tends to enumerate specific functions that give him difficulty, such as turning a doorknob, rising from a chair, stumbling, chewing, or caring for hair, rather than stating vague complaints of being weak, tired, fatigued.

When muscle weakness is detected, the involved muscles are carefully inspected for atrophy or unusual bulk, tenderness, fasciculations, and tone. Muscle weakness is indicative of pyramidal pathway disturbance in the cerebrum, brainstem, or spinal cord; in peripheral nerves; at the neuromuscular junction; or in the muscle itself.

The foregoing systematic assessment of the muscle groups helps the nurse examiner to define specifically which muscle functions are weak and to grade the weakness. The nurse examiner is also concerned about the functional abilities of the patient for such things as activities of daily living. This is determined by observing the patient get out of bed, brush his teeth, dress, and eat and so on, or by having the person describe his functioning in these activities.

Joint Function   To examine an extremity is to study the elements of it—reflexes, muscles, joints, skin, subcutaneous tissue, and related vascular and nervous structures. Joint and bone examinations are integrated into the examination of each extremity.

Any bony structure or joint(s) implicated by the patient's history or the physical findings should have a detailed examination.

Bones are assessed for angulation, masses, tenderness to palpation or percussion, and structural integrity. Joints are inspected and palpated, and bilateral comparisons are made of alignment, shape, circumference, range of motion, state of joint fluid (effusion), stability, scars, draining sinuses, warmth and redness of overlying skin, presence of swelling, wasting of adjacent muscles, and tenderness.

The patient is asked to move affected or selected joints through as full a range of motion as he can. If there are limitations, passive range of motion is done by the examiner. The limb is supported above and below the joint, and the patient's face is observed for expressions of pain during the test. Joint range of motion is estimated in terms of degrees of the arc of a circle. The neutral position (no flexion, no abduction, and so on) of the extremity or trunk is used as a starting point. It is considered 0 degrees. Any flexion, abduction, or hyperextension is measured in degrees from there. *Measuring and Recording of Joint Motion,* published by the American Academy of Orthopaedic Surgeons, contains criteria by which the measurements can be obtained for specific joints. A simple instrument called a goniometer helps one to make more accurate measurements.

A variety of terms is used to describe deformities of the extremities. The use of the terms *varus* (toward midline) and *valgus* (away from midline) has been frequently confused. They are correct only for describing deformities. The terms *adduction* and *abduction* are used in descriptions both of deformities and of normal range of motion. Deformities resulting from fractures are described by the relationship of the distal portion to the proximal. A "posterior dislocation of the elbow" means that the ulna and radius are dislocated posterior to the humerus. The angulation of bone, such as might occur with a fracture, is sometimes described by the direction in which the apex of the abnormal angle points, i.e., posterior, lateral, medial, anterior. Proximal, middle, and distal contractures should be described in specific detail, e.g., "a flexion adduction contracture of left hip." Extremity lengths should be measured for objective comparisons when the examiner is uncertain of variations. The measurement is taken between two bony prominences, with the extremities in symmetric, extended positions. The crest of the anterior superior iliac spines to the medial malleoli of the ankle are the lower extremity landmarks, and the acromion of the shoulder to the radial styloid projection above the thumb are landmarks for the arms.

Effusion, or increased synovial joint fluid, causes a uniform swelling of the joint and obliterates the normal landmarks. A sense of fluctuation can be felt. To elicit fluctuation in the knee, it is extended, and the pouch above the patella is squeezed toward the joint with one hand. In the presence of effusion this hand feels an expanding impulse when the lateral aspects of the knee are squeezed with the opposite hand. Effused joints are usually held in flexion, and attempts to extend it cause pain.

Roughened joint surfaces or bone fractures may produce a grating (crepitus) that can be heard or felt over the moving joint or fracture. Bony overgrowths (nodules) occasionally may be felt along the margins of large joints like the knee and the elbow or the distal phalanges of the fingers.

Flexibility of the upper spine is assessed by instructing or assisting the patient to tip his head backward (hyperextension) and forward (flexion), toward each shoulder, and then to turn it from side to side (rotation). Bending over to touch the toes and rotating the shoulders from the pelvis tests the flexibility of the lower spine. The patient should be able to accomplish these movements easily in the absence of disease and changes of aging.

Backache is an affliction frequently seen in today's society. Evaluation of the complaint is difficult because objective symptoms often are not found. This does not negate the symptom, and careful evaluation of spinal function and obtaining data on occupational and other activities provide salient clues to the probable cause and severity of the problem. Appraisal of spinal motion is done in conjunction with the examination of the upper and the lower extremities.

In radiculopathies (disease of the nerve roots), flexion, extension, and rotation of the cervical lumbosacral spine may produce pain, and movement may be limited in one or more directions. In compression of lumbar or sacral nerve roots from a herniated disc, the patient's pain may be reproduced by the straight leg raising test. With the patient supine, the legs are kept straight and raised one at a time by the examiner. The degree of leg elevation from the bed at which the patient feels pain, which leg is affected, and the site of the pain should be noted. Dorsiflexion of the foot by the examiner while the leg is raised to a 45-degree angle stretches the nerve even more and may reproduce the pain that straight leg raising alone did not. Sharp pain radiating down the leg is indicative of sciatic nerve irritation; whereas the discomfort from muscle tightness is not. Back pain symptoms are correlated with the muscle strength, reflex, and sensory findings of the lower extremities.

When observing a side view of an erect, well-developed person with good postural habits, one should, figuratively speaking, be able to draw a perpendicular line that begins at the lobe of the ear, goes through the shoulder, the trochanter of the femur, the center of the knee, and to the front of the ankle. The spinal silhouette should have a gentle C curve of the cervical spine with the concavity posterior, the dorsal spine with a convex curve to the posterior, and the lumbar spine curving forward and then back at the sacral spine. The head should be held back and the chin up, so that the chin is not projected beyond the same line as the chest. The abdomen should be flat.

When viewed from the back the iliac crests should be at the same level and the shoulders squared and of equal height while the arms hang easily at the sides. The scapular wings should be even and move symmetrically, and the spinous processes of the vertebrae should be in a vertical line. Deviations from a straight vertical line may be seen more readily by putting a mark on each spinous process. Lateral curvature of the spine is called *scoliosis;* round shoulders and exaggerated posterior curvature of thoracic spine is called *kyphosis* and an increased lower back (lumbar) curvature is called *lordosis.*

Muscle Stretch Reflexes

Voluntary muscles contain stretch-sensitive receptors which, when stimulated by mechanical stretching, send impulses through the afferent fibers in peripheral nerves and dorsal roots to anterior horn cells of the spinal cord. The anterior horn cells are excited at the same cord segment and send efferent impulses via the anterior root and motor nerve to the same muscle, leading to a brief contraction of the muscle. This is a simple monosynaptic reflex that may be diminished or lost with interruptions of afferent (sensory) fibers. It is also diminished with extensive destruction of efferent (motor) fibers and anterior horn cells. Release of this monosynaptic reflex from the influence of higher levels of the pyramidal tract and cerebral motor cortex produces hyperreflexia (exaggerated reflexes). Extreme hyperreflexia leads to clonus.

Only a discrete mechanical stimulation (i.e., a quick blow of the reflex hammer) can elicit muscle stretch reflex (MSR). To produce a brisk and consistent stroke with the reflex hammer, it is held loosely between the thumb and index finger, and the swing is made from the wrist, allowing the hammer to fall by gravity against the tendon. The broad head of the hammer is used to strike accessible tendons (e.g., the Achilles) and the pointed end for smaller, less accessible tendons (e.g., the biceps). Complete relaxation of the patient and a proper degree of muscle tension are the other two factors that must accompany an adequate stretch stimulus to elicit consistent muscle stretch reflexes. These two factors are basically dependent on proper positioning of the patient and the extremity. When seated, the patient should be comfortable and have both the arms and legs in a relaxed position with the forearms on the thighs and the feet on the floor or dangling freely. With too little or too much muscle stretch, a reflex cannot be elicited. Usually, positioning midway between full extension and full flexion obtains the proper degree of tension. Practice helps in determining this degree. Palpating the tendon helps identify the exact location to be tapped.

If these measures do not produce muscle stretch reflexes, reinforcement techniques may help. These involve instructing the patient to contract muscles other than the one being tested. For instance, have him interlock his fingers and pull while the reflexes of the lower extremities are being tested, and squeeze the knees together while the upper extremities are being tested.

The biceps, triceps, brachioradialis, patellar, Achilles tendons, and jaw reflexes are the common reflexes tested in general physical examinations. Methods of testing some of these reflexes are shown in Figure 13-3.

To test the biceps reflex (cervical nerves [C] 5 and 6) the examiner places the

Figure 13-3.
Technique of obtaining
muscle stretch reflexes.
(Reproduced with
permission from J. F.
Simpson and K. R. Magee.
*Clinical Evaluation of the
Nervous System.* Boston:
Little, Brown, 1973.)

tip of his thumb or index finger over the biceps tendon at the antecubital space, pressing firmly to produce slight tension, then strikes a sharp blow on the finger with the reflex hammer. The patient's arms should be positioned symmetrically. This is achieved in the recumbent patient by placing both hands in identical position on the abdomen. When the patient is sitting, his elbow is supported by the examiner's hand, and his hand is placed on the examiner's forearm or the pronated forearm is placed on the patient's thigh. The reflex response is flexion of the arm (Fig. 13-3A).

The triceps reflex (C 6, 7, and 8) is tested on the supine patient with the forearm flexed on the anterior chest and the tendon struck directly above the elbow. With the patient in the seated position the arm may be supported at the upper arm. This tendon is short and difficult to percuss without hitting muscle fibers too. The reflex response is extension of the arm (Fig. 13-3B).

The brachioradialis reflex (C 5 and 6) is tested by striking the distal radius just above the thumb with the patient's forearm midway between pronation and supination and the elbow at a right angle. The tendon can be located by asking the person to flex the thumb; tap the area where the tendon movement occurred. The patient's hands are on the abdomen when he is in a recumbent position, but on the knees or held by the examiner when the patient is sitting. The response is flexion of the forearm on the arm and usually also flexion of the fingers and hand [1] (Fig. 13-3C).

The quadriceps reflex (knee jerk) (lumbar nerves [L] 2, 3, and 4) is elicited by striking the tendon just below the patella when the patient is seated with legs dangling. The patient should sit far enough forward to allow the legs to swing freely with knees apart. To help evaluate the extent of the response, the examiner's hand may be placed on the patient's knee. When the patient is supine, the knees are bent slightly (about 20 degrees) by lifting the thighs, to create slight muscle stretch. The reflex response is quadriceps contraction and knee extension (Fig. 13-3E).

Achilles reflex testing (ankle jerk, sacral nerves [S] 1 and 2) requires that slight stretch be placed on the tendon. Several positions can be used. In all positions, slight dorsiflexion should be induced by gentle pressure on the ball of the foot. For access to the Achilles tendon of the bedfast patient, the foot and ankle can be placed on the opposite shin by flexing the knee and externally rotating the hip. With the prone patient the knees are bent to a 90-degree angle; the ambulant patient may kneel in a chair with feet and ankles suspended over the edge of the chair. The Achilles tendon is struck directly, and plantar flexion is the reflex response (Fig. 13-3F).

Jaw reflex (pons, cranial nerve V) is elicited by having the jaw relaxed and partially opened with one finger pressing downward on the chin; the finger is then tapped with the hammer. Closure of the jaw is the response. Normally, this is difficult to obtain and so, if it is obtained without reinforcement, it is likely that hyperreflexia is present.

In general, if one receives no response when attempting to elicit a muscle stretch reflex, be sure to (1) locate the tendon, (2) strike the blow crisply, and (3) alter the muscle tension by adjusting the position of the extremity, changing the finger compression of the tendon, or using reinforcement.

In hyperreflexic states of the legs, clonus may be elicited by slightly flexing the knee and then briskly jerking the foot upward and slightly outward and holding it. With the continued application of pressure to the sole of the foot, the foot oscillates between flexion and extension. This continues for as long as the pressure is applied. Only clonus sustained beyond a few jerks is pathologic.

Superficial Reflexes   Other motor cortex and pyramidal tract reflexes can be elicited by stimulating surface receptors in skin. The abdominal reflex (upper and lower) is tested in all four quadrants with a brisk stroke toward the umbilicus. The response is movement of the umbilicus toward the quadrant stimulated. The supine relaxed position is used. Upper motor neuron lesions and abdominal distention are causes of absence of the reflex. The cremasteric (L 1 and 2) reflex is tested in males by stroking the inner surface of the upper thigh. The normal response is quick upward movement of the ipsilateral testicle.

The anal reflex (S 3, 4, and 5) should be evaluated when there is low back pain, possible cauda equina lesions, or sacral nerve root compression. The patient is placed on his side and the buttocks spread. The perianal area is then scratched or pricked. There should be an obvious quick contraction of the external sphincter. This may also be evaluated by feeling the contraction when a finger is inserted into the rectum.

Pathologic Reflexes   Except in infants, the Babinski reflex is pathognomonic of motor area dysfunction of the brain or corticospinal pathway disease. With the patient in a relaxed, recumbent position and legs extended, a firm stroke is applied with an object like the thumb, a key, or an orange stick against the sole of the foot (Fig. 13-4). The stroke is begun at the lateral aspect of the heel, moved slowly up-

Figure 13-4. Technique of eliciting the Babinski reflex. The sole is stroked firmly along the path indicated. (Reproduced with permission from J. F. Simpson and K. R. Magee. *Clinical Evaluation of the Nervous System.* Boston: Little, Brown, 1973.)

ward toward the little toe, and then across the ball of the foot toward the large toe. The normal response is plantar flexion of the toes. The pathologic Babinski response consists of extension of the big toe and flexion and spreading of the small toes. Flexion of the leg may even occur. The response may be equivocal and therefore difficult to evaluate when there is voluntary withdrawal that is not pathologic. The voluntary withdrawal is faster and associated with rapid withdrawal of the leg. The Babinski sign is slow and usually disappears quickly when stimulation ceases. The examiner should strive to achieve a consistent response. This may require varying the stroke pressure, speed, and length.

The Hoffmann reflex is tested by flicking the nail of the middle finger (Fig. 13-3D). Normally there is little if any response. In hyperreflexia there is a flexion of the thumb and finger.

Symmetric reflexes should be compared immediately; e.g., one Achilles reflex is tested and then the other, for immediate comparison. Asymmetry and discrepancy between one part of the body and another is assessed. Any isolated reflex change, either hyporeflexia or hyperreflexia, requires consideration by the examiner and correlation with muscle bulk, strength, and sensory findings. Decrease of muscle stretch reflexes occurs when the reflex arc is interrupted. The interruption can be in the spinal cord, the sensory or motor nerves, or the muscle. Exaggerated reflexes frequently represent upper motor neuron disease located anywhere from the cerebral cortex to the appropriate anterior horn cell.

Reflexes are graded on a 0 to 4+ scale and recorded on a stick figure (Fig. 13-5).

Figure 13-5.
Stick figure for recording
muscle stretch reflexes.

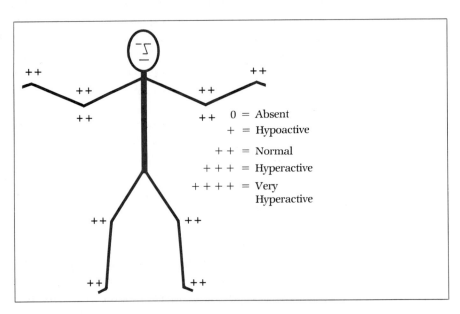

Coordination and Equilibrium

Coordination and equilibrium are achieved by the integrative functioning of the cerebellum, posterior columns of the spinal cord, and the vestibular mechanism of the ear. Injury to the proprioceptive system—the receptors and nerve pathways for the sense of movement and position of body parts—produces incoordination, ataxia, and imbalance.

Coordination

Coordination is the synergistic action of muscles functioning in proper sequence to produce a smooth, purposeful movement. Incoordination occurs because of improper programming of the involved muscles, which causes errors in the speed and the dexterity of movement as it is performed. These can be evaluated by the use of some simple tests.

The finger-to-nose test is performed with the patient in a sitting position with his arms extended forward; then, using alternating hands, the patient touches the nose with the forefinger and returns the arm to the extended position. This test is done first with the eyes open and then with the eyes closed. The patient should be observed for smooth movements and the maintenance of proper body posture.

Another test is forefinger approximations. The patient extends his arms out at the sides and then brings them forward until the forefingers meet at the midline. This test is done first with the eyes open and then with the eyes closed.

Diadochokinesia, or "diametrically opposite hand movement," is evaluated using several different tests. With the patient in a sitting position, the palms of his hands are placed downward on top of the knees and he is then asked to alternate the hands rapidly from pronation to supination. The hands are compared for equality of movement. Another test is to have the patient place the heels of his hands on top of the knees and then ask him to tap his knees with his fingers, using a rapid motion. Coordination is also demonstrated by touching the tips of the forefinger and the thumb in a series of rapid approximations. While observing the performance of these tests it is important to remember that the very young and the elderly may perform less well than young and middle-aged adults.

The heel-to-knee test demonstrates coordination of the legs. In a supine position, the heel of one foot is placed on the patella of the contralateral leg. The heel is slid down the skin toward the foot without removing the heel from the skin surface. Any deterioration in the quality of the movement should be noted.

While the tests are being performed, some specific observations should be made concerning the initiation of the movement, the direction the extremity takes toward the goal, and the manner in which the extremity is returned to the resting state or end point. Normally, the beginning of the movement should be promptly initiated and show no evidence of slowness or hesitation. The movement should be smooth, purposeful, and reach the goal directly and accurately without taking circuitous routes. The return to the original resting position should be performed smoothly, without evidence of past pointing or extraneous movements.

Equilibrium

Equilibrium is tested by asking the patient to stand erect with his feet together. This is done first with the eyes open and then with the eyes closed. With his eyes open, the patient may then be asked to walk, first naturally, and then in tandem fashion (placing the heel in front of the toe). The nurse examiner should remain near the patient and be ready to prevent injury in case the patient should begin to fall. Normally, the patient should be able to maintain his balance (even on one leg alone) and to walk tandem with the eyes open or closed. The patient who cannot stand steadily with the feet together and who has increasing difficulty with the eyes closed is said to have a positive *Romberg sign*. This is positive only if there is actual loss of balance, causing a shifting of the feet in order to restore balance. Swaying of the trunk alone is not regarded as a positive Romberg sign.

While the patient is performing tests of coordination, care must be taken to prevent him from injuring himself. Patients with disequilibrium may lose their balance easily. When lack of coordination is present, the muscles are not working synergistically, and they may be operating at the wrong time. To compensate for this, the movements become jerky and have increased force. Thus, in the finger-to-nose test, the patient, when attempting to touch his nose, may hit his face.

Abnormal Movements

Ordinarily, movements of the musculoskeletal system are under voluntary control. However, certain pathologic conditions of the extrapyramidal tracts produce muscle movements over which voluntary control is inhibited or ineffective. These involuntary movements may involve only a single muscle fiber or may extend to include multiple muscles in the limbs, trunk, and head. Some of the more common abnormal movements are fasciculations, tremors, chorea, and tics.

Certain types of abnormal movements occur at complete rest, with increased muscle tonus, or at the completion of a movement. Description of the involuntary movement in relation to these three phases is most helpful in properly identifying the movement. Movements occurring at complete rest can best be observed with the patient in a supine position during maximum muscle relaxation. To initiate movements produced by increased muscle tension, the extremities may be actively held in a stationary position of extension and adduction. The extremity may also be flexed and gently tapped with a percussion hammer. Abnormal movements occurring at the termination of an activity can be observed by having the patient drink from a cup, reach for an object, or do any of the coordination tests.

Characteristics of the abnormal movement pattern should be assessed in a systematic way. Identify the location and degree of muscle involvement. Some movements, such as tics and fasciculations, begin in the region of the head and shoulders and involve only parts of muscles. Other involuntary movements frequently begin in distal extremities, gradually progressing toward the trunk and including more muscle to produce more extensive movement. The onset of the involuntary movement may be slow or so abrupt as to endanger equilibrium. The amplitude of the movement can be grossly visible or so fine that it is barely detectable. Fasciculation is an example of a movement of such a low amplitude that it appears wormlike. Movements of low amplitude are more difficult to observe in an obese or muscular person. Fascicular reflections on wet skin from a good light can help make them more clearly visible, but care should be taken to keep the patient warm. Shivering caused by cold can resemble and be mistaken for fasciculations. Fasciculations can be palpated and auscultated. A light tap on the muscle mass with a percussion hammer can initiate fascicular muscle movements.

Involuntary movements may have a rhythmic quality, as is characteristic of tremor, or may be jerky, like chorea. Some movements are repetitive, like the pill-rolling tremor in parkinsonism, whereas other involuntary movements are dissimilar one to another. The components of the motor exam are summarized in Table 13-4.

SENSORY FUNCTION EXAMINATION

The function of three areas of the central nervous system is assessed by testing sensory discrimination. These areas are the posterior columns and the spinothalamic tract of the spinal cord and the sensory cortex of the parietal lobe.

The posterior columns transmit deep-structure sensitivities, which consist of vibration, position sense, and deep-pressure pain. The fibers enter the spinal cord through the dorsal roots and ascend on the same side of the posterior columns to the medulla. In the medulla the fibers cross and ascend through the thalamus to the sensory cortex on the side of the brain opposite to the area stimulated.

The pathways for superficial cutaneous sensations of light touch, superficial pain, and sensitivity to temperature enter the spinal cord through the dorsal roots and cross over to the ventral surface of the opposite side of the cord. After crossing, the impulses travel upward in the lateral spinothalamic tract to the thalamus and from the thalamus to the sensory cortex of the parietal lobe.

Vibratory and position sense, deep and superficial pain, and tactile and thermal sensitivity are thus dependent on intact receptors, peripheral nerves, spinal cord pathways, and thalamic and sensory cortex function. Fine discrimination of sensory stimuli is the function of the sensory cortex. When cortical sensitivity is lost, the basic sensation is recognized, but there is little discrimination of its qualities.

The sensory part of routine health assessment is a head-to-toe survey of the

Table 13-4. Motor Function	Area of Assessment	Assessment Method	Normal Response
	Muscle		
	Bulk	Inspect size, contour, symmetry	Symmetric Comparable to one's concept of normal muscle bulk
	Tone	Palpate, shake extremities and feel degree of resistence ROM Observe swing of extremities	Symmetric Mild even resistance to movement through entire range
	Strength	Flexion and extension of major joints against resistance	Symmetric Smooth steady counterpressure. Joint movement as applied pressure increased (score 3 to 5 on scale)
	Joint function	Inspect, palpate, manipulate form ROM, shape, fluid, discomfort, etc.	Freely moveable without discomfort
	Posture	View from side	Perpendicular line from ear lobe to shoulder to hip trocanter to center of knee to front of ankle
		Anterior-posterior view	Shoulders, scapulae, iliac crest are same height
	Muscle stretch reflexes	Quick tap with hammer to:	
	Biceps	Anticubital area	Flexion of arm
	Triceps	Above elbow	Extension of arm
	Brachioradialis	Wrist above thumb	Flexion of forearm, hand
	Patellar	Knee just below patella	Leg extension
	Achilles	Posterior ankle	Plantar flexion of foot (Score + + on scale)
	Superficial reflexes		
	Abdominal	Stroke each quadrant of abdomen	Umbilicus moves toward quadrant stroked
	Cremasteric	Stroke inner thigh	Upward movement of ipsilateral testicle
	Anal	Stroke perianal area	Quick contraction of sphincter
	Pathologic reflexes		
	Babinski	Stroke sole of foot	Plantar flexion of toes
	Hoffman	Flick nail of middle finger	Little if any finger flexion
	Coordination	Finger-to-nose Forefinger approximation Rapid alternating movements Heel-to-shin	Prompt initiation of smooth, purposeful, accurate movements
	Equilibrium	Walk naturally and tandem	Tandem walk and maintain balance with eyes open or closed

Table 13-4.
Continued.

Area of Assessment	Assessment Method	Normal Response
Involuntary movements	Stand with feet together, with eyes open, and with eyes closed Observe faee, extremities, trunk in resting and active states	Absence of extra purposeless movements

patient's ability to perceive superficial and deep sensations and to make fine sensory discriminations. All are checked in a brief fashion to exclude the presence of a sensory deficit. A pin and cotton are used to test for pain and touch on the face, trunk, forearms, upper arms, thighs, and lower legs. The hands and feet are tested for vibration sensitivity with the tuning fork, and also for position sense. The examination may be limited to these tests when the patient's history has aroused no suspicion of sensory involvement of any kind. A painstaking assessment is done of any areas expected to show impairment from the history related by the patient.

Both sides of the body and the proximal and distal parts are compared for equality of reaction by testing back and forth between the areas with each sensory stimulus and comparing thresholds and responses.

Under normal conditions, a person has sensory responses to all stimuli, and sensations over the body surface are felt equally on both sides of the trunk, extremities, and face. Abnormal reactions that follow anatomic divisions indicate a disruption somewhere along the pathways from the receptors to the sensory cortex of the cerebrum.

The sensory examination is likely to be difficult when the examiner is attempting to map out the margins of the areas of sensory loss and to compare thresholds to stimuli, because this procedure involves a subjective reaction from the patient, and the patient is suggestible to a significant degree. This suggestibility stems from clues that inadvertently are given with the application of the sensory stimulus; for example, the way questions are phrased or the visual clues received by the patient. All sensory testing should be carried out with the patient's eyes closed or his face screened so that he cannot see the body part being tested or the examiner's movements or facial expression. The application of each stimulus should be in a random, unpredictable order, purposefully designed to prevent the patient from anticipating any particular site sequences or intervals between applications of the stimulus. The intervals between stimulus administration should be varied slightly so that stimulation is not rhythmic. This will help to maintain the patient's attention and prevent predictability.

Reasonably definitive results can be gained provided the patient is clearly told what is going to be done and how he is to answer. A brief practice demonstration with the patient's eyes open may facilitate comprehension and avoid unclear results. Only consistent, demonstrable sensory abnormalities on several examinations are acceptable. It may be necessary to check and recheck to map out margins and to compare thresholds. Diminutions in sensation occur more than does total loss, so watch for gradual as well as abrupt changes. The sensory section of the examination may be repeated later if there are questionable changes. It should not be done when the patient is fatigued, because it requires that he be alert, attentive, and cooperative. The foregoing applies to sensory testing in general, as do the following:

1. Test from the decreased area to the normal areas.
2. Test across dermatomes, i.e., up the trunk, across the midline, and across the dorsa of hands and feet (Fig. 13-6).
3. Test the length of the body, both sides, and all four extremities.
4. Test the saddle area (the buttocks and genitalia).

Vibration   Vibratory perception is tested by applying a vibrating tuning fork (128 cps) to bony points such as the ankle, knee, hip, wrist, elbow, and shoulder on both sides of the body. Begin at the periphery and work toward the center. If the response is normal in the distal site, it is normal in the proximal areas. Ask, "Do you feel the buzz," as the tuning fork buzz is demonstrated. Then test by instructing the patient to report each time he feels the buzzing and when it stops. Strike and apply the fork with a consistent degree of force and firmness. Since the patient hears the tuning fork being struck to set it vibrating, strike the fork before each application, but vary the stimulation as follows: (1) sometimes stop the vibration of the fork with the hand before applying it, and (2) sometimes after applying it for varied intervals; (3) sometimes let it run down. Squeeze the vibrating ends to stop it. Compare thresholds in various areas by the length of time the vibrations are discernible to the patient while the fork runs down.

Normal function is recognition of the vibration and awareness of its cessation. Persons over 60 may have diminished vibratory sensation in their feet and lower legs. The level of bone sensory perception corresponds with sensory level in the overlying skin.

Proprioception   Proprioception, the sense of movement and of position of body parts, is tested in all four extremities. First, the patient is instructed to say "Up," or "Down," as digits are passively extended or flexed. One hand supports the patient's completely relaxed foot or hand, while the other hand grasps a digit by its sides and wiggles it up and down. Then movement is stopped in one direction or the other randomly. Do the exercise five times, as the probability of success by chance is 50 percent [2]. Take care not to use a different tone of voice or to ask a question between the up and down positions or to apply different pressures. The patient may respond to these associated stimuli.

Figure 13-6.
Arrangement of
dermatomes. (Reproduced
with permission from J. F.
Simpson and K. R. Magee.
*Clinical Evaluation of the
Nervous System.* Boston:
Little, Brown, 1973.)

Anterior   Posterior

Figure 13-6. Arrangement of dermatomes. (Reproduced with permission from J. F. Simpson and K. R. Magee. *Clinical Evaluation of the Nervous System.* Boston: Little, Brown, 1973.)

Once the patient understands the test he should easily detect movements of a few millimeters and be able to identify which toe is being manipulated and the direction of the position at the end of the movement. Recognition of position and direction of movement permits coordinated movements.

Deep Pain   Deep pain is pain from deep-lying muscle, fascia, bone, and ligaments. Firm squeezing of the structures causes an unpleasant pain. The areas squeezed are usually the Achilles tendon and the muscle at the junction of the thumb and first finger. Other areas are the calf and forearm muscles, the trapezius at the sides of the neck, the testicles, and the supraorbital notch. Note the amount of pressure required to elicit pain. Normally, these parts are tender to pressure, and as the patient becomes conscious of firm and prolonged pressure, he will rise slightly in protest, grimace, withdraw, or resist. This may be the only sensory testing that can be done in the obtunded patient.

Light Touch

Light touch (superficial tactile sense) of the skin surfaces is tested by stroking them with a wisp of cotton or with the finger; cotton tests a finer response. The patient is instructed to say "Now" and "Right" or "Left" each time he is touched. Avoid asking, "Do you feel this?" as this is too suggestive. Sometimes, do not touch him when he expects you to. Periodically, ask him to point with a finger to the exact site of the stimulation. Normal skin has various areas with different thresholds to touch. Hairy and thin skin is more sensitive than horny skin. Lines are drawn on the skin to map out the regions of the loss. Diminished sensation is called *hypesthesia;* increased sensation, *hyperesthesia;* complete loss of sensation, *anesthesia.* Record the specific stimulus and the elicited sensation exactly.

Superficial Pain and Temperature

Superficial pain is elicited by pricking the skin with a pin hard enough to cause an unpleasant sensation. This can be determined on your own hand. Demonstrate "sharp" and "dull" respectively with the point and head of a safety pin. Then apply the sharp and blunt ends in random order, and ask the patient to stipulate whether the stimulus is sharp or dull. Again, avoid asking, "Is this sharper than that?" Rather ask, "Is there a difference between this and that?" If the response is affirmative, ask, "What is the difference?" You may sometimes state the opposite of the actual situation to test suggestibility; for example, "Is this sharper than this?" when it is actually duller.

Pain thresholds vary over different body surfaces, but pain can be perceived on all surfaces. Complete loss of pain sensation is called *analgesia. Hyperalgesia* and *hypalgesia* are the terms for increased and diminished pain respectively. In hyperalgesic states the patient winces the moment the area is touched with the pin.

Superficial pain and temperature pathways are so close anatomically that testing one evaluates the pathways of the other. Pain sensation is tested in the routine health assessment, and, if it is altered, sensory response to temperature is assessed. Sensitivity to temperature is effectively tested by the random application and alternation of two test tubes, one filled with hot water and the other with ice water. The tuning fork may be used instead by heating one prong with hot tap water. The temperatures used for testing must differ from skin temperature and the temperature of the environment. Excessive heat or cold causes a painful, not a thermal, response. The patient is instructed to state "hot" or "cold" each time he is tested. The skin should be observed for signs of loss of sensation such as trauma and cigarette burns on the fingers and irritation of the feet by the shoes.

Mapping The Area of Loss

Mapping the exact distribution of sensory loss is done in order to determine whether it is confined to a peripheral nerve, has a dermatomal distribution, or involves one entire side of the body.

In organic lesions the margins can be defined with reasonable reproducibility and are compatible with the anatomy of the nervous system. Bizarre, non-anatomic distributions occur with functional disturbances. These may be most quickly seen by having the patient draw on his own skin the area of numbness.

To delineate the margins of sensory changes, the area of sensory loss is marked on the skin with a ball-point pen during the testing of each type of stimulus. A different-colored line is used for the different stimuli. A sketch of the affected areas or a sensory dermatome chart may be a helpful way of recording the involved arrangement. The overall picture of the patient conforms to the sensory dermatome chart or sketch, but he may have certain minor variations in distribution.

Stereognosis

Stereognosis is the use of tactile sensation to identify objects in the hand. With the patient's eyes closed, the examiner places a series of small objects in the patient's hand one at a time, and the patient is asked to identify each one. The objects can be anything from the examiner's pockets, such as scissors, coins, pen, pencil, paper clips, or safety pin. Usually, most of the work of identification is done not with the palm but with the fingers, which will hold the object and feel and manipulate it. If the patient demonstrates inability to handle the object well with the fingers and instead holds it in the palm of his hand, he frequently may be unable to name the object correctly. This may be due to peripheral neuropathy, posterior column disease, or parietal involvement.

Graphesthesia

Graphesthesia tests the patient's ability to identify numbers or letters traced on the skin. It is especially helpful in identifying sensory loss when the patient has poor coordination or cannot make fine movements of the hand for stereognosis sensory tests. Although the test is most often performed on the hands, other body parts such as the sole of the foot and the truncal area also can be used. The patient is instructed to close his eyes; then, one at a time, single digits or letters are written on the skin. On the hand, the characters should initially be drawn 0.5 cm high; on the arm, 1.5 cm high; and on the trunk, 2 cm high. If the patient cannot identify what was written, the height is increased with each subsequent trial. Normally, the letters or numbers should be identified as rapidly as when written on paper.

Two-Point Discrimination

Two-point discrimination is a more precise evaluation of tactile sensation than the tests previously described. The patient should be able to differentiate between being touched with one point or two points. If touched with two points simultaneously, the distance between the two points is important to quantify. With the fingers and toes, a distance of 5 mm between the two points is normally sufficient to distinguish two points. If a greater distance is needed, a sensory defect is present. If the dorsum of the lower leg (shin) is used, the normal distance at which two-point discrimination is made is 10 cm [4].

The test is conducted using either a pair of calipers or two pins held to simulate a compass. The procedure is explained to the patient, and the one- and two-point stimuli are demonstrated. With eyes closed, the patient is then asked to tell whether the stimulus has one or two points. The stimuli are applied in random fashion, sometimes touching the skin with one point and at other times with both points. When applying two-point stimulation, the examiner should make sure that both points make skin contact at the same time; otherwise, each point is experienced as a separate stimulus. If, when using two points, the stimuli are not recognized as being two, the distance between the

Table 13-5.
Sensory System

Area of Assessment	Assessment Method	Normal Response
Superficial sensations		
Touch and pain	Pin and cotton testing of face, arms, legs, trunk	Perception and accurate identification of all stimuli; equal bilaterally; threshold may vary but touch, pain, temperature perceived on all body surfaces
Temperature	Random application of two test tubes—one filled with hot water the other with ice water	
Deep structure sensitivities		
Vibration	Vibrating tuning fork applied to bony prominence of feet and hands	Recognition of vibration and awareness of its cessation
Position sense	Digits on all 4 extremities passively extended and flexed	Detect movement of few millimeters and identify which digit is manipulated and the direction
Deep-pressure pain	Firm squeezing of Achilles tendon, thumb and first finger junction, trapezius, supraorbital notch	Tender to pressure as indicated by grimace, withdrawal, etc.
Stereognosis	Identify objects in the hand with eyes closed	Name object correctly
Graphesthesia	Numbers or letters traced on the skin	Identified as rapidly as when written on paper
Two-point discrimination	Touch with two points simultaneously	Differentiate between being touched with 1 or 2 points: fingers and toes 5 mm and shin 10 cm; distance between the two points distinguished
Extinction phenomenon	Two identical simultaneous stimuli (touch) applied bilaterally	Perception of both stimuli

points should be increased until the patient makes the discrimination. This distance is then recorded. If the shin is used, the examiner can use his fingers. The normal distance between which the two points are felt simultaneously varies depending on which part of the body is being tested. A general rule of thumb is that the trunk, arms, and legs do not have so fine a touch discrimination as do the hands and feet.

Since sensory abnormalities are related to disturbances in the nerve supply to the different parts of the body, some knowledge of peripheral and central pathways is indispensable in interpreting the abnormalities. Considering the sensory findings along with the patient's complaints, reflex changes, and motor weakness may make apparent a pattern that will enable localization of the defect. As previously mentioned, the objective of this chapter is merely to help the nurse examiner distinguish normal from abnormal findings. She needs other resources to enable her to localize lesions. The components of the sensory examination are summarized in Table 13-5.

SYMPTOMS ASSOCIATED WITH CENTRAL NERVOUS SYSTEM DISORDERS
Headache

Headache (cephalalgia) is one of the most common symptoms encountered in routine as well as neurologic examinations. In many cases the source of headache can be suspected from the patient's history. All types of pain of the head and face are described by patients as headache regardless of the cause. The pain may be from the teeth, sinuses, nose, throat, or temporomandibular joint. The guidelines that follow are primarily for chronic headaches, but they can be helpful in evaluating other types of head pain. Chronic headaches are primarily caused by vascular dilatation (migraine) and sustained tension of the muscles of the head and neck.

As a screening question, in a routine examination, it is best to ask the patient if he has severe or frequent headaches, not if he has headaches. Everyone has occasional, mild, short-lived headaches which are of little consequence. What is significant is the chronic recurring headache.

The first step is to learn from the patient how many types of headaches he has and then to obtain a general outline of the history of each headache in regard to onset, duration, progression of severity, frequency, location, extent, and its episodic or constant nature. This is followed by assessment of the following: possible relationships to the time of day, season, emotional status, or bodily positions; the nature of the pain, e.g. "throbbing," "bandlike," or "vise-like"; the presence of associated symptoms of nausea, vomiting, scotoma, aura (such as mood changes), effect on sleep, allergies, vertigo, lightheadedness, tinnitus, family history, emotional instability, and impaired memory. The muscles of the head and neck are palpated for the presence of tenseness.

If the reason for the examination is the complaint of headache, asking the person why he sought help for the headache at this particular time may bring out important recent changes in symptoms that the person has forgotten to mention in the barrage of questions. A willingness to let the patient talk about other aspects of himself, his lifestyle, and activities of daily living as well as his immediate symptoms might help in relating these to his symptoms and providing data for estimating the emotional and physical demands confronting him.

If the assessment of a headache is approached with a preconceived idea about the patient or the diagnosis, there may be subconscious rejection of symptoms that do not fit this diagnosis. The absence of organic findings does not rule out the presence of a health problem.

Pain   Pain of neurologic origin may originate from irritation of a peripheral nerve, a spinal nerve root, the thalamus, or a sensory tract. Mechanical compression or inflammation of a peripheral nerve or of a dorsal (spinal) nerve root irritates pain and other sensory fibers. The pain and paresthesia from these lesions are perceived by the patient as occurring along the anatomic distribution of the affected nerve. The area of skin supplied by one dorsal nerve root is a dermatome, and pain of a dermatome distribution is known as radicular pain. Charts depicting dermatomes such as that appearing in Figure 13-5 help in determining which dermatomes are involved. Charts of cutaneous fields of the principal peripheral nerves are used for lesions of peripheral nerves.

If the pain has a radicular distribution, it should be determined whether it is aggravated by coughing, sneezing, straining (as with defecation), or the straight leg raising test previously described.

Thalamic and sensory tract pain distribution depends on the level at which the pathway is affected. It can be over the whole side of the body or limited to large contiguous portions of the body.

The profile of the patient's pain includes many aspects—topographic, quantitative, temporal, qualitative, and the associated physiologic and behavioral and psychologic processes. The evaluation is much the same as for headache pain.

Meningeal Irritation   Meningeal irritation causes a stiff neck from the muscle contraction of the extensor muscles of the neck. The degree of irritation and defensive muscle spasm is determined with the patient in the recumbent position and the examiner passively flexing the neck so that the chin rests on the chest. Little resistance is met in the patient free of musculoskeletal defects and meningeal irritation. Marked resistance is encountered (nuchal rigidity) in meningeal irritation; at times, it may be so powerful that the back is arched (opisthotonos), and the patient can be raised off the bed like a board by lifting his head. Blood or bacteria in the cerebrospinal fluid can cause meningeal irritation.

Seizures   Brain cells that have sustained some type of injury, or have a constitutional predisposition for alterations in electrical activity, are capable of producing seizures. The repetitive dysrhythmic bursts of electrical activity from the brain cells may be localized to a specific area of the cerebral cortex or may spread to involve more cerebral and subcortical areas, manifested by loss of consciousness and generalized involvement of the whole body.

A generalized seizure often progresses in the following way: A premonitory sign or aura foretelling the advent of the impending seizure may occur seconds, minutes, or hours prior to the onset of the convulsion. The tonic phase of the convulsion begins with an audible involuntary cry, falling to the ground, loss of consciousness, stiffening of the body and extremities, and temporary cessation of respiration. The clonic phase is characterized by severe jerking movements of the extremities and labored respirations which may last for minutes. When a seizure is occurring, bed covering should be thrown off so that the patient's entire body can be observed for the extent of the involvement.

The tongue may be bitten, and urinary incontinence may occur. During the postictal period (time immediately following the seizure) the patient may be drowsy or confused and experience aphasia, temporary paralysis, headache, and fatigue. The period of time required to recover from the seizure is dependent on its severity, the areas of the brain involved, medications administered during the seizure, and the general physical condition of the patient.

To obtain an accurate and detailed history that will provide necessary information about the seizures, the examiner may need to question not only the patient, but also friends, relatives, and others who can provide firsthand observations. Because of the stigma surrounding convulsive disorders and the nature of the seizure itself, the patient may be hesitant to provide information or actually may not know the details of the seizure if he has been rendered unconscious at the onset.

In eliciting the characteristics of the convulsions, the examiner must not accept ambiguous words and phrases used by the patient and must obtain a precise interpretation and clarification of the meaning with him. In talking to the patient and significant others about his seizures it is helpful to use whatever terminology for the seizures the patient uses; it may not be understood, for example, that "convulsion" and "seizures" are synonymous.

The patient can be asked directly about the frequency of seizures, the time of day they occur, and precipitating factors. Note the date and time of the last seizure. Seizures frequently occur during the day, usually shortly after arising. About one-third of the patients have a convulsion during the night, frequently in the early hours of the morning. Some patients have seizures both day and night, in which case most occur during the daytime. Precipitating factors initiating seizures vary widely and may include sudden loud noises, music, flickering light, fatigue, worry, and premenstrual changes, to name just a few.

The presence of an aura and its characteristics should be determined. The time relationship of the aura to the initiation of the seizure should be known. The type of seizure may help to locate the epileptogenic focus in the brain. The aura may be a visual, auditory, gustatory, or olfactory hallucination.

When evaluating the patient's functional return during the postictal period, it is necessary to remember that any medications given him during the seizure may be influencing his recovery, that is, his level of consciousness and ability to move around.

Medications being taken for seizure control and the frequency and times of their administration are important for the examiner to ascertain. Asking the patient the name of each medication, its action, side effects, dosage, and time and method of administration provides background information on how well the patient understands his medications and adheres to the regimen prescribed.

Vertigo   The patient probably talks about being dizzy. Dizziness and vertigo are not synonymous. There are several types of dizziness; true vertigo is only one type of dizziness.

Vertigo is a condition in which the person is aware of an altered spatial relationship between his body and the surrounding environment. This may be manifested as a sensation that the environment is rotating around him, or that he is whirling around and the environment is stationary. Movements and positioning of arms and legs may also be somewhat unsteady. The patient with vertigo talks about being "dizzy," "spinning," or "the room spinning around him."

The onset of vertigo may be sudden and unrelated to movement, or it may be precipitated by a change of head position. Body movement and changes in the position of the head affect existing vertigo and may precipitate its occurrence. Such movements and positions and their effects should be identified. Flex and extend the head and rotate it in the horizontal plane.

The eyes should be checked for nystagmus during episodes of vertigo. The patient is questioned as to the occurrence of diaphoresis, nausea, and vomiting. To help differentiate labyrinthine dysfunction from brain center impairment, tinnitus and impaired hearing, if present, should be evaluated to determine whether they are unilateral or bilateral.

SUMMARY   Physical assessment of neuromuscular functioning can be extensive, too extensive for a complete assessment in all situations. The two general types of situations in which the nurse is involved in detecting alterations in neuromuscular functioning are screening and monitoring. The screening may be a general health assessment or a special assessment of neuromuscular functioning. Monitoring frequently involves an intracranial lesion or spinal cord lesion.

To help the nurse examiner determine pertinent components for appropriate efficient neuromuscular assessment in each situation, the key areas of assessment are identified in the cue cards.

NEUROMUSCULAR FUNCTIONING- ASSESSMENT GUIDE

	Screening		Monitoring	
	General Health Assessment Examination	Neuromuscular Screening Examination	Monitoring of Acute Intracranial Lesion	Monitoring of Acute Spinal Cord Lesion
Mental Status	General behavior Other areas if behavior or history arouses suspicion	General behavior Memory Intellect Other areas if responses or history arouse suspicion: Orientation Language Responsiveness	General behavior Orientation Responsiveness Memory and concentration Language	Dependent upon site of lesion and general behavior Other areas if associated intracranial lesion is possible Responsiveness Orientation
Cranial Nerves	Cranial nerves II to XII Not necessarily all modes of testing each nerve, e.g., omit taste	Cranial nerves I to XII	Initial exam: Cranial nerves I to XII Frequent periodic monitoring Pupillary reflex Corneal reflex Gag reflex Facial movements Fundoscopic	
Motor System	Gait General coordination and ease of movement Posture Muscle stretch reflexes Equilibrium Symmetry	Muscle bulk, tone, strength Joint function Posture Muscle stretch reflexes Coordination Equilibrium Involuntary movements Other areas if responses arouse suspicion: Superficial reflexes Pathological reflexes	Muscle stretch reflexes Babinski Muscle tone and strength Ulnar drift	Muscle tone and strength below lesion Muscle stretch reflexes below lesion Superficial reflexes Cremasteric Abdominal Anal
Sensory System	Head-to-toe survey of superficial and deep sensations Pain Touch Position sense Vibratory	Head-to-toe survey of Pain Touch Position sense Vibratory Other areas if responses arouse suspicion: Temperature Stereoginosis Graphesthesia Two point Extinction Map area if sensory deficits found	Head-to-toe survey of Deep and superficial pain	Identify sensory level and survey below for Touch Pain Vibration Position

	Screening		Monitoring
Other	Vital signs	Depending on level
	TPR	of lesion
	BP	Muscles of
	Airway patency	respirations
	Respiratory pattern	Bladder function
	Associated symptoms	
	Headache	
	Seizure	

REFERENCES

1. Alpers B. J., and Mancall, E. *Clinical Neurology* (6th ed.) Philadelphia: Davis, 1971.
2. De Myer, W. *Technique of the Neurologic Examination, a Programmed Text* (3rd ed.). New York: McGraw-Hill, 1979.
3. Judge, R. D., and Zuidema, G. D. (Eds.). *Methods of Clinical Examination: A Physiologic Approach* (3rd ed.). Boston: Little, Brown, 1974.
4. Van Allen, M. W. *Pictorial Manual of Neurologic Tests.* New York: McGraw-Hill, 1969. RC 348, V 22.

SUGGESTED READINGS

Alexander, M., et al. Neurological examination. Parts 17 and 18. *Nursing* 76:6, 1976.
Beetham, W. P. *Physical Examination of the Joints.* Philadelphia: Saunders, 1965.
Brain, W. R. *Brain's Clinical Neurology* (3rd ed.) (Rev. by Roger Bannister). New York: Oxford Medical Publications, 1969.
Daniels, L., et al. *Muscle Testing: Techniques of Manual Examination* (3rd ed.). Philadelphia: Saunders, 1972.
Debrunner, H. *Orthopedic Diagnosis.* Edinburgh: Livingstone, 1970.
De Jong, R. *The Neurologic Examination* (4th ed.). New York: Harper & Row, 1979.
Dodd, M. J. Assessing mental status. *Am. J. Nursing* 78:1501, 1978.
Mechner, F. Neurological Examination. *Am. J. Nursing.* Part 7, 75: P.I. 1, 1975; Part 8, 75: P.I. 1, 1975; Part 9, 76: P.I. 1, 1976.
Plum, F., and Posner, J. *Diagnosis of Stupor and Coma* (2nd. ed.). Philadelphia: Davis, 1972.
Renfrew, S. *An Introduction to Diagnostic Neurology* (vols. I and II). Edinburgh: Livingstone, 1964.
Salibi, B. Levels of consciousness in acute head injuries. *Wis. Med. J.* 62:375, 1963.
Walleck, C. Neurological assessment for nurses—A part of the nursing process. *J. Neurosurg. Nurs.* 10:13, 1978.
Weintraub, M. L. Hysteria: A clinical guide to diagnosis. *Clin. Symp.* 29:2, 1977.

III. Age Group Considerations in Physical Assessment

14. The Newborn

GLOSSARY

acrocyanosis Cyanosis of the hands and feet.

brown fat Mass of tissue in neck and scalp region of the newborn and capable of greater thermogenic activity than ordinary fat, especially in periods of cold stress; also called *interscapular gland.*

congenital choanal atresia Congenital obstruction between the posterior nares (choana) and the pharynx.

cretinism Condition produced by the complete absence of thyroid secretion from birth.

gestational age Number of completed weeks from the first day of the last menstrual period.

glabella Smooth depressed area between the two superciliary arches (point between the top of the bony orbit).

harlequin color change Vasomotor phenomenon of unknown origin and lasting only a few minutes in which, with infant on its side, the upper half is pale and the lower half is pink and red, with a clear line of demarcation; if the infant is turned, changes occur in 1 to 2 minutes. It appears more frequently in the immature.

hypospadias Anomalous position of the urethral meatus on the ventral portion of the glans penis, rather than in its center.

kernicterus Deposit of unconjugated and unbound bilirubin in brain cells, the most serious complication of neonatal hyperbilirubinemia.

Klippel-Feil syndrome Shortness of the neck resulting from reduction in the number of cervical vertebrae or fusion of their spinal processes

perinatal Period between 28 weeks gestation and 4 weeks after delivery.

supraorbital ridges Anterior limit of the frontal bone that forms the top of the orbit.

torticollis (wryneck) Spasmodic contraction of the neck muscles, drawing the head to one side with the chin pointing to the other side.

tracheoesophageal fistula (TEF) Congenital anomaly that usually takes one of three forms: (1) esophageal atresia with fistulous connection between the lower esophageal segment and the trachea; (2) esophageal atresia with normal respiratory tract; (3) normal esophagus and trachea connected by a fistula.

Turner's syndrome Retarded growth and sexual development associated with absence of one sex chromosome.

vascular rings Congenital anomalies of the aortic arch and its tributaries, forming a ring about the trachea and esophagus and causing various degrees of compression of these passages.

HISTORY

THE history of a newborn is that of past generations, especially of his parents. Since a newborn cannot be interviewed, past information is gained mainly from his medical record and from his mother. It is of utmost importance that this information be accurate. If any pertinent data appear invalid or missing, another source should be sought when possible.

There are four major areas to be considered in the history of this new person: the family history, mother's obstetric history, and prenatal and perinatal events. Positive and negative findings anywhere within this history may affect the outcome of this newborn's life.

Family History

The family history covers the same areas as in the adult. Therefore only a few of the most significant influences will be indicated here. A family history of diabetes, congenital heart disease, hypertensive cardiovascular disease, sickle cell anemia, thyroid disorders, renal disease, chromosomal defects, or heredi-tary central nervous system disorders may have profound consequences for the infant. The economic status, race, national origin, or height and weight of his parents may create special problems. The mother's general health, nutritional status, smoking, drinking, and drug habits, or marital status also influence the neonate's well-being [6].

Obstetric History The general obstetric history should include the number of pregnancies, the number and type of deliveries, length of labors, and size of the infants. The *high-risk areas* that should be investigated include: premature labor, pro-longed labor, fetal loss before and after 28 weeks, infertility, maternal age of less than 16 or more than 40 years, previous Rh sensitization, toxemia, bleeding during a pregnancy, multiple pregnancy, hydramnios, and obesity.

Prenatal Data The amount and quality of prenatal care and other specific prenatal conditions and events have a direct bearing on the health of the infant. Some of the facts that affect the outcome are: last menstrual period; first visit to the physician and number of visits; laboratory finding (e.g., blood type, VDRL*); vital signs (blood pressure, weight gain, fetal heart tones [FHT]); type of pelvis; drugs taken; illnesses exposed to or contracted during pregnancy (rubella, influenza, syphilis, streptococcal or staphylococcal infection, radiation); nutrition (good, poor, pica, starch). The *high-risk areas* are similar to those under Obstetric History, but include, in addition, hospitalization of the mother and special tests (e.g., amniocentesis, estriols).

Labor and Delivery Events during labor and delivery have a direct influence on the fetus. Basic information related to these events should always be readily available in a nur-sery area. These facts include the following:

1. How labor started (spontaneously, induced).
2. Length of labor (less than 3 hours, average, prolonged).
3. Length of time membranes were ruptured (less or more than 24 hours).
4. Color of amniotic fluid (clear, cloudy, meconium-stained).
5. Drugs taken during labor and how close to delivery.
6. Status of fetus during labor (FHT patterns, activity).
7. Presentation (cephalic, breech, transverse).
8. Anesthesia (general, local, pudendal, paracervical, caudal, spinal).
9. Type of delivery (normal spontaneous delivery [NSD], low forceps delivery [LFD], midforceps delivery [MFD], cesarean section).
10. Complications (toxemia, abruptio placentae, placenta praevia, shoulder dystocia, hemorrhage, pneumonia, nuchal cord, multiple birth, major anomaly or injury).

*Venereal Disease Research Laboratory blood test.

Table 14-1.
Apgar Score for Reactions
of the Newborn*

Score	0	1	2
Heart rate	Absent	100	100
Respiratory effect	Absent	Weak cry, hypoventilation	Good strong cry
Muscle tone	Limp	Some flexion of extremities	Well flexed
Reflex irritability (response of skin stimulation to feet)	No response	Some motion	Cry
Color	Blue or pale	Body pink, extremities blue	Completely pink

*The score is computed at 1 and 5 minutes after delivery by assigning a value (0, 1, or 2) for each aspect and totaling them. Thus a score of 0 indicates a moribund or dead infant; a score of 10 indicates optimum condition. (Adapted from Apgar, V., et al. Evaluation of the newborn infant—second report. *J.A.M.A.* 168: 1935, 1958. By permission of the authors and publisher.)

11. Resuscitation needed (time before first breath, oxygen, drugs, ear bulb, De Lee suction trap, laryngoscope).
12. Routine drugs (silver nitrate 1% in eyes, intramuscular vitamin K).
13. Number of vessels in cord (three is normal).
14. Elimination (time of first stool and voiding).
15. Apgar score (Table 14-1).

General Assessment at Birth

The major factors in success of adjustment of a newborn to extrauterine life are inherent vitality, his state of maturity, and the degree of any pathologic condition that interferes with normal events (Table 14-2). Before the infant leaves the delivery room, a gross assessment should be done. Choanal atresia should be ruled out by observing breathing while holding the infant's mouth closed. A catheter should never be routinely passed. Some authorities feel a stomach tube should be passed and the contents measured to rule out tracheoesophageal fistula and obstructions, and that this catheter should also be used to test for a patent anus. Certainly, the infant should be observed for any signs of distress or anomalies that require special care.

Table 14-2.
General Assessment at Birth

System or Anatomical Part	Observations	Significance
Gross Assessment Based on Major Concepts of Growth and Development		
Body proportions	Head to rump	1:4 is normal
	Crown rump	Equal to head circumference
	Head to chest	12½–31.1 cm.
	Head circumference	Baseline 13½ in. (34.3 cm.)

Table 14-2. Continued.	System or Anatomical Part	Observations	Significance
		Length	Baseline 18–21 in. (45.7–53.3 cm.)
	Estimate of gestational age	Charts	Term or immature
		Avery (Usher) Battaglia Dubowitz	Special care needed for preterm, small-for-dates, and postmature infants
	Sensory motor responses	Rooting and sucking	Needed for feeding; if absent: immature or brain damage
		Setting-sun sign	If positive: brain damage (Kernicterus)
			Absent or partial: immature or CNS damage
			Partial: paralysis, dislocation, fracture
		Tonic neck	No early significance
		Grasp	If negative: paralysis, fracture, or immature
		Deep tendon	Generalized response knee jerk, functional reflex arch
		Moro	If partial: paralysis, dislocation, fracture
			If absent or partial: immature or CNS damage
		Babinski	Positive is normal
		Dancing	Normal
		Blinking, yawning, sneezing, hiccupping	Protective
		Tactile sensations	
		Touch	Infant should respond
		Pressure	Infant should respond
		Temperature	Reaction greater to cold than to heat
		Pain	May indicate pathology
	Body temperature regulation	97°–99° (cool)	Stable, brown fat metabolism, acidosis, hypoglycemia, sepsis, increased mortality
	Physical Assessment		
	Head	Symmetry	Normal moulding
		Asymmetry	Excessive trauma
		Fontanelles	Microcephalas, hydrocephalas, dehydration
		Lacerations	Potential infection
		Caput succedaneum	Normal
		Cephalhematoma	Possible skull fracture, increased bleeding, possible jaundice later
	Face	Symmetry	Facial paralysis
		Contorted features	Distress, chromosomal or genetic disorders

Table 14-2. Continued.	System or Anatomical Part	Observations	Significance
	Eyes	Conjunctivitis	Silver nitrate reaction, infection
		Subconjunctival hemorrhage	Normal; due to labor/ delivery
		Pupil reaction to light	Absent or unequal: brain damage
		Cornea, anterior chamber	If not clear: cataract If steamy or enlarged: congenital glaucoma
		Retina	If hemorrhage present: severe trauma
	Nose	Breathing	Inability to nose breathe, difficulty in feeding: congenital choanal atresia
		Milia	Normal
		Saddle nose	Congenital syphilis
		Severe asymmetry	Fracture
	Mouth	Lips Sucking blister on lips	Normal
		Harelip	Congenital
		Gums	Pink, intact
		Tongue	If large: Down's syndrome, rhythmic protrusion: increased cranial pressure
		Frenulum linguae	Adequate depth
		Palate	Intact: normal cleft palate:
		Epstein's pearls	Normal
		Thrush	Fungus (C. albicans)
		Growths	Cysts, tumors
		Taste	Inability to refuse toxic substances
	Cries	Nature, pitch, intensity, frequency, effort	Normal: normal pitch, loudness varies Abnormal: high-pitched, shrill, shriek, hoarse, low intensity, sluggish, mewing of a cat, strong to weak intensity
	Ears	Normal shape	Normal
		Lack of cartilage	Immaturity
		Low placement	Renal anomalies, chromosomal disorders
		Preauricular fistullas or tubucles	Congenital
		Hearing	Difficult to test in newborns
	Neck	Short and weak	Normal
		Masses	Goiter, tumor
		Decreased mobility	Anomaly of vertebrae, Kleppel-Fiel syndrome
		Webbing	Turner's syndrome
		Masses on sternocleidomastoid muscle	Hematoma, congenital torticollis

Table 14-2. Continued.

System or Anatomical Part	Observations	Significance
Skin	Turgor and elasticity	Normal
	Acrocyanosis	Normal
	"Boiled lobster" look	Normal
	Milia, lanugo, erythema, toxicum, Mongolian spots, superficial Telangiectasia, vernix caseosa	Normal
	Generalized cyanosis	Cardiac or respiratory problem
	Ashen gray cyanosis	Septic shock
	Pallor	Blood loss, shock, erythroblastosis, hypoglycemia
	Jaundice	If present during first 36 hrs.: usually pathological (Rh, ABO, congenital defect, sepsis) After 36 hrs.: usually physiological (immature liver with RBC breakdown)
	Harlequin color change	Immaturity
	Patechiae	Normal: fast or long labor nucal cord Abnormal: clotting defect
	Rashes	Normal: toxic, erythema, heat, diaper Abnormal: pustular
	Dryness	Normal Abnormal, excessive: congenital syphillis postmature
	Edema	Normal: local Abnormal: local, dosa of head and feet: Turner's syndrome general: hydrops fetalis, respiratory distress syndrome, congestive heart failure
Back	Ribs, vertebrae	Anomalies palpable
	Tufts of hair along intact spinal column	Pathology beneath
	Open, vertebral body	Spina bifida, meningocele
	Masses	Cysts, tumors
	Deep coccygeal dimple	Dermoid cyst
Extremities	Excess or limited motion	Fractures, dislocations, local nerve damage, CNS damage
	Bowlegged, flat footed, cold extremities	Normal

	System or Anatomical Part	Observations	Significance
Table 14-2. Continued.			
		Abrasions	Activity
		Polydactyly (extra digits)	Possible bone involvement, X-ray may be necessary; increased incidence in Blacks
		Hip abduction	Dysplasia, dislocation
		Intact extremities	Possible congenital absence or abnormality
	Thorax	Cylindrical	Normal
		Symmetrical	Normal
		Hypertrophy of breasts	Normal
		Ribs flexible	Normal
		Xyphoid cartilage palpable	Normal
		Asymmetrical	Funnel chest, pigeon breasts
		"Knot" felt on clavicles	Fracture
	Respiration	Diaphragmatic, irregular, 30–60/ min.	Normal
		Excessive mucus	TEF
		Expiratory grunt, generalized cyanosis, flaring of nostrils, shallow respiration, sternal retraction, periods of apnea, Cheyne-Strokes breathing, tachypnea, rales	Respiratory distress
	Circulation	Methods: inspection, palpation, percussion, auscultation	
		Apical impulse displaced	Pneumothorax, diaphragmatic hernia, dextrocardia
		Cyanosis or pallor, tachycardia, enlarged heart (X-ray)	Heart disease
		Prominent brachial pulse with weak or absent femoral pulse	Coarctation of aorta
		Feeble or absent femoral pulses	Congenital heart disease
		Bounding pulses	Patent ductus arteriosis, aortic valve insufficiency
	Abdomen	Contour	Normal: cylindrical Abnormal: distention, local bulging, congenital

Table 14-2. Continued.	System or Anatomical Part	Observations	Significance
			absence of abdominal musculature, diaphragmatic hernia
		Umbilicus (cord)	Bleeding, infection, hernia
		Masses	Tumor, cyst
		Vomiting	Obstruction
		Anus	Abnormal: imperforate, absent
	Genitalia	Urine	Normal: productive by 24–48 hrs., clear, dilute, uric acid crystals
		Structures	Normal; Abnormal: sex ambiguity
		Female:	
		Gaping vulva	Normal
		Prominent labia majoria	
		Hymenal tag	
		Bloody mucus discharge	
		Vagina present one fingertip length between introitus and anus	
		Absence of vagina	Abnormal
		Male:	
		Penis and scrotum vary in size	Normal
		No circumcision or healing circumcision	
		Testes in scrotum	
		Hypospadias	Abnormal
		Hydrocele	
		Torsion of testis	

When the newborn's appraisal is done in the hospital, records are readily available. However, an appraisal may happen to be done in the home or elsewhere in the community, and in these situations, information sources may be nonexistent or limited to an interview with the parent or parents or to material from a public health agency referral.

CONDITIONS FOR EXAMINATION

After collection of the pertinent data in the history of a newborn, the physical assessment can take place. The assessor should be properly attired according to the nursery rules and should follow the accepted handwashing technique. All equipment used should be clean or sterile, and the examining room should be properly lighted and warm enough. A detailed examination should *not* be done on a newborn immediately after birth, when he is in distress, or immediately before or after a feeding. Proper precautions for safety would include having at least an ear bulb available, closing of safety pins, and never leaving or turning from the newborn while he is on an open surface. Needed equipment should be collected before starting (if not routinely in the crib) and should include the following:

1. Ear bulb
2. Stethoscope with small diaphragm
3. Penlight or ophthalmoscope and otoscope
4. Infant tongue blade
5. Tape measure
6. Bell (or appropriate substitute)
7. Pacifier or bottle of water
8. Finger cot or catheter

The examination of a newborn requires patience, gentleness, and flexibility in routines of procedure. First, observe the neonate undisturbed. Quickly note the infant's position, color, facial expression, breathing pattern, depth of sleep, and spontaneous activity. One should now note such gross characteristics as an enlarged head, prominent abdomen, or short extremities. If the infant is relaxed, you may wish to listen to the heart or palpate the abdomen first.

Parents may or may not be present during the examination. They should, however, always be kept informed about the findings, whether normal or abnormal. If the findings are questionable, the nurse may plan to re-examine the newborn at some later time or to consult with another colleague. If a more serious problem is suspected or apparent, medical consultation, referral, or both is mandatory. Follow-up public health nurse referral should also be considered. All findings warrant careful recording for use in making later comparisons. Finally, when the examination is completed, the newborn is replaced safely and comfortably in his crib.

MAJOR CONCEPTS OF GROWTH AND DEVELOPMENT
Body Proportions

The newborn's head-to-body proportion is 1 to 4. Several measurements should be made to rule out anomalies, to provide baseline data for future comparisons should complications arise, or to demonstrate normal growth. These measurements vary with the general size of the baby.

The head circumference average is 13½ in. (34.3 cm) and is measured by placing a metal, paper, or cloth tape firmly over the glabellar and supraorbital ridges anteriorly and, posteriorly, over the part of the occiput that gives the maximum circumference. The chest circumference averages about one inch less than the head (12½ in., 31.7 cm) and is measured at the level of the xiphoid cartilage or substernal notch in a plane at right angles to the vertebral column. The chest should be measured when the neonate is in a recumbent position and at mid-respiration. The neonate's length varies from 18 to 21 in. (45.7 to 53.3 cm). The easiest approach to measuring length is to have the infant supine. Lay the tape measure next to the baby. First measure crown to rump. This measurement is usually comparable to the circumference of the head. Then extend the neonate's leg and continue the measurement to the heel.

Estimate of Gestational Age

Since many menstrual histories are inaccurate, it is important to make an objective estimate of gestational age (Figs. 14-1 to 14-3). Some specific observations that aid in making this estimate are shown in Table 14-4 and Figures 14-1, 14-2, and 14-3. It should be noted that new research appears to show that sole creases may not be a good criterion for gestational age in the black neonate [4]. A scoring system for external criteria is cited by Dubowitz, Dubowitz, and Goldberg [5]. It includes skin texture, color and opacity, lanugo, edema, and labia majora development.

The absence of vernix caseosa means either a very immature infant or a postmature infant. The presence and completeness of reflexes also helps one judge the gestational age (see section on reflexes). The size of newborns is variable. However, size may be related to specific complications in the mother; for example, a large infant in a diabetic mother or a small infant (in relation to term) in a mother who has toxemia or is a smoker (Fig. 14-4).

It is important to remember that any position of posture that is not charac-

Figure 14-1. Intrauterine growth status by birth weight at various gestational ages. (From F. C. Battaglia and L. O. Lubchenco. *J. Pediat.* 71:159, 1967. By permission.)

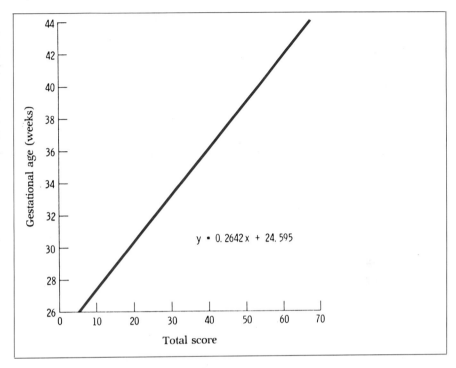

Figure 14-2. Gestational age based on total score derived from evaluation of neurologic signs and external characteristics. (From L. M. S. Dubowitz, V. Dubowitz, and C. D. Goldberg. *J. Pediat.* 77:1, 1970 [5]. By permission.)

$y = 0.2642x + 24.595$

teristic may be the result of an inherent problem, such as fracture, dislocation, nerve damage, narcosis, or asphyxia. A full range of motion can be observed as the newborn moves spontaneously during the assessment. Total flaccidity is considered abnormal and needs further investigation.

The concept of symmetry can be applied throughout the assessment where appropriate (e.g., to movements, reflexes, observations of the face and extremities).

Neuromuscular Development

Testing neurologic signs related to maturity encompasses another important series of observations, which are detailed in Table 14-3 and Figure 14-3.

SENSORIMOTOR RESPONSES

The neurologic examination of the newborn requires skilled observation. It should never be attempted when the infant is hungry or sound asleep. The quality of nervous system functioning is revealed by the neonate's activity, readiness of response to stimuli, spontaneous alertness, strength and character of cry, comparative use of all four extremities, vigor of feeding, and degree of postural muscle tone. You may observe some fine rapid tremors during the first few days after birth, especially on stimulation, but these usually disappear. Athetoid movements, coarse tremors even at rest, generalized stiffening, or opisthotonus are considered pathologic.

Figure 14-3.
Testing of neurologic signs
related to maturity guides
another important series of
observations. (From L. M.
S. Dubowitz, V. Dubowitz,
and C. D. Goldberg. *J.
Pediat.* 77:1, 1970 [5]. By
permission.)

Neuro- logical sign	SCORE					
	0	**1**	**2**	**3**	**4**	**5**
Posture						
Square window (wrist)	90°	60°	45°	30°	0°	
Ankle dorsi- flexion	90°	75°	45°	20°	0°	
Arm recoil	180°	90°- 180°	(90°			
Leg recoil	180°	90°- 180°	(90°			
Popliteal angle	180°	160°	130°	110°	90°	(90°
Heel to ear						
Scarf sign						
Head lag						
Ventral suspension						

Reflexes   Reflexes may be elicited all at one time, or, more ideally, in a head-to-toe sequence as the general assessment is completed. Specific reflexes to test for are:

1. *Rooting.* Stroke the cheek and lips, or place a finger right above the upper
lip. The infant should search for the finger.

2. *Sucking.* Place a nipple or clean finger into the baby's mouth, being sure to
touch the palate. The infant will suck. (If sucking is present, the swallow and
gag reflexes are also functional.)

3. *Ciliary.* Touch the eyelashes lightly while the infant is in a supine position.
He should close one or both eyes.

Table 14-3.
Some Notes on Techniques
of Assessment of Neurologic
Criteria*

Posture
Observed with infant quiet and in supine position. Score 0: Arms and legs extended; 1: Beginning of flexion of hips and knees, arms extended; 2: Stronger flexion of legs, arms extended; 3: Arms slightly flexed, legs flexed and abducted; 4: Full flexion of arms and legs.

Square Window
The hand is flexed on the forearm between the thumb and index finger of the examiner. Enough pressure is applied to get as full a flexion as possible, and the angle between the hypothenar eminence and the ventral aspect of the forearm is measured and graded according to diagram (see Fig. 14-3). (Care is taken not to rotate the infant's wrist while doing this maneuver.)

Ankle Dorsiflexion
The foot is dorsiflexed onto the anterior aspect of the leg, with the examiner's thumb on the sole of the foot and other fingers behind the leg. Enough pressure is applied to get as full flexion as possible, and the angle between the dorsum of the foot and the anterior aspect of the leg is measured.

Arm Recoil
With the infant in the supine position the forearms are first flexed for 5 seconds, then fully extended by pulling on the hands, and then released. The sign is fully positive if the arms return briskly to full flexion (Score 2). If the arms return to incomplete flexion or the response is sluggish it is graded as Score 1. If they remain extended or are only followed by random movements the score is 0.

Leg Recoil
With the infant supine, the hips and knees are fully flexed for 5 seconds, then extended by traction on the feet, and released. A maximal response is one of full flexion of the hips and knees (Score 2). A partial flexion scores 1, and minimal or no movement scores 0.

Popliteal Angle
With the infant supine and his pelvis flat on the examining couch, the thigh is held in the knee-chest position by the examiner's left index finger and thumb supporting the knee. The leg is then extended by gentle pressure from the examiner's right index finger behind the ankle and the popliteal angle is measured.

Heel To Ear Maneuver
With the baby supine, draw the baby's foot as near to the head as it will go without forcing it. Observe the distance between the foot and the head as well as the degree of extension at the knee. Grade according to diagram. Note that the knee is left free and may draw down alongside the abdomen.

Scarf Sign
With the baby supine, take the infant's hand and try to put it around the neck and as far posteriorly as possible around the opposite shoulder. Assist this maneuver by lifting the elbow across the body. See how far the elbow will go across and grade according to illustrations. Score 0: Elbow reaches opposite axillary line; 1: Elbow between midline and opposite axillary line; 2: Elbow reaches midline; 3: Elbow will not reach midline.

Head Lag
With the baby lying supine, grasp the hands (or the arms if a very small infant) and pull him slowly towards the sitting position. Observe the position of the head in relation to the trunk and grade accordingly. In a small infant the head may initially be supported by one hand. Score 0: Complete lag; 1: Partial head control; 2: Able to maintain head in line with body; 3: Brings head anterior to body.

Ventral Suspension
The infant is suspended in the prone position, with examiner's hand under the infant's chest (one hand in a small infant, two in a large infant): Observe the degree of extension of the back and the amount of flexion of the arms and legs. Also note the relation of the head to the trunk. Grade according to diagrams (see Fig. 14-3).

If score differs on the two sides, take the mean.

*From Dubowitz, L. M., Dubowitz, V., and Goldberg, C. Clinical assessment of gestational age in the newborn infant. *J. Pediat.* 77:1, 1970.

Table 14-4.
Estimation of Gestational Age*

Characteristic	Below 37 weeks	37 to 38 weeks	Above 38 weeks
Sole creases	Anterior transverse crease only	Occasional creases in anterior two-thirds	Sole covered with creases
Diameter of breast nodule	2 mm	4 mm	7 mm
Scalp hair	Fine and fuzzy	Fine and fuzzy	Coarse and silky
External ear	Pliable, no cartilage	Some cartilage	Stiffened with thick cartilage
Testes and scrotum	Testes in lower canal, scrotum small, few rugae	Intermediate	Testes pendulous, scrotum full, extensive rugae

*Adapted from Usher, R., McLean, F. and Scott, K. E. Judgment of fetal age. II. Clinical significance of gestational age and objective method for its assessment. *Pediatr. Clin. North Am.* 13:835, 1966; by Avery, Kraybill, and Mullick [2].

Figure 14-4.
Three babies of the same gestational age. Weights are 600, 1400, and 2750 gm respectively. (From S. Korones. *High-risk Newborn Infants* (2nd ed.). St. Louis: Mosby, 1976. By permission.)

4. *Doll's eyes.* Turn the infant's head from side to side. You should expect to see the eyeballs move in the opposite direction. (This reflex is difficult to test and disappears after 10 days of age.)

5. *Setting-sun sign.* If the trunk is raised and then quickly lowered to a supine position, the eyes slowly drift downward. You would *not* expect to see this sign except with cerebral damage (e.g., in kernicterus).

6. *Moro.* With the infant in a supine position, support the head and shoulders a few inches off the mattress. Then suddenly let the head drop. The reaction should be a symmetric extending then abducting of both the arms and legs with the fingers spread (embrace). The infant may or may not cry out. This should not be confused with a startle reflex or elicited by simple banging of the crib. Absence or asymmetry of this reflex is abnormal, and the possibility of fractures, a dislocation, paralysis, or central nervous system damage should be investigated. (However, be sure to repeat this reflex test at another time for verification.)

7. *Tonic neck.* The infant, when placed in a supine position, spontaneously assumes a "fencing position." As a demonstration of an immature nervous system, his head turns to one side with the arm and leg on that side extended. The opposite arm and leg are flexed. If the infant's head is passively turned, the reversal of extremity positions occurs. This reflex may normally be absent or incomplete, but if it is still present by the second or third year, this is pathologic.

8. *Grasp (palmar).* Place small objects (e.g., fingers) into the neonate's palms. He should hold on with enough force to be gently pulled to a sitting position. (Pressure on the balls of the feet elicits a grasping attempt with the toes.) The responses should be symmetric, with definite flexion tone in the arms.

9. *Deep tendon.* Gently tap the patellar tendon with your fingers. This reflex may be difficult to obtain or may create a more generalized response (i.e., whole leg jerks, both legs jerk). Mass responses are attributed to immaturity. (Only the knee jerk is important to test routinely in the neonate.)

10. *Babinski (plantar).* Stroke the lateral plantar surface (bottom of the foot on the side of the small toe), not the ball of the foot. The neonate should respond with an upward fanning of the toes (positive response). There is, however, no clinical significance to its presence or absence in early infancy, but it should disappear about the ninth month. Its presence thereafter is a sign of abnormality.

11. *Dancing.* If the infant is held upright with his feet touching a surface, he usually makes stepping or dancing movements.

12. Other normal reflexes are blinking, yawning, sneezing, and hiccups.

Table 14-5 Some Infant Reflexes	Reflex	Age Present (weeks)	Age When Disappears (month)
	Rooting	Good at 32	9
	Sucking	Strong at 34	9–12
	Moro	Complete at 28	2–3
	Tonic neck	? at 32	2–3
	Grasp	Solid at 32	6
	Dancing	Weak at 34	2–3

Table 14-5 serves as a helpful guide for added information about some of the reflexes.

Tactile Sensations   The skin sensations of touch, pressure, temperature, and pain are all present at birth or shortly afterward, The lips are hypersensitive, while the skin of the trunk, thigh, and forearms tends to be hyposensitive. Cold appears to elicit a more pronounced and prompter reaction than does a heat stimulus. During the first few days of a neonate's life he is only weakly sensitive to pain. However, the soles of the feet or the lips react much more positively to pain than do the body, hands, or feet. The presence or absence of pain should be observed for, not tested, during the assessment. Its presence may indicate a pathologic condition.

Temperature Regulation   The neonate's temperature regulation system is in poor equilibrium due to an immature hypothalamus. Heat loss is extreme and heat production low because of wetness in the delivery room, large body surface, inactivity during the first few days of life, and a low rate of metabolism. Heat is lost from the body surface by radiation, evaporation, convection, and conduction. The neonate does not appear capable of shivering or perspiring. If the environment is conducive to the neonate (70° to 75° F), his temperature usually stabilizes between 97° and 99° F, and his supply of brown fat is helpful in this process. The more immature the infant, the less stable his temperature. A cool environment is biochemically detrimental to the neonate and may result in metabolic acidosis, hypoglycemia, and increased mortality.

A rectal or axillary temperature may be taken as a part of the assessment, but the pattern of temperature recorded on a chart, if available, would probably be more helpful.

GENERAL ASSESSMENT Head   The head is examined for size (see Body Proportions), shape, symmetry, and character of the fontanelles. Any molding usually returns to its normal shape within a few days (Fig. 14-5). Soon after delivery the presentation or type of delivery may be evident from the molding: cephalic—sloping upward from the forehead; breech—flat top of head, cesarean section—round. The sutures may be felt to overlap.

Figure 14-5.
Molding. *A.* and *B.*
Molding immediately after
birth. Note overriding of
sutures which help the
head conform to the birth
canal. *C.* and *D.* return to
normal within the first
week. (Courtesy of Mead,
Johnson and Company.)

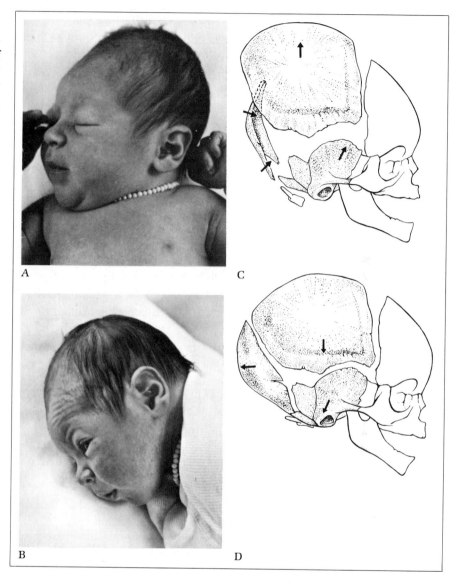

If there is any extreme displacement of the cranial bones, the examiner
should look for signs of intracranial hemorrhage. These signs are variable. Ap-
neic episodes and other signs of respiratory distress are common. The most
common neurologic signs are hypotonia, diminished spontaneous movement,
convulsions, coma, and lethargy. If the head is abnormally large or asymmetric, it should be transilluminated. Transillumination is performed as follows:
The neonate is taken to a completely dark room. A bright flashlight (fitted with
a rubber cuff) is held tightly against the infant's head, moving it to various
spots on the head. Normally, a faint halo of light, 1 to 2 cm wide, is seen in

the scalp just around the cuff. If the halo is large and irregular, or if light can be transmitted from one side of the head to the other, the diagnostic possibilities include hydranencephaly, severe hydrocephalus, or a large porencephalic cyst.

The anterior and posterior fontanelles should be palpated. When the examiner passes her fingers over the fontanelles, they should feel soft but not bulging or depressed. The anterior fontanelle should be *at least* as large as the tip of the little finger and is diamond-shaped and located between the parietal and frontal bones. The posterior fontanelle is located between the parietal and occipital bones, is triangular in shape, and may be almost closed at birth.

While inspecting the head, any lacerations, abrasions, or skin defects of the scalp should be noted. While palpating along the sagittal suture, especially the posterior portion of the parietal bones, it is possible on some infants to be able to indent the bone easily with light pressure. You will have the sensation of pressure on a ping-pong ball. The shape is resumed when the pressure is removed. This indicates the presence of craniotabes, which is probably due to mechanical factors, along with a generalized deficiency in calcium metabolism. It never occurs in breech presentations and is more common in nonwhite infants.

If the neonate is 24 hours old or less, he may have *caput succedaneum*, a local area of edema, congestion, and petechiae on the scalp (presenting part); this crosses suture lines. A *cephalhematoma*, which is a hematoma under the periosteum and usually over the parietal bone, does not cross suture lines. It tends to appear on the second or third day, to be firmer to the touch than an edematous area (like touching a water-filled balloon), and disappears over a period of weeks or months.

The amount of hair may be noted, but is of little consequence except to the mother. The hairline is low over the forehead, and lanugo may be present on the ears and shoulders.

Face   The face is small and round, and the lower jaw appears to recede. The face should be observed for symmetry (eye creases equal), and to see that the mouth remains on a level plane when the infant sucks or cries and that neither side of the face is motionless; if these are not observed, facial paralysis is suspected. Note the facial expression, which may indicate distress or serenity. Down's syndrome, as well as some other chromosomal and genetic disorders, may be identified by characteristic facial features.

Eyes   The neonate has almost no eyebrows, but may have long eyelashes. Eye color is usually blue or gray in the Caucasian baby, but may be darker in the nonwhite infant. The newborn has no protective blink. As a result of the instillation of silver nitrate 1 percent as a preventive against gonococcal conjunctivitis, the eyes may appear swollen (puffy) and red, with some purulent-appearing drainage. The drainage may be considerable, but it is important to differentiate an infection from this normal reaction. Tears are seldom seen before the thirteenth to sixteenth day of life.

Subconjunctival hemorrhages due to labor and delivery pressures are common and not significant. Pupils should react equally to light. Eye motion is generally random and lacking in coordination. The eyes of the neonate appear able to converge for short periods of time and are especially drawn to contours. If he is shown a black triangle on a white field, his eyes hover near the sides of the triangle, where the contrast between black and white is maximal. The infant may react to the examiner's eyes because of a like dark-light contrast. He probably has binocular vision and can see in color, seeing best at about 8 in (20 cm). If the eyes oscillate back and forth and rotate in a peculiar searching manner, the nurse should suspect partial or total blindness.

The following observations can be made with the naked eye, but are more satisfactorily made with an ophthalmoscope. The cornea and anterior chamber should be crystal-clear; otherwise, a cataract is suspected. If the cornea is enlarged or steamy in appearance, congenital glaucoma is suspected. Retinal hemorrhage may only be seen with an ophthalmoscope and is a sign of severe birth trauma. The neonate is not too cooperative in opening his eyes, and so patience is required. It may be helpful to place the baby in a supine position, raising his head slightly and shading his eyes from a bright light. Another maneuver that may work is to rock the whole body from an upright to a horizontal position several times.

Nose   The most pertinent observation related to the nasal passages is congenital choanal atresia (see the section on assessment at birth). Dried mucus or lint in the nose may cause sneezing, noisy breathing, or both. The nose may be flattened due to delivery. This corrects itself in a few days. Milia, small white nodules that are clogged sebaceous glands, are usually found over the surface of the nose and sometimes elsewhere on the face. A severely stuffy nose or saddle nose are indications of congenital syphilis.

The sense of smell is well developed in the newborn. Some reactions of the neonate when exposed to strong odors (e.g. ammonia, acetic acid) are crying, squirming, grimacing, sucking, and a changing respiratory rate. However, there is a wide range of individual differences in these reactions, as well as varying reactions in the same infant.

Mouth   The lips appear dry but pink. A harelip should be noted. By the end of the first week of life a sucking blister may start to develop. The mouth can be forcibly opened, but is best examined when the infant is crying. A tongue blade may be useful. The gums should appear a healthy pink; tooth buds should be visible. Rarely, erupted teeth are seen. If present, it is better to remove them to avoid trauma or aspiration, or both, since they are usually loose. There should be no cysts or tumors of the mouth. The tongue should not appear too large for the mouth. A continued rhythmic protrusion of a normal-sized tongue suggests increased intracranial pressure. The frenulum linguae should be of adequate length. The palate should be visualized and palpated with a clean finger or finger cot, to be sure it is intact. Epstein's (epithelial) pearls, small shiny whitish-yellow nodules, may be seen at the junction of the soft and hard palate. These should not be mistaken for thrush, which is a yeastlike fungus (*Candida albicans*) infection of white patchy exudate on the tongue, palate, and other mucous surfaces of the mouth and pharynx.

The newborn appears to have a more developed sense of taste than of sight or hearing. He reacts to a sweet taste with contented sucking. If offered fluid with a salty, sour, or bitter taste, his reactions are mainly negative, that is, he appears to show discomfort. However, the newborn probably would not refuse harmful fluids because of the taste, and so care that nothing toxic is given to the infant is essential.

Infant Cries   The neonate usually cries spontaneously during the examination. If not, he may be stimulated to cry by slapping the bottom of his foot. Crying is the beginning of vocalization. When a neonate cries, he holds his head in the midline position, and there is mass activity. The cry should be observed for its nature, pitch, intensity, frequency, and effort.* Listening carefully, the nurse can distinguish a normal from an abnormal cry.

Normal Cries

The normal cry has a normal pitch; loudness varies with breathing and can increase when the baby wants it to do so. A normal cry of discomfort at first is monotonous in pitch, staccato-like, and intermittent. It will increase in its incessantness. A cry of pain rises in pitch. A cry of rage is longer, the breath is held, and the face often becomes purplish. Gasping sounds usually accompany the rage cry.

Abnormal Cries

A cry indicating illness goes from strong to weak. The cry in central nervous system damage is a high-pitched, shrill shriek. A normal but extra sound at the end of a cry or a hoarse, high-pitched inspiratory crow indicates a laryngeal problem. The cry in creatinism is hoarse, not loud or frequent, of low intensity, and sluggish. The cri-du-chat cry, like the mewing of a cat, is indicative of a chromosomal abnormality. The infant whose mother is drug-addicted has a high-pitched cry.

*Feingold, M. *Baby Cries: The Differential Diagnosis* (audio production tape). Medcom, Inc., New York, N.Y.

Ears   The ears may temporarily be misshapen by intrauterine positioning, but rapidly assume their normal configuration. In the full-term infant, cartilage formation gives firmness and support to the structure. If the ears are placed low or if some malformation is present, renal anomalies or chromosomal disorders should be suspected. Preauricular fistulas or tubercles may be present. Visualization of the canal and drum may be difficult because of the angle of the canal and the presence of vernix caseosa. However, an attempt to examine the canal and drum with an otoscope should be made to rule out infection and anomalies.

Hearing is possible for the neonate after the eustachian tubes become aerated, which occurs about 24 hours after birth. If a bell is rung or an electric device sounded, the infant may react by cessation of activity, increased movement of the body, limbs, or eyes, and blinking [8]. However, deafness cannot be diagnosed with certainty in the newborn.

Neck   The neck is short and weak (see the section on neuromuscular development). Because of this, skin folds are deep and moist and a common site of pustules. The neck should be inspected and palpated for masses or a goiter. Although an immature infant's head can be rotated so that the chin goes well beyond the acromial tip, the normal newborn's chin stops at the acromial tip. Abnormally decreased mobility of the neck may occur if there is an anomaly of the vertebrae (e.g., Klippel-Feil syndrome). Webbing of the neck is a feature of Turner's syndrome. Congenital torticollis may be due to a maldevelopment or to hematoma of the sternocleidomastoid muscle. It is most commonly seen in breech or difficult cephalic deliveries. Diagnosis is seldom possible in the newborn period. A firm, circumscribed noninflamed or discolored mass felt on the sternocleidomastoid muscle of an infant at about two weeks of age would be a hematoma.

Skin   The skin should be inspected in its entirety. There is a loose attachment of the epidermis to the underlying dermis. Turgor and elasticity are to be expected. Depression of the fontanelles may be one sign of dehydration.

At birth the skin is a purplish red, and acrocyanosis is present. Within hours, only the palms and soles still appear cyanotic. To differentiate poor peripheral circulation from true cyanosis, vigorously rub the palm or sole. Normally, it quickly turns pink. Generalized cyanosis is abnormal (see Chaps. 9 and 10). An ashen-gray cyanosis may indicate septic shock. Within 24 hours, some babies have a "boiled-lobster" look. This very red appearance is a normal reflection of a high hematocrit and thin subcutaneous fat layers. Pallor may indicate blood loss, erythroblastosis, or cutaneous vasoconstriction (shock, heart failure), and the medical staff should be alerted.

Jaundice that appears during the first 24 hours is abnormal and usually indicates hemolysis or sepsis. If physiologic jaundice, which appears after 24 to 36 hours, is severe, further investigation is also indicated (i.e., bilirubin level). Jaundice can best be observed in daylight. Press your finger against the infant's nose or abdomen. On release, the skin appears yellow, not white, if jaundice is present. On nonwhite babies' skin, jaundice can be more easily detected by observing the color of the palate and sclera.

Pigmentation is variable and usually dependent on racial origin. Mongolian spots, which are blue or blue-black spots of varying size, are found especially in the sacral area. The majority are in Oriental or black infants but, rarely, may appear in the Caucasian infant also. In the black infant, pigmentation is most prominent in the nail beds and genitalia. Generally, these babies may not reach their regular pigmentation for several weeks. A harlequin color change may be observed but is more apt to occur in an immature infant.

The newborn has many skin "markings" that are normal but peculiar to him. These are as follows:

1. *Milia* (clogged sebaceous glands) are usually present on the nose and maybe the cheeks for several weeks and appear as "whiteheads" (Fig. 14-6).
2. *Lanugo* is fine downy hair found on the forehead, ears, and shoulders. Although it is more noticeable in the premature, it is not necessarily a sign of prematurity.
3. *Erythema toxicum* is a transient maculopapular rash which appears to be

Figure 14-6. Milia. (Courtesy of Mead, Johnson and Company.)

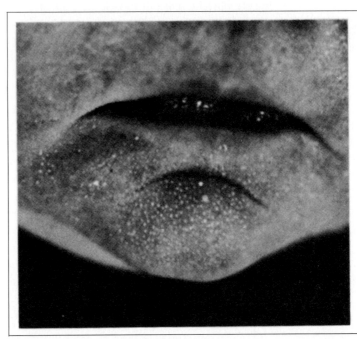

urticarial with a blanched, wheal-like appearance. At times, the center has vesicles of clear fluid which should not be mistaken for impetigo, which is purulent (Fig. 14-7).

4. *Petechiae* may be found and usually relate to a long labor or rapid delivery. They may indicate intrauterine infection or thrombocytopenia. (Any increase in bruising should be noted.) Generally, a routine injection of vitamin K helps to control any bleeding tendency of the young neonate before the coagulation processes become established on about the fifth day.)

5. *Superficial telangiectasia*, reddened, vascular unraised areas, are found in the nape of the neck (stork bites), or on the upper eyelids or upper lip (flame nevi). These disappear within the first year and should be differentiated from larger, bright red or dark purple, often elevated hemangiomas which often persist. (Examples of these are the port-wine stain and strawberry and cavernous hemangiomas.)

Vernix caseosa, the whitish, cheesy, greasy protective material found on the skin at birth, is eventually absorbed, but may still be seen after several days in skin folds, especially the labia. A yellow discoloration of the vernix is abnor-

Figure 14-7.
Erythema toxicum.
(Courtesy of Mead, Johnson and Company.)

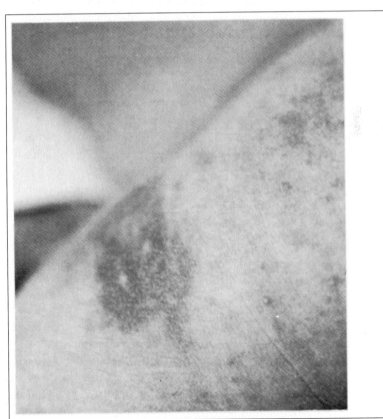

mal, and some fetal pathologic process can be assumed (e.g., erythroblastosis, anoxia, postmaturity). The skin usually becomes dry in the first weeks, but the dryness is more extreme in the postmature neonate or one who was malnourished in utero. These infants need to be watched for signs of hypoglycemia (low blood sugar), manifested by apnea, cyanosis, rapid and irregular respirations, tachypnea, jitters, tremors, twitches, lethargy, convulsions, coma, abrupt pallor, upward rolling of the eyes, sweating, weak cry, and refusal to eat. Extensive desquamation of the palms and soles, together with radiation fissures around the mouth, pustular rash, and nasal discharge, is an early sign of congenital syphilis.

Localized edematous areas (e.g., caput succedaneum) are normal. Generalized edema is abnormal and might indicate hydrops fetalis, hyaline membrane disease, or congestive heart failure. Localized edema of the dorsa of the hands and feet may be the only clue to Turner's syndrome during the newborn period.

Back   Turn the neonate on his abdomen and inspect the back. The ribs and vertebrae can easily be palpated for anomalies. Large openings in the vertebral body cause herniation of the contents of the canal. These are cystic masses and must be differentiated from a more solid tumor. Look for tufts of hair along an intact spinal column; these may indicate a pathologic condition beneath. Inspect a deep coccygeal dimple for a dermal sinus with perhaps a dermoid cyst at the end of the sinus.

Extremities   With the neonate lying on his back, evaluate all four extremities for gross deformities and activity. Observe and test the range of motion at all joints (see Reflexes). Intrauterine positions may influence the "position of comfort" assumed, but should be distinguished from a pathologic condition. The lower extremities in a breech presentation may take several weeks to assume a normal position. Injury to the brachial plexus causes the arm to assume a characteristic position of extension, adduction, internal rotation, and pronation. All newborns are bowlegged, flat-footed, and have cold extremities. The active infant may have abrasions on his knees, ankles, or toes.

Polydactyly (extra digits) should be checked for on both the hands and the feet. Polydactyly, especially of the hands, is relatively common in the black population. It should be established by x-ray examination if there is bone involvement. The presence or absence of webbing should also be determined.

It is important to find a dysplasia of the hip or a dislocated hip as early as possible. With the baby still on his back, flex his thighs, one at a time, outward and downward to the table or mattress. If one thigh does not easily abduct, suspect the diagnosis. Also listen for a consistent sharp click heard on the affected side during abduction and high or extra creases in the affected thigh. Dysplasia may be diagnosed by Ortolini's sign, as follows: Active attempts are made to subluxate the femoral head in and out of the acetabulum by a firm anteroposterior pushing and pulling with the pelvis fixed with the other hand. If dysplasia is present, one can feel and often see the head slipping in and out of the acetabulum, and triple diapering should be used to keep the hips in a partially flexed and abducted position.

Thorax   The thorax is cylindrical, having equal anteroposterior and lateral diameters (see Body Proportions). Hypertrophy of the breasts may be present in both females and males as a result of estrogen from the mother crossing the placenta. Signs of inflammation should not be present. Supernumerary nipples may be present. The ribs are flexible. The xyphoid cartilage may be felt and often can be seen below the sternum in the epigastrium. The fingers should be passed over the clavicles to rule out the most commonly seen fracture in the newborn; it feels like a "knot," but may not be felt until the third or fourth day of life. One should also observe for evidence of pain on pressure, asymmetry of angulation, and a complete Moro reflex (see Reflexes). Common congenital deformities of the chest include: (1) funnel chest, in which the lower portion of the sternum is depressed and (2) pigeon breast, in which the sternum, together with the costal cartilages, is prominent, and the lateral walls of the thorax are correspondingly depressed.

Respiration   The respiratory pattern should be observed before the infant is disturbed. In the normal neonate, respiratory movements are predominantly diaphragmatic. The abdomen rises and falls with inspiration and expiration, while the thoracic cage remains relatively immobile. If intercostal muscles are being used to any extent, a pathologic condition should be suspected. Normal breathing rate varies between 30 and 60 respirations per minute, but tends to be more rapid during the first hours after birth and with activity. The normal respiratory pattern varies considerably. Irregular, shallow respirations, short periods of apnea, breathing of the Cheyne-Stokes type, followed by several deep breaths, are all common in the neonate. Transient tachypnea may normally occur, especially in an infant born by cesarean section or in a breech presentation. If tachypnea (over 60 respirations per minute) is at a sustained rate, it is abnormal.

Other signs of distress include generalized cyanosis, respiratory grunt, retractions of the chest on inspiration and flaring of the nostrils on inspiration. Inability to handle mucus can cause a problem to the neonate, especially in his "second period of reactivity" after birth [1].

Gentle percussion gives a resonant note over the lung fields. If done heavily, data are inaccurate. It is difficult, especially for the inexperienced, to learn much about the lungs by percussion. Although the lungs and heart should be examined simultaneously, they are discussed in separate sections for clarity of understanding.

Proper stethoscope technique is vital if accurate data are to be obtained (see

Chaps. 9 and 10.) For example, rapid respirations may produce a sound which on auscultation may be confused with a heart murmur. An adult-size diaphragm is not ideal for auscultation because it covers too large an area of the baby's chest wall and fails to conform to the curvature of his chest.

Auscultatory signs in the lungs are of less value in the neonate than in other pediatric age groups. . . . Diminished breath sounds occur in hyaline membrane disease, atelectasis, emphysema. . . . Fine rales are produced in terminal bronchioles and alveoli by the rush of air through fluid within them. These rales are classically described as crackling in character. . . . Rales are heard in some infants with hyaline membrane disease, pneumonia, pulmonary edema and occasionally in normal babies immediately after birth. They are sometimes audible only after deep inspiration, which must be induced by stimulating a cry [6].

If labored breathing is noted, it may be due to abnormalities of the respiratory system or other systems of the body. Choanal atresia, anomalies of the epiglottis and larynx, or vascular rings should be suspected if there are signs of upper airway obstruction.

Circulation The methods used in examining the cardiovascular system of the newborn are observation, palpation, percussion, and auscultation (see Chap. 10 for techniques).

Inspection
Inspect the chest wall at about the fifth intercostal space in the midclavicular line for local pulsations on the chest wall. Pulsations are more prominent in small babies. If pulsations are prominent in the epigastrium, the heart is probably considerably enlarged.

Palpation
To identify the normal apical impulse, feel at the fifth intercostal space. Detection of an abnormal heart position early in the examination is an important initial step in establishing a correct diagnosis and of particular importance with a dyspneic infant. In *pneumothorax*, the apical impulse moves away from the affected side owing to the shift of the mediostinum. In *diaphragmatic hernia*, the apical impulse is displaced to one side of the chest. In *dextrocardia*, the apical impulse is in the right chest. (Compare the right and left chest.)

Percussion
The size and configuration of the heart may be judged by percussion, but in the neonate they are difficult to estimate by this method.

Auscultation
Auscultation is the most informative component of the physical examination of the heart when done by a skilled nurse practitioner. In the neonate the first and second heart sounds resemble the syllables "toc-tic" and are normally well

defined and clear. The second sound is somewhat sharper and higher-pitched than the first. Murmur at birth does not necessarily mean heart disease. It may be a late-closing ductus arteriosus. Only after several weeks will a murmur assume its normal intensity. Therefore only the ones that persist and increase in intensity are most likely to be significant. If present, these require medical follow-up, together with x-ray examination of the chest and an electrocardiogram. Localization of a murmur in the newborn may be difficult. Most murmurs are systolic and occur after the first sound and at or before the second sound. Continuous murmurs extend beyond the second sound into diastole. Arrhythmias are most often observed during deep sleep. The nurse needs considerable practice with the stethoscope to make accurate observations [7].

The heart rate of a newborn varies with crying, activity, sleeping, and feeding. However, a persistent rate below 100 or above 180 beats per minute is abnormal and should be investigated.

An instinctive feeling that "something is not quite right about the baby" may be a first indication of a problem, causing the nurse to reassess certain areas.

Cyanosis or pallor are often the first signs of heart disease. If cyanosis increases with crying, this is much more suggestive of heart disease than of a respiratory problem, which crying usually helps. Other signs of heart disease may include tachypnea, failure to feed well, breathlessness during or after feeding, irritability, tachycardia (gallop rhythm), edema of the face and feet, enlarged heart (cardiomegaly on x-ray examination), hepatomegaly (liver more than 3 cm below the right costal margin), abnormal electrocardiogram, and abrupt and unexpected weight gain of several ounces.

Peripheral pulses should always be examined by simultaneously palpating the brachial and femoral pulses. A strikingly prominent brachial pulse, coupled with a weak or absent femoral pulse, suggests coarctation of the aorta. In congestive heart failure the femoral pulses are feeble or absent; infants with patient ductus arteriosus or aortic valve insufficiency have bounding pulses [3].

Taking the blood pressure is usually not considered routine in examination of the newborn. However, if any condition that might affect the blood pressure is suspected, pressure should be taken in both an arm and a leg. The cuff should cover two-thirds of the upper arm or leg. The method used may be the ausculation, palpation, or the flush method. The neonate's pulse may be difficult to palpate. In the flush method:

Apply but do not inflate the cuff. Elevate the extremity and massage to produce blanching. Then raise the cuff pressure to above the expected systolic pressure. Lower the extremity to heart level and slowly lower the pressure in the cuff. The point at which a flush appears in the limb is the approximate systolic pressure. (Normal is 60 mm Hg at birth and 80 mm Hg after one week [2].)

Abdomen The contour of the abdomen is noted first. Ordinarily it is cylindrical and slightly protuberant. Some gross abnormalities such as distention, localized bulging, or congenital absence of abdominal musculature are apparent on inspection alone. The umbilicus is routinely inspected for the healing of the cord. A scaphoid or turnip-shaped abdomen is suggestive of a diaphragmatic hernia and requires immediate surgery.

Percussion may help localize masses in the abdomen and may demonstrate gaseous distention of the bowel. Palpation should be gentle (only one to two fingers may be required in a premature). The best findings are obtained when the infant is quiet and relaxed. The following may be palpated:

1. Xiphoid process—prominent.
2. Liver—2 cm below costal margin.
3. Spleen—usually not felt, but the tip at the costal margin may be felt.
4. Kidneys—found deep at the lower poles (larger flank masses: hydronephrosis, Wilms' tumor, neuroblastoma).
5. Umbilical or inguinal hernia.
6. Bladder—distention: pressure on pubic area may force male to urinate so that you can observe for a forceful stream.

Other points of importance to note are vomiting, excessive mucus (TEF), eating habits, first stool by 24 hours after birth, and normal color, consistency, and odor of stools. A rectal examination is done with the little finger (or catheter) to rule out imperforate anus and pelvic masses.

Genitalia   It is important to recognize ambiguity of sex in the genitalia so that a mistaken gender is not assigned. The neonate should void within 48 hours of birth. Uric acid crystals may normally be found in the neonate's urine and appear as a dusty red, clay-colored stain on the diaper. It should not be mistaken for hematuria. Normally, the urine is not concentrated, cloudy, or hematuric. In a breech presentation, the genitalia may be bruised and edemateous for several days after birth. The following are observations to be made:

Female.   Gaping vulva; labia minora more prominent than labia majoria; clitoris varies in size; hymenal tag; clear milky and bloody vaginal discharge; one fingertip length between anus and introitus (question ambiguity of sex if not present).

Male.   Penis and scrotum vary in size; prepuce covers entire glans of penis; testis is in the scrotum or can be induced there; forceful urinary stream; healing of circumcison if performed. Watch for hypospadias, hydrocele (transilluminates well), and torsion of testes (firm, swollen, discolored).

THE NEWBORN-ASSESSMENT GUIDE

A. History - family, obstetric, prenatal, labor/delivery.
B. General Appraisal at Birth - Apgar score, estimate of gestational age, vitality.
C. Physical Examination

1. Body proportions: head to rump, crown rump, head to chest, head circumference, length.
2. Head: symmetry, fontanelles, lacerations, caput succedaneum, cephalhematoma.
3. Face: symmetry, features.
4. Eyes: conjunctivities, subconjunctival hemorrhage, pupil reaction to light, cornea and anterior chamber, cornea, retina (with ophthalmoscope).
5. Nose: nose breathing, milia, saddle nose, asymmetry.
6. Mouth: lips, gums tongue, frenulum linguae, palate, Epstein's pearls, thrush, growths, taste.
7. Cries: nature, pitch, intensity, frequency, effort.
8. Ears: shape, cartilage, low placement, preauricular fistulas or tubucles, hearing.
9. Neck: short and weak, masses, decreased mobility, webbing, mass on sternocleidomastoid muscle.
10. Skin: turgor and elasticity, acrocyanosis, generalized cyanosis, "boiled lobster" look, pallor, jaundice, Harlequin color change, milia, erythema toxicum, Mongolian spots, superficial Telangiectasia, vernix caseosa, petechiae, rashes, dryness, edema.
11. Back: ribs and vertebrae, tufts of hair along intact spinal column, open vertebral body, masses, deep coccygeal dimple.
12. Extremities: motion, bowlegged, flat footed, cold extremities, abrasions, polydactyly (extra digits), hip abduction, intact extremities.
13. Thorax: cylindrical, symmetrical, asymmetrical, hypertrophy of breasts, ribs flexible, xyphoid cartilage palpable, "knot" felt on clavicles.
14. Respiration: diaphragm, irregular (30-60/min), excessive mucus, exspiratory grunt, generalize cyanosis, flaring of nostrils, shallow respiration, sternal retraction, periods of apnea, Cheyne-Strokes breathing, tachypnea, rales.
15. Circulation: apical impulse displaced, cyanosis or pallor, tachycardia, enlarged heart (x-ray), prominent brachial pulse with weak or absent femoral pulse, feeble or absent femoral pulses, bounding pulses.
16. Abdomen: contour, umbilicus (cord), masses, vomiting, anus.
17. Genitalia: urine, structures.

REFERENCES

1. Arnold, H., et al. The Newborn: Transition to extrauterine life. *Am. J. Nurs.* 65:77, 1965.
2. Avery, G., Kraybill, E., and Mullick, U. Examination of the newborn infant. *G. P.*36:78, 1968.
3. Black, J. A. *Neonatal Emergencies—and Other Problems.* New York: Appleton-Century-Crofts, 1972.
4. Damoulaki-Sfakianaki, E., Robertson, A., and Cordero, L. Skin creases on the sole of the foot as a physical index of maturity: Comparison between Caucasian and Negro infants. *Pediatrics* 50:483, September, 1972.
5. Dubowitz, L. M. S., Dubowitz, V., and Goldberg, C. Clinical assessment of gestational age. *J. Pediatr.* 77:1, 1970.
6. Korones, S. B. *High-risk newborn infants. The Basis for Intensive Nursing Care* (2nd ed.). St. Louis: Mosby, 1976.
7. Nadas, A., and Fyler, D. *Pediatric Cardiology* (3rd ed.). Philadelphia: Saunders, 1969.
8. Shimek, M. L. Screening newborns for hearing loss. *Nurs. Outlook* 19:115, 1971.

SUGGESTED READINGS

Clark, A., and Affonso, D. *Childbearing: A Nursing Perspective* (2nd ed.). Philadelphia: Davis, 1979.
Clausen, J., Flook, M., and Ford, B. *Maternity Nursing Today* (2nd ed.). New York: McGraw-Hill, 1977.
Cochran, W. Guide to visual diagnosis in the newborn. *Hosp. Med.* 8:38, 1972.

Harding, P. G. R. The metabolism of brown and white adipose tissue in the fetus and newborn. *Clin. Obstet. Gynecol.* 14:685, 1971.

Hodgemen, J. E. Clinical evaluation of the newborn infant. *Hosp. Pract.* 4:70, 1969.

Hott, K. S. Neurological examination of the newborn. *Hosp. Med.* 8:86, 1972.

Kelley, V. (Ed.). *Brennemann's Practice of Pediatrics* (vol 1, part 2). Maryland: Prior, 1972. Chaps. 80 and 83.

Miller, M., and Brooten, D. *The Childbearing Family: A Nursing Perspective.* Boston: Little, Brown, 1977.

Moore, M. L. *The Newborn and the Nurse.* Philadelphia: Saunders, 1972.

Moore, M. L. *Realities in Childbearing.* Philadelphia: Saunders, 1978.

Nelson, W., Vaughan, V., McKay, R., and Behrman, R. *Textbook of Pediatrics* (11th ed.). Philadelphia: Saunders, 1979.

Parmelee, A. H. *Management of the Newborn* (2nd ed.). Chicago: Year Book, 1959.

Reader, S., Mastroianni, L., Martin, L., and Fitzpatrick, E. *Maternity Nursing* (13th ed.). Philadelphia: Lippincott, 1976.

Roach, L. Color changes in dark skins. *Nursing '72* 2:19, 1972.

Smart, M., and Smart, R. *Infants: Development and Relationships* (2nd ed.). New York: Macmillan, 1978.

Waechter, E., and Blake, F. *Nursing Care of Children* (9th ed.). Philadelphia: Lippincott, 1976.

Suzanne Brunner
Barbara A. Sachs

15. Infancy, Childhood, and Adolescence

GLOSSARY

Brushfield's spots Scattered white flecks found around the circumference of the iris, usually indicative of Down's syndrome.

bruxism Grinding of teeth.

clubbing Rounding of the fingernails or toenails, progressing to thickening and shininess of the terminal phalanx.

croup Acute obstruction of the larynx caused by allergy, foreign body, infection, or new growth and characterized by resonant barking cough, hoarseness, and persistent stridor.

cryptorchidism Failure of one or both testes to descend into the scrotum.

cyanosis Bluish discoloration of specific surfaces of the body due to inadequate oxygenation of the blood.

dentition Process that moves the tooth from its developmental position into the oral cavity in occlusion with its antagonist; tooth eruption.

development Maturation of systems, acquisition of skills, adaptability, responsibility, and creative expression.

dyspnea Deep, labored, difficult respirations.

encopresis Incontinence of feces in a child who has achieved bowel control previously, not caused by organic defect or physical illness.

fusion Development of binocular vision by cerebral combination of the two retinal images to produce a single image.

hydrocele Scrotal cystic mass filled with clear fluid.

hypoxia Inadequate amount of oxygen.

macule Discolored spot on the skin that is not elevated above the surface.

nodule Small, solid node that can be palpated.

papule Small, circumscribed solid elevation of the skin.

paradoxical respirations Respirations in which a lung or portion of a lung is deflated during inspiration and inflated during expiration.

pustule Small elevation of epidermis filled with purulent fluid.

regurgitation Nonforceful expulsion of small quantities of food or liquid.

rumination Voluntary or habitual regurgitation of previously swallowed food.

squatting Bending of the knees so that the buttocks are close to or rest on the heels.

strabismus Tendency of the eye to deviate due to poor muscle control.

stuttering Speech disorder in which rhythm and continuity of diction is broken by spasms of muscles used in speech mechanism.

vesicle Small, cystlike circumscribed elevation of the epidermis containing fluid.

vomiting Forceful expulsion of gastric contents accompanied by contractions of the abdominal muscles.

wheal Edematous, short-lived elevated area on the skin which can vary greatly in size.

We approach all problems of children with affection. Theirs is the province of joy and good humor. They are the most wholesome part of the race, for they are the freshest from the hands of God.

Charles Stewart Mott
C. S. Mott Children's Hospital Plaque
Ann Arbor, Michigan

T HE purpose of this chapter is to present the important considerations of physical assessment in the child. As the child's cognitive, psychologic, and social development is a significant indicator of physical well-being, a brief overview of these areas is provided for each age group. It is not possible to include a complete survey of all the components of child development that need to be assessed. The reader is referred to comprehensive child health references for further assistance in understanding the many indices of health in children.

GENERAL CONSIDERATIONS

Child health care is, to a large extent, aimed at promoting the health of the child and preventing illness and disability through early identification of problems.

The examination of the child is ideally carried out over an extended period of time in a planned sequential pattern. The dynamic changes that occur in the normal growth and development of the child require the practitioner to carefully assess the increments in growth; the changes in physiologic function; and the development of cognitive, social, and motor skills of the child during each examination.

It is by comparing the individual child's current growth achievements and parameters of health with those found in previous examinations and by comparing the child with other normal healthy children that the health of the child is determined. The child should be seen more frequently during infancy, when the growth changes are most rapid and dramatic, and then at less frequent intervals throughout the childhood years [8].

The examination of the child also gives consideration to the environment in which the child lives and to the parental concerns in child-rearing. The adults responsible for the child's care often have concerns about the development of the child and about their own ability to manage. They need respect, support, and guidance that encourage them to express the concerns they may have and to discuss their needs and the needs of the child. The mother is usually the person most familiar with the child's health and is the one most likely to detect changes, both normal and abnormal, that go unnoticed by others, including the health practitioner. The health practitioner should also be alert to any signs of stress between the mother and child. A mother who is concerned, anxious, or angry about a child's behavior or physical condition is showing evidence of stress that may interfere with the mother-child relationship and ultimately with the development of the child. Therefore, consideration is given to the needs of the mother or other adults caring for the child as well as to those of the child.

The attitude of the practitioner should always demonstrate respect for both the child and the parent, a willingness to listen to problems, and a concerned interest in finding adequate solutions. Both the child and the parent are sensitive to the attitudes of the practitioner and respond according to the impressions they receive (Fig. 15-1). In essence, the examiner needs to be sensitive to the child as a growing, developing human being who is ever changing.

Figure 15-1.
Both parents and their
children are sensitive to the
attitudes of the practitioner,
and the kind of health care
experience they have
depends on the respect and
concern the practitioner
shows. (Courtesy of
Harvard Community Health
Plan.)

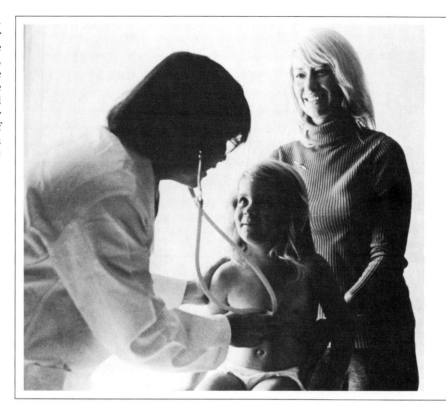

CULTURAL CONSIDERATIONS

The relationship of cultural patterns to the child-rearing process must be of concern to the nurse who approaches the physical assessment of the child. Human beings need order and exploration during the experiences of child-bearing and parenting. Each culture has its own health and healing belief systems, of which the parenting process is a component. Its members and the forms of the systems vary from culture to culture. Knowledge about these cultural forms and how they interrelate with the social environment is necessary for the nurse who wishes to work in transcultural health care settings. For such an experience the nurse must have the skill to cope with ambiguity and translate beliefs, values, and actions that are multiculturally based to clients who seek assistance for themselves and their children [2].

NUTRITIONAL CONSIDERATIONS

Nutrition plays a major, often underappreciated, role in the preservation of health at all ages, particularly in childhood. In addition, nutrition in infancy has to be scrutinized in relation to its immediate as well as later effects. The long-term harmful consequences of malnutrition are increasingly recognized in the form of defective brain development, physical stunting, impaired immunocompetence, and even more unexpected changes, such as lens damage and cataracts [10]. More recently the potential long term effects of overnutrition (or unbalanced nutrition) are becoming evident or suspected. For example, the role of calorie overdosage in infancy and childhood in the pathogenesis of obesity in adult life seems to be increasingly likely. The significance of abnormally low intake of cholesterol in vegetable oil-fortified formulas in conditioning the body's metabolism to deal with cholesterol in adulthood is also under investigation. Although a variety of conflicting and overlapping opinions exist, it is important for the nurse to gradually develop a system of nutritional data based on a blend of modern science, knowledge, an awareness of successful time-tested approaches, and the human being's ancient biologic mammalian heritage. Specific tools for the assessment of nutritional status appear later in this chapter.

APPROACH TO THE PHYSICAL ASSESSMENT OF THE CHILD

The pediatric history provides the opportunity to interview both the child and the parent in order to gather information about the child's health, development, relationships with others, and care. [8] It also provides the opportunity for the child to become acquainted with the practitioner before being examined. The informant for the history may be a parent, a relative, a guardian, or the child. It is useful for the child, to participate in the interview, to volunteer information and to develop a relationship with the nurse. The data collected during the interview and examination must be guided by some predetermined, organized framework to ensure that the assessment will be thorough and that the data needed will be obtained (see Chap. 5).

The physical examination of the infant or child varies according to the age, development, and behavior of the child. The organization is changed to accommodate the individual child. If consideration is not given to the child's age and development, the examination is likely to be incomplete.

When carrying out a pediatric examination, the examiner should keep in mind that each visit for health care is a learning experience for the child. The child's experience may result in increased self-confidence and trust of others, or the child may experience feelings of failure and distrust in health care providers. Thus, it is most productive to provide opportunities for the child to develop positive relationships during the visits for routine health care. It is also important to remember that any separation from the parent may be anxiety-provoking and may increase the child's level of fear and distrust. It is therefore important to encourage the parent to participate in the examination in order to support the child. The older child may be able to participate more freely without the parent present. Most parents recognize the child's developing independence and encourage this participation. Finally, for greater cooperation on the part of the child and parent, it is important to prepare both for any new or painful procedure. This requires the examiner to have a special appreciation for the feelings of children and parents.

Little difficulty is encountered in the performance of the physical examination of the infant in the first six months of life, since the infant has little fear of strangers. The infant often enjoys having his clothes removed and is easily distracted by the parent or the examiner with repetitive vocal sounds and smiles. However, the examination of the ears and mouth may cause distress and should be done as the last part of the examination. It is wise to take advantage of the opportunities that are offered. If the infant is quiet or sleepy, it is best to start with the auscultation of the thorax; if the infant is playful and active, it is easier to start with the extremities and wait for a quieter moment to examine the thorax.

During the second half of the first year of life, the infant experiences an increasing fear of strangers; thus, it is often profitable to conduct the entire examination while the infant is held on the parent's lap. Even under the best of circumstances, it may not be possible to create a situation that is ideal. The infant may remain resistant throughout the examination, requiring the examiner to carry out the examination expeditiously and with minimal restraint of the infant. The parent often experiences discomfort or embarrassment because of the infant's behavior and needs reassurance that the infant is behaving normally. The situation is ideal for helping the parent to understand normal development and the needs of the infant at this age.

The child under the age of four is a challenge to even the most experienced examiner. The child is learning how his body works and to manipulate and experiment with all aspects of the environment. Any restraint in the pursuit of his desired activities may be seen by the child as an interference, resulting in his unhappiness or frustration. The child at this age is getting much pleasure from recently acquired skills such as walking and talking and enjoys the ability to manipulate objects such as doors and wastebaskets. At the same time, the child is still unsure of strangers and needs the parent's presence in order to feel safe. The two- or three-year-old child may be charming and cooperative, or difficult to examine; whichever the case, the examiner is required to make many modifications in the organization of the examination. The child may be examined in a standing position or on the parent's lap. Removal of all clothing at one time is unpleasant for the child, but often cooperation is gained if only one article of clothing is removed at a time as the examination is carried out. The child also needs the opportunity to handle and use the examining instruments. The opportunity may be enjoyable, but may also be rejected if the offer is too fear-provoking. Intrusive procedures (entering body orifices) are especially frightening to the young child, and time should be taken to explain candidly the necessity of performing them. Despite the difficulties in examining the child of this age, the ability of the child to relate more positively at each subsequent visit can be rewarding and profitable for the examiner.

At four or five years of age, the child is usually able to understand and cooperate during the examination. Anxious to please, the child is usually a delightful participant. Although the child has better control of his feelings and behavior than the younger child, control may still be lost if fear is great. He should receive recognition of his efforts to participate, to enhance self-image. This child especially enjoys trying out the examiner's equipment (Fig. 15-2)

Figure 15-2.
The child needs the
opportunity to become
familiar with examining
instruments.

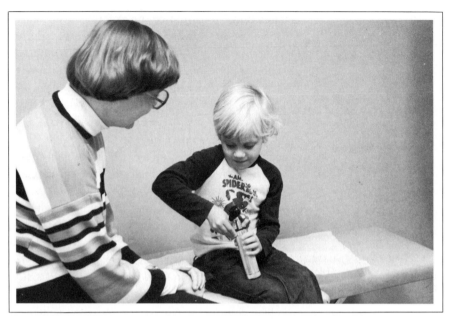

and is likely to demonstrate his new learning in future play activities; this is a way to incorporate the role of the examiner and master his fears.

The school-age child may be approached in a much more forward manner. However, he may be extremely shy and modest. If the child is distressed about removing clothing, this modesty should be respected and attempts made to conduct the examination with as little exposure as possible.

Usually the school-age child can be examined without the parents being present, but the nurse needs to be alert to the child's needs and permit the parents to remain in the room if the child wishes. If the child is willing to be examined without the parent, this is an ideal time for the nurse to gather a history from him. The child often provides information about hobbies, friends, and school achievements and relationships which adds to the nurse's understanding of him.

Parents accompanying adolescents for health care visits may be invited to join their child for the initial interview. At the time of examination, however, it is advisable to see the adolescent alone, allowing sufficient opportunity to discuss his symptoms and problems privately. Rapid acceleration of growth and body changes coupled with newly aroused sexual drives may stimulate a variety of fantasies and fears in an adolescent who previously felt comfortable with his physical self.

**INFANCY
Interview**

Interviewing during the infancy period naturally involves only the parents directly. However, considerable information can be obtained by observing the parent-infant relationship as the history is obtained. The nature of touch, holding, and body contact between parent and child provides significant clues to the parents' security with the infant and to the degree of trust the infant has in them. The nurse must be aware of the concept of bonding and approaches to its assessment.

A history of specific developmental achievements and behavior, as well as of sleeping, feeding, and play habits, is essential. When feeding problems are a major concern, the parent can be asked to offer a feeding in the nurse's presence, thereby providing an opportunity to assess the parent's comfort and skill, as well as the infant's response.

Whenever possible, it is desirable to have both parents present for interviewing and examination. Concerns expressed by the father are often different from those voiced by the mother. When the infant is ill, however, the nurse should proceed directly to the examination, obtaining essential information during the procedure.

Developmental Achievements of the Infant

Parents may express concern about the normalcy of their baby's growth and development during the first year. Questions and anxiety levels of experienced and inexperienced mothers vary. Parents need information about the demanding behavior of infants and need to have outlets to release their own feelings appropriately, since controlled anger or permissiveness can be frightening to the child seeking limits. The nurse must be aware of the wide latitude of normal behavior, and the pattern of each child's growth and development over an extended period of time, thereby focusing on factors that influence his development. If the day-to-day changes in the child's development can be pointed out to the parents, anxiety can be decreased, and the parents can begin to enjoy the wonders of their child.

The crucial developmental task of the first year is the development of a sense of trust. The infant, who begins life as an individual with reflexive behavior, gradually learns that cries of hunger, discomfort, or need for attention are answered. As these needs are met, the infant gradually associates pleasure and security with his mother's care and begins to develop a sense of trust. This trust is further developed as he learns to move about his environment, to do things independently, and to interact with significant persons.

During the first year (especially in the first six months), physical growth and maturation are rapid, with increasing adequacy of physiologic processes and, particularly, with rapid development of the nervous system. Birth weights for full-term infants usually double by five months and triple in one year. Length increases from a range of 18 to 21 in (45.7 to 53.3 cm) to a range of 27 to 31 in (68.6 to 78.7 cm). Head circumference at birth is 35 cm, increasing to between 46 and 47 cm at one year.

Development throughout infancy and childhood is orderly and sequential, proceeding in a cephalocaudal direction. For example, head control precedes control of the upper extremities, which is followed by control of the lower extremities. Also, development in the extremities progresses in a proximal-distal direction, with control of the arms preceding finger control.

The gross motor skills of an infant advance on a continuum: from lifting and gradually controlling the head to lifting head and chest; rolling over; sitting with support; sitting steadily without support; creeping; pulling to a stand; standing alone; and walking.

The fine motor skills of an infant advance through stages of eye-hand coordination: following objects with the eyes; bringing the hands together at the midline; grasping offered objects; reaching for objects; swiping at objects; transferring objects from hand to hand; radial-palmer grasp and pincer grasp.

Language, which begins at birth with the infant's first cry, progresses to small throaty sounds, coos, laughs, squeals, and repetitive sounds; then, by the end of the first year, to several words, mostly names.

In the personal-social realm, the infant progresses from staring at surroundings to smiling (first responsively, then spontaneously) and to having some separation anxiety when the parents leave him. The infant plays "peekaboo," waves "bye-bye," and begins to self-feed finger foods and drink from a cup.

Special Developmental Considerations for the Infant

Nutrition. Nutrition is a major concern for mothers of young infants. Frequency and amounts of bottle and breast feedings vary with the growth pattern of the infant. Feeding schedules need to be flexible, allowing time for the infant to satisfy sucking needs. Additional information on infant feeding is presented in the section on nutrition.

Weaning. The infant can usually be weaned directly to the cup for juices between the ages of four and eight months. Cup feedings can then gradually replace breast or bottle feedings. The bedtime feeding is usually the last bottle to be relinquished and may need to be given as late as 14 to 15 months of age.

Sleeping Patterns (1 to 3 Months). Sleeping patterns in the first three months are as follows:

At 1 Month. Sleeps most of the time. Sleep not always quiet. May make sucking motions; opens and closes eyes; breathes unevenly.

At 2 Months. Awake for portions of day; sleeps most of night; beginning to give up night feeding; requires late evening and early morning feeding.

At 5 Months. Sleeps well when wakeful times have been interesting. Likes bright toys hanging over crib. Enjoys social attention; likes to hear voices and see household activities.

Nap Patterns. Nap patterns evolve in the following manner.

At 1 to 6 Months. Has two to three naps per day, with range of 1 to 4 hours.
From 6 to 10 Months. Has two naps per day.
From 10 Months to 2 Years. Has one nap per day, usually in the afternoon.

Teething. The infant may be irritable and fussy and have increased salivation as teeth erupt. A clear nasal discharge, reddened gums, and occasionally a nonspecific facial rash may be noted. Fever is not usually present. Chewing on a blunt, firm object or cracked ice wrapped in a cloth may relieve pain.

Eyes. Strabismus is present to varying degrees in many infants during the neonatal period. The infant's eyes can focus accurately when awake and alert, and slight deviations of eye movement may occur when he is tired. Should irregular movements persist, the parents should consult an ophthalmologist.

Handling the Genitals. Around six months of age, infants discover their genitals and handle them in the same way they handle their fingers and toes. Curiosity and exploration are aspects of healthy learning and should not be forcibly prohibited. Distracting the infant with a toy is possible and allows completion of dressing procedures.

Immunizations. Only healthy children should receive immunizations. Children with acute infection or skin infection should be immunized after the problem has resolved. Those with seizures, those with blood or lymph diseases, and those receiving corticosteriods or immunosuppressive drugs should be referred to their physician for advice. Patients with a history of allergy to egg or fowl should not receive vaccines prepared with these tissues. A schedule approved by the American Academy of Pediatrics for active immunization and tuberculin testing of normal infants and children appears in Table 15-1.

Table 15-1
Recommended Schedule for
Active Immunization of
Normal Infants and
Children*

2 mo	DTP[1]	TOPV[2a]
4 mo	DTP	TOPV
6 mo	DTP	[2b]
1 yr		Tuberculin test[3]
15 mo	Measles,[4] rubella[4]	Mumps[4]
1½ yr	DTP	TOPV
4-6 yr	DTP	TOPV
14-16 yr	Td[5]—repeat every 10 years	

[1]DTP—diphtheria and tetanus toxoids combined with pertussis vaccine.
[2a]TOPV—trivalent oral poliovirus vaccine. This recommendation is suitable for breast-fed as well as bottle-fed infants.
[2b]A third dose of TOPV is optional but may be given in areas of high endemicity of poliomyelitis.
[3]Frequency of repeated tuberculin tests depends on risk of exposure of the child and on the prevalence of tuberculosis in the population group. For the pediatrician's office or outpatient clinic, an annual or biennial tuberculin test, unless local circumstances clearly indicate otherwise, is appropriate. The initial test should be done at the time of, or preceding, the measles immunization.
[4]May be given at 15 months as measles-rubella or measles-mumps-rubella combined vaccines (see Rubella, section 9, and Mumps, section 9, for further discussion of age of administration).
[5]Td—combined tetanus and diphtheria toxoids (adult type) for those more than 6 years of age, in contrast to diphtheria and tetanus (DT) toxoids which contain a larger amount of diphtheria antigen. *Tetanus toxoid at time of injury:* For clean, minor wounds, no booster dose is needed by a fully immunized child unless more than 10 years have elapsed since the last dose. For contaminated wounds, a booster dose should be given if more than 5 years have elapsed since the last dose.
Concentration and Storage of Vaccines
  Because the concentration of antigen varies in different products, the manufacturer's package insert should be consulted regarding the volume of individual doses of immunizing agents.
  Because biologics are of varying stability, the manufacturer's recommendations for optimal storage conditions (e.g., temperature, light) should be carefully followed. Failure to observe these precautions may significantly reduce the potency and effectiveness of the vaccines.
*Modified from the Report of the Committee on Infectious Diseases (18th ed.), American Academy of Pediatrics. Evanston, Ill., 1977. Table I-2, pp. 3 and 11. ©Copyright American Academy of Pediatrics, 1977. [11]

TODDLER, PRESCHOOL, AND SCHOOL-AGE CHILD Interview

The nurse should be sensitive to individual differences and plan the interview and examination sequence accordingly. Accurate assessment may be obtained by conducting the health interview with the parent and assessing the child over several visits. Usually, interviewing begins after rapport is established among the nurse, child, and parent. Engaging the child in simple play or allowing the child to explore some of the examining equipment promotes cooperation and provides an opportunity to begin assessing growth and development and the parent-child relationship.

The initial interview is concerned with essential information. Additional history should be delayed until after the examination. Conduct the detailed interview without distractions from the child, if possible. Because the "parenting person" possesses the most detailed information about the child, it is important to interview that person. The history obtained during the interview should include the prenatal and neonatal information mentioned in Chapter 14, general development, immunizations received, and communicable diseases contracted.

The school-age child can comprehend more detailed verbal explanations of the nurse examiner's purpose. The 6-year-old has a short attention span, but can be expected to sit quietly or play while a cursory history is obtained. In the later school years it may be beneficial to interview the child separately from the parents to gain additional insights into the history and assessment, including school adjustment and achievement.

Developmental Achievements of the Toddler and Preschooler

Although physical growth slows after the first six months of life, development continues at a rapid pace. The major task of the second and third years is development of autonomy, which leads to the toddler's familiar "No!" The child generally first develops bowel control, then bladder control. Skills the child learns include feeding, undressing and dressing, and walking, climbing, riding a tricycle, and throwing objects. The child expresses needs and desires through a rapidly expanding vocabulary, used with increasing skill. The 4-year-old is developing sexual identity and shows an intense attraction for the parent of the opposite sex. The child relates to the world in a concrete but egocentric manner. By five years speech patterns are clear, sentence structure has increased in complexity, and the child is able to both comprehend and express thoughts more clearly and accurately. Gross motor skills include more difficult maneuvers such as hopping, balancing on one foot, tandem walking, and jumping rope. Although attention span is limited, the four- to five-year-old child likes to draw, color, and work with scissors and paste. There is more social awareness, seeking out other children and playing cooperatively with them.

A helpful tool for evaluating development of the infant through the age of six years is the Denver Developmental Screening Test (DDST) (Fig. 15-3). [4] When the test is administered, the child's parents should be informed that it is a screening instrument and that no child is expected to accomplish every item. The nurse must be thoroughly familiar with the manual describing its use. The

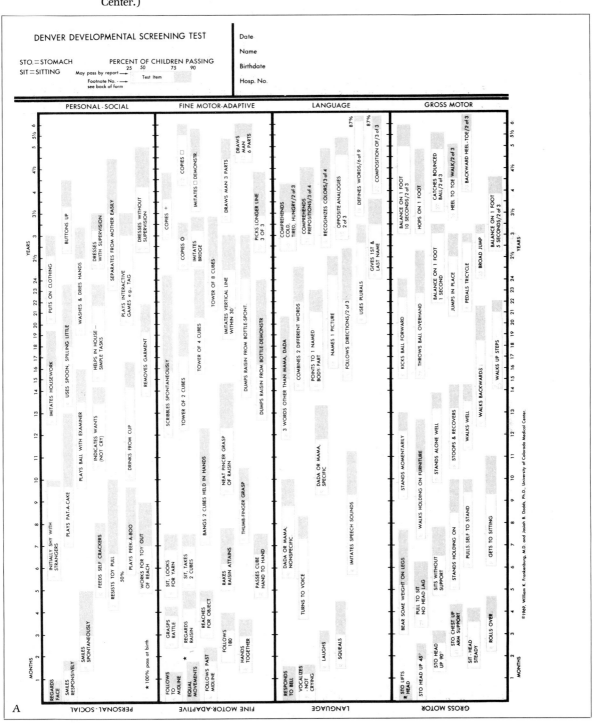

Figure 15-3B.
Continued.

1. Try to get child to smile by smiling, talking or waving to him. Do not touch him.
2. When child is playing with toy, pull it away from him. Pass if he resists.
3. Child does not have to be able to tie shoes or button in the back.
4. Move yarn slowly in an arc from one side to the other, about 6" above child's face. Pass if eyes follow 90° to midline. (Past midline; 180°)
5. Pass if child grasps rattle when it is touched to the backs or tips of fingers.
6. Pass if child continues to look where yarn disappeared or tries to see where it went. Yarn should be dropped quickly from sight from tester's hand without arm movement.
7. Pass if child picks up raisin with any part of thumb and a finger.
8. Pass if child picks up raisin with the ends of thumb and index finger using an over hand approach.

9. Pass any en-closed form. Fail continuous round motions.
10. Which line is longer? (Not bigger.) Turn paper upside down and repeat. (3/3 or 5/6)
11. Pass any crossing lines.
12. Have child copy first. If failed, demonstrate

When giving items 9, 11 and 12, do not name the forms. Do not demonstrate 9 and 11.

13. When scoring, each pair (2 arms, 2 legs, etc.) counts as one part.
14. Point to picture and have child name it. (No credit is given for sounds only.)

15. Tell child to: Give block to Mommie; put block on table; put block on floor. Pass 2 of 3. (Do not help child by pointing, moving head or eyes.)
16. Ask child: What do you do when you are cold? ..hungry? ..tired? Pass 2 of 3.
17. Tell child to: Put block on table; under table; in front of chair, behind chair. Pass 3 of 4. (Do not help child by pointing, moving head or eyes.)
18. Ask child: If fire is hot, ice is ?; Mother is a woman, Dad is a ?; a horse is big, a mouse is ?. Pass 2 of 3.
19. Ask child: What is a ball? ..lake? ..desk? ..house? ..banana? ..curtain? ..ceiling? ..hedge? ..pavement? Pass if defined in terms of use, shape, what it is made of or general category (such as banana is fruit, not just yellow). Pass 6 of 9.
20. Ask child: What is a spoon made of? ..a shoe made of? ..a door made of? (No other objects may be substituted.) Pass 3 of 3.
21. When placed on stomach, child lifts chest off table with support of forearms and/or hands.
22. When child is on back, grasp his hands and pull him to sitting. Pass if head does not hang back.
23. Child may use wall or rail only, not person. May not crawl.
24. Child must throw ball overhand 3 feet to within arm's reach of tester.
25. Child must perform standing broad jump over width of test sheet. (8-1/2 inches)
26. Tell child to walk forward, heel within 1 inch of toe. Tester may demonstrate. Child must walk 4 consecutive steps, 2 out of 3 trials.
27. Bounce ball to child who should stand 3 feet away from tester. Child must catch ball with hands, not arms, 2 out of 3 trials.
28. Tell child to walk backward, toe within 1 inch of heel. Tester may demonstrate. Child must walk 4 consecutive steps, 2 out of 3 trials.

DATE AND BEHAVIORAL OBSERVATIONS (how child feels at time of test, relation to tester, attention span, verbal behavior, self-confidence, etc,):

DDST may also be used to evaluate school readiness for either nursery school or kindergarten. The parent may require guidance in preparing the child for the school experience. The nurse may find the use of the DDST form of help in assisting parents to establish appropriate preschool expectations for their child.

Special Developmental Considerations for the Toddler and Preschooler

As the child matures, behavior patterns change, resulting in different parental concerns about former issues, such as nutrition, sleep, and elimination. Parents may express new concerns as well.

Nutrition. Nutrition is a major developmental concern for parents of children between one and five years of age. With the normal decrease in physical growth during these years, appetite diminishes. Parents who have been providing for the nutritional needs of the rapidly growing infant often become anxious over seeming anorexia in the toddler. Problems are exaggerated by forcing intake or creating struggles at meals. Reassurance can be offered that a decreased appetite is normal and that an active toddler who demonstrates a weight gain of several pounds and skeletal growth of several inches each year is progressing satisfactorily. Parents with children who are chronically ill or have acute infections also need to understand that illness further decreases appetite.

Sleep Disturbances. Sleep disturbances are usually exhibited in children between two and six years of age and may be related to the frequent occurrence of nightmares in this period. The child needs both reassurance and limits. The child should be comforted, and the nature of the nightmares should be explored. A night light or an open door may be helpful. Children who have recently experienced emotional trauma may also show exacerbation of sleeping problems. The possibility of pinworms should be investigated if sleeping disturbances are accompanied by rectal itching and bruxism.

Nocturnal Enuresis. Nocturnal enuresis occurs in many three- and four-year-olds who have good bladder control when awake. This occurs most frequently in males and often has an emotional basis. Sleep reduces inhibitions, and tension and aggression toward parents may be expressed through enuresis. Poor bladder training, anomalies of the urinary system, developmental lag, and regression should also be considered. Recommendations include: limiting the child's fluids for several hours before bedtime; thoroughly awakening the child at several intervals during the night to walk to the bathroom; attempting to reduce the child's anxiety; and putting less pressure on the child in the form of high expectations. Soiled linen should be changed without a punitive attitude.

Bowel Training. Bowel training is accomplished much earlier than bladder control because myelinization of the spinal cord innervating the rectal sphincters occurs earlier than development of the portion of the spinal cord innervating bladder sphincters. Constipation can develop between the ages of two and three years as a part of the negative behavior of the toddler. While striving for autonomy, the child expresses independence by withholding feces from the parents. Encopresis may indicate developmental lag or serious behavior disturbances.

Thumbsucking. Thumbsucking usually occurs between 12 and 18 months and is related to unsatiated oral need, boredom, or anxiety. Prolonged thumbsucking in the preschool years can cause some alteration in jaw formation and minor dental problems. Parents should attempt to establish reasonable expectations for the anxious child and provide appropriate attention, to help alleviate the problem.

Temper Tantrums. Temper tantrums begin around one year of age, reaching a peak at about 18 months of age. They are usually symptoms of frustration, which the preverbal child cannot adequately express. Relief of immediate frustration and direction of the child toward more acceptable expressions of emotions are recommended. Neither retaliation nor appeasement is a workable means of coping with this behavior.

Masturbation. Masturbation may be marked during the fourth and fifth years of life (the Freudian oedipal stage of development). A second period of frequent genital play occurs in the preadolescent years. No damage results from masturbation. Shaming the child and increasing guilt should be avoided.

Stuttering. Stuttering, a common speech disorder, may appear at various intervals in the life cycle, but occurs primarily during the preschool years, at the time of entry into school, and at puberty. Its cause is believed to be anxiety. The severity of the problem may be increased by overly concerned parents. The child may feel rejected and unworthy and avoid contact with others. Management should be directed toward relieving anxiety, reducing the parents' concern, and helping them to develop a patient, accepting, nonstressful approach toward their child.

THE SCHOOL-AGE CHILD
Developmental Achievements

The tasks of middle childhood are successful school adjustment, development of a time-space concept, and a development of a sense of justice and morality (superego). Intellectual development with abstract thinking and reasoning ability is an important part of the school child's mental processes. The child also develops more independence and begins to feel secure while away from home and parents for extended periods of time.

During the school-age years, appetite gradually returns, muscle mass increases, and fine motor skills become developed to a degree that permits greater manual dexterity. Hormonal changes stimulate skeletal growth and the development of secondary sexual characteristics.

The school-age child develops hobbies that are often short-lived. Between the ages of eight and ten years, collections of stamps, baseball cards, beer cans, dolls, comic books, records, and stuffed animals are of paramount interest. Social relationships revolve around rule-oriented games and gang activities. A recent healthy development has been the promotion of participation of boys and girls in sporting activities during childhood.

One should assess development in the school-age child by ascertaining school performance, activities, and hobbies, and by evaluating motor and social skills demonstrated during the interview and examination. Few screening tests exist for evaluating school-age development. Specific testing for areas of concern should be done by referral to a clinical psychologist.

Special Developmental Considerations for the School-age Child

Nutrition. In general, the school-age child prefers plain food and sometimes sweets. The child may be reluctant to try spicy foods or those with sauces and may dislike fruits, vegetables, and salads. Trying new foods in small quantities should be encouraged. Mealtime struggles do not improve dietary patterns and should be avoided. In the early school years, a child tends to dawdle at the table, prolonging the meal. By the age of nine, food is bolted, so that the child can rejoin friends in play. Parents can be assured that both behaviors are temporary.

Respiratory Infections. The body's immunologic system does not fully develop until the early school years. Infections, especially those spread by droplet and affecting the respiratory system, are common occurrences in the young school-age child. Therefore there is a high susceptibility to the many organisms to which the child is exposed at school. A frequent concern of parents of the young school-age child is the number of colds and other respiratory infections suffered in the first several years of school attendance. Treatment is symptomatic. Infection rates improve chronologically with age and maturity of the immune system.

Anxiety. Nail-biting usually indicates anxiety and has no serious consequence. Tics most commonly occur between the ages of five and ten years. Although usually a sign of emotional problems, they are sometimes caused by local irritation. Treatment should address the cause. Ritualistic behavior occurs frequently in the six- to eight-year-old when the child is developing a conscience. The child with poorly controlled conscience may develop elaborate rituals in an attempt to repress socially unacceptable feelings. If these rituals interfere with normal activities, professional consultation is indicated.

Aggression/Withdrawal. Sibling rivalry, feelings of inferiority, or inconsistent parenting may result in aggression and/or withdrawal. Careful determination of the cause should precede education directed at more acceptable expression of feelings. Excessive fear or dependency may result from a child's being urged toward too much independence too early or from overprotection. School phobias most frequently occur in girls in the early school years. A wide variety of symptoms may be presented, but the origin can often be traced to school pressures and social maladjustment, such as mutual dependence of mother and child. Careful evaluation should be done to rule out organic disease.

Delinquency. Delinquency is more than the occasional petty larceny that occurs during the middle school years when gang influence is strong. It consists in the ongoing illegal activities of a child or adolescent. The incidence of delinquency is increasing in America, and the crimes committed by children are becoming similar to those of adults.

If a child exhibits illegal behavior, ego strength, relationship to authority, neurotic guilt, and need for punishment require evaluation. Parents' fluctuation between overindulgence and high expectations should also be noted. The child usually harbors feelings of depression and of being unloved and has low self-esteem. Management is directed toward developing consistent external controls to assist the weak internal controls (conscience, or superego) of the child.

ADOLESCENCE
Interview

Approaches to interviewing the adolescent require the same sensitivity to individuality as in other age groups. Since the adolescent can be classified as neither a child nor an adult, emphasis should be placed on understanding development during this period, including fluctuations between dependent and independent behavior.

It is imperative that the interviewer convey sincere interest in the adolescent and the myriad problems of this age. A sense of trust between the practitioner and the patient is essential and will require varying lengths of time to establish. Direct, truthful responses to questions and assurance that all information will remain confidential promote the development of trust and rapport.

Unlike the adult, the adolescent does not usually present orderly information about illnesses or complaints. An adolescent may not recognize the specific problem, or may be reluctant to reveal or discuss concerns. The adolescent is usually resentful of individuals who have an authoritative manner, and may sometimes appear angry or withdrawn when coping with feelings of fear and discomfort. There may be rejection of the nurse for several visits. Occasionally, an adolescent may openly and instantly share feelings and problems. It is important to allow extended time during such an interview in order to gain significant information that may not be repeated at a later visit. The patient may find anxiety-provoking subjects difficult to talk about directly and then suddenly bring up a sensitive topic for discussion during the physical examination, when less attention is focused on verbal communications.

Adolescents attempt to conform to their peer group in appearance and actions, and they are greatly concerned with other's perceptions compared with their self-image. Varying degrees of hypochondriasis may occur because the adolescent is concerned with physical perfection. Nevertheless, it is essential for the practitioner to complete a careful history and examination to determine the presence of any specific disease.

When interviewing adolescents, it is important to be attentive, to avoid interruptions, and particularly to avoid offering unsolicited advice. Careful observations of the adolescent are essential throughout the interview. Mannerisms, tics, restlessness, and a variety of signs of uneasiness may be apparent when specific subjects are discussed. A rigid posture, grimaces, stuttering, excessive modesty, and inability to face the interviewer are all signs of anxiety and insecurity to be considered in the assessment of the patient. Finally, the manner of self-expression of the adolescent is critical. Depth of feeling and choice of words are as important as the content of the conversation (Fig. 15-4).

When parents accompany the adolescent for health care it is important to carefully observe the interaction between the parent and child. Whenever possible, parents should be invited to visit the practitioner a day or two in advance of their child's visit. This allows for adequate amounts of individual time with both parents and child.

There are a number of areas of psychosocial development that should be explored with each adolescent. They include self-concept, body image, manner of coping with life stresses, relationships with peers, feelings for others, with particular attention to heterosexual relationships, future vocational goals, and progress toward independence from the family.

Developmental Achievements of the Adolescent

Adolescence is a time of major developmental changes. It is the period that marks the termination of childhood and the development of the foundations for adult life. Changes occur in physical, social, cognitive, and moral realms. The most significant physical changes are achievement of linear bone growth with epiphyseal closure, and completion of the development of secondary sexual characteristics. The pattern of sexual development is found in Tables 15-2 and 15-3.

The physical growth spurt signals the initiation of social change as well. The adolescent begins to develop into a fully sexual person. General role development is a major social task, with sexual role a part of self-identity. Dating

Figure 15-4.
Interviewing the adolescent requires sincere interest and sensitivity to individuality.

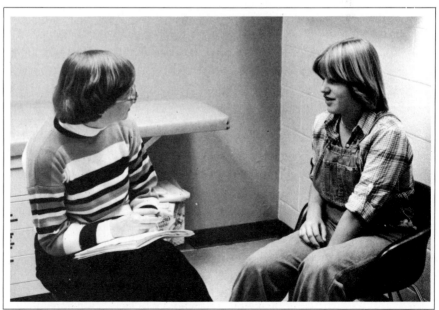

Table 15-2.
Average Time of
Appearance of Sexual
Characteristics in American
Girls

Pelvis	Female contour evident in early childhood and becomes well established by 8–10 years
Breasts	I. Preadolescent
	II. Bud stage:nipple and areola enlarged, small mound beneath, 9–11 years
	III. Nipple enlarged and areola forms mound above the surrounding skin of breast, pigmentation apparent. 12–13 years
	IV. Nipple projects but aerola is level with surrounding skin, glandular tissue palpable, histologic maturity. 14–17 years
Vagina	Some thin milky secretion often begins a year before menarche; glycogen content in cells and epithelial changes on smear, 11–12 years
Pubic hair	I. Initial appearance, 11–12 years
	II. Mainly labial, darker and coarser than body hair, 12–13 years
	III. Well-formed triangle, curly and dark, 13–14 years
	IV. Thick, spreads to thighs
Menarche	13 years
Axillary hair	Initial appearance, 12–14 years
	Increases in amount until early adulthood
Acne	Varies in severity and duration, usually precedes menarche

Modified from Lowrey, G. H. *Growth and Development of Children* (6th ed.). Copyright© 1973 by Year Book Medical Publishers, Inc., Chicago. Used by permission.

marks efforts toward heterosexual role development. Social acceptance by peers is crucial, as is autonomy from parents and family.

Cognitively the adolescent should be moving from concrete operations to formal thought, characterized by abstract thought, generation and testing of hypotheses, and deductive problem-solving. The adolescent should be moving from moral judgments which are rigid and based on societal rules and authority to internalized values and rules of conduct.

Adolescents are faced with vocational choices, too. The young man or woman begins to explore potential educational and employment opportunities.

Table 15-3.
Average Time of
Appearance of Sexual
Characteristics in American
Boys

Breasts	Some hypertrophy often assuming a firm nodularity, 12–14 years
	Disappearance of hypertrophy, 14–17 years
Testes and penis	Increase in size begins, 10–12 years
	Rapid growth, 12–15 years
Pubic hair	Initial appearance, 12–14 years
	Abundant and curly, 13–16 years
Axillary hair	Initial appearance, 13–16 years
Facial and body hair	Initial appearance, 15–17 years
Acne	Varies considerably, 14–18 years
Mature sperm	Average, about 14–16 years

From Lowrey, G. H. *Growth and Development of Children* (6th ed.). Copyright © 1973 by Year Book Medical Publishers, Inc., Chicago. Used by permission.

Part-time jobs during leisure hours provide both experience in evaluating the working world and some economic independence for the young person.

Adolescent behavior vacillates between fierce independence and dependence. Passage through the developmental stages is neither smooth nor always in a forward trajectory. Frequently adolescents reject parental values and established societal practices. This may be viewed as part of the identity crisis the young person is experiencing. The adolescent can be assisted by firm, consistent behavior by adults.

Special Developmental Considerations for the Adolescent

Self-image. The parents and the adolescent are mutually perplexed by the rapid physical and emotional changes they are experiencing. It is helpful to review developmental changes with both parents and adolescent, stressing the emergence of the secondary sex characteristics and the accompanying changes in impulses and desires that occur. Adolescents often feel lonely and uncertain, but mask their insecurity with bold, aggressive behavior. Parents can also be helped to evaluate their child more favorably when provided with information about developmental progression during adolescence.

Acne Vulgaris. Acne vulgaris is present in varying degrees in 75 to 90 percent of adolescents under 18 years of age [7]. The seriousness of acne for this age group cannot be overestimated, for even mild acne can affect popularity and self-confidence at a time when attractiveness and friendships are essential. Acne is related to overproduction of oil from sebaceous glands controlled by hormones that are predominantly androgenic. Other causes include infection, familial predisposition, endocrine gland imbalance, poor diet, lack of sleep or exercise, excessive sweating, and emotional conflicts. Frequent thorough cleansing of the face with a detergent soap is the recommended treatment. Adolescents with severe acne should be referred to a dermatologist.

Obesity. Obesity is seen throughout childhood, with peaks during the first four years of life and between seven and 11 years of age. It is a difficult problem in adolescence, a time when the individual is most sensitive to appearance and approval from peers. Lawrey [7] suggests that any child who weighs 20 percent or more above the mean compared to height should be considered obese.

Obesity in adolescence is usually caused by poor dietary habits, frequently related to emotional stress. Eating becomes a source of satisfaction and comfort when coping with anxiety and tension. Treatment is often difficult and prolonged, consisting of a counseling program in exercise and dietary restriction. Results are entirely dependent on the adolescent's degree of motivation, but frequently are disappointing. Referral for psychiatric counseling may be helpful.

Dysmenorrhea. Dysmenorrhea is a common adolescent problem and may be severe enough to cause frequent absences from school. Complaints vary considerably and may include cramping, lower abdominal fullness, headaches, nausea and vomiting, irritability, and frequently, gastrointestinal symptoms. A careful history, physical examination, and pelvic examination should be completed to rule out a pathologic pelvic condition. In adolescence, psychogenic factors associated with menstrual pain are prevalent and may be due to fears and fantasies based on misconceptions and misinformation. A detailed explanation of the menstrual cycle is essential for the premenarchal girl, as is information on other aspects of puberty, including anticipated secondary sexual developments.

Venereal Disease. It is most important that examinations and cultures for venereal disease be done on patients thought to be sexually active. There appears to be no satisfactory explanation of the increased incidence in venereal disease among adolescents. Lack of adequate sex education has been mentioned as a possible influence, as well as the preoccupation with sex in our society. The availability of abortions, decreased parental supervision, and a changing morality are other possible contributing factors.

Adolescents may refuse to seek treatment because of the sensitive nature of the problem. An understanding attitude is essential when working with adolescents with suspected venereal disease. Some adolescents fear their parents will be notified of their condition. Few states require parental permission prior to rendering care for venereal disease. Syphilis and gonorrheal infections are required to be reported to the health department. The nurse needs to be informed of public health codes governing these practices, remembering that confidentiality must be maintained. Education and counseling should be an integral part of health care provided for suspected venereal disease.

Contraception. Like venereal disease, contraception is a sensitive issue for adolescents. Those who seek such services are demonstrating responsible behavior. They should be treated with understanding and provided with information about the various methods of birth control, so that they can make an informed decision about what is best for them.

Drug Abuse. Drug abuse is a chronic problem in modern society. Although a variety of drugs are used, alcohol abuse has recently increased among the young. Education for parents and other adults who work with adolescents is needed. Nurses can help by familiarizing parents with behavior patterns suggestive of drug abuse. The reader is referred to Suggested Readings for resources providing a discussion of this subject.

PHYSICAL ASSESSMENT
General Appearance

The child's general appearance must be observed quickly but carefully. Posture, activity, and verbalizations including cry are pertinent observations that can assist in determining the degree of health of the child. The smiling, playful child usually is not acutely ill or seriously ill. In the preverbal child the strength, pitch, and frequency and duration of the cry may provide valuable clues to the child's health status.

Table 15-4.
Respiratory Rates

Age	Rate
Premature	40–90
Newborn	30–80
3 years	20–30
5 years	20–25
10 years	17–22
15 years	15–20

(Modified from Lowrey, G. H. *Growth and Development of Children* [6th ed.]. Copyright 1973 by Year Book Medical Publishers, Inc., Chicago. Used by permission.)

Measurements

Following the observation and inspection of the child's general appearance, vital signs should be obtained. Because the insertion of a rectal thermometer may cause the child to become agitated it is advisable to obtain the respiratory rate first, followed by the pulse rate and then the temperature. Respiratory rates vary widely in infants and young children, and should be noted when the child is quiet. In the child under six years of age, the respirations are abdominal, with little thoracic movement. Variations in the infant may include short periods of apnea. Therefore, it may be necessary to observe the breathing patterns for more than one minute to obtain an accurate respiratory rate. Table 15-4 illustrates ranges of respiratory rates for children of different ages. The quality and characteristics of respirations are discussed in the chapter on the adult respiratory system.

Heart rates in children vary greatly with exercise, crying, excitement, and illness. In infants and young children apical pulses should be obtained; in older children radial pulses may be evaluated. Whenever possible, heart rates should be obtained when the child is quiet. Table 15-5 illustrates resting heart rates in infants and children.

Blood pressure readings provide useful data and should be obtained on most infants and children. A proper-sized cuff is essential for accurate measurement. The width of the cuff should cover approximately two-thirds of the length of the child's upper arm—or thigh, if a leg pressure is being measured. The bladder of the cuff should encompass at least three-fourths of the circumference of the extremity. An infant's blood pressure can be obtained by the flush method,

Table 15-5.
Resting Heart Rates (per minute) at Different Ages

Age	Average	Standard Deviation
Newborn	120	40
1–12 months	110	30
1–5 years	95	15
6–10 years	85	15
11–15 years	75	15

which is performed as follows: Place an appropriate-sized cuff on the extremity. Wrap the extremity with an elastic bandage beginning at the distal end and working proximally. Inflate the pressure in the cuff slightly above the anticipated reading and note the systolic reading at the time of flush, as normal color returns to the extremity when the cuff is released and the bandage removed. Another method of obtaining blood pressure in young children, when auscultation of pulsation is not possible, is to locate the radial pulse, inflate the blood pressure cuff behind the point at which the pulse is obliterated, then release the pressure in the cuff. The systolic pressure is the reading at which the pulse returns. These readings are slightly lower than those obtained by the usual procedures. Many young children show interest in the mechanics of the sphygmomanometer and become cooperative once the equipment and the procedure have been explained. Average blood pressure values are found in Table 15-6.

Children under five years of age should have rectal or axillary temperatures taken. Reliable oral temperatures usually can be obtained from children over five who are able to cooperate. Normal temperatures vary widely in children. Infections may be characterized by either subnormal or elevated temperatures, and vigorous activity, excitement, or anxiety may cause temperatures to rise.

Convulsions may accompany high temperatures in children between the ages of six months and five years, especially if the rate of elevation is rapid. Five percent of children in this age group experience at least one seizure, with approximately 40 percent suffering their first convulsion with a fever. If prolonged and accompanied by significant hypoxemia, febrile convulsions may result in

Table 15-6. Normal Blood Pressures for Various Ages (mmHg)

Age	Systolic	2 S.D.	Diastolic	2 S.D.
Infants*				
1st day	52			
4th day	70			
10th day	80			
2nd month	95			
8th month	95			
1 year†	96	30	65	25
2 years	99	25	65	25
4 years	99	20	65	20
6 years	100	15	60	10
8 years	105	15	60	10
10 years	110	17	60	10
12 years	115	19	60	10
14 years	118	20	60	10
16 years	120	16	65	10

(Modified from Lowry, G. H. *Growth and Development of Children* [6th ed.]. Copyright © 1973 by Year Book Medical Publishers, Inc., Chicago. Used by permission.)
*The figures for infants represent averages by the flush method described in the text.
†From 1 year on, the figures in the columns represent the average for systolic and diastolic pressure and 2 standard deviations. Diastolic pressure is indicated by the first change in auscultatory sound.

brain damage. Children who experience repeated seizures should be referred to a physician for management. Additional guidance for parents should be directed toward prevention and control of fevers.

Nurses should be familiar with centigrade (Celsius) temperatures, because health care agencies are gradually changing to that system. Since parents are able to understand Fahrenheit values more readily, readings should be converted to Fahrenheit when they are shared with parents.

The height or length of the child should be measured each time the child is seen and values should be accurately recorded on standard growth charts (Fig. 15-5) to provide data for continuing evaluation of general patterns of growth. Infants are measured in the supine position with the neck and lower extremities extended as much as possible. The length is then marked on the examination table sheet and the length determined in centimeters after the infant has been removed from the sheet.

Children who can stand may be measured on a scale equipped with a measuring device or by standing against a wall-mounted height chart. Although most measuring devices are calibrated in the metric system, parents are interested in height or length measurements in the more familiar inches and feet.

Infants should be weighed nude on infant kilogram scales. Young children may be permitted to keep their underpants on for the weighing process on balance scales, and older children should be weighed wearing only underpants and the examination gown. As was true of height, weight must be carefully recorded in the appropriate growth charts to provide a longitudinal pattern of growth. Serious deviations from average values should be evaluated carefully.

Although head circumference is part of the neuromusculoskeletal examination, the measurement is often obtained prior to any other part of the assessment. The head circumference should be obtained routinely at every examination until the child is at least two years old. In childhood, head circumference should be measured whenever the head size appears suspicious. Measurements should be taken at least twice on each infant or child. The largest circumference is measured by placing the tape over frontal and occipital prominences. Although a paper tape is adequate, a nonstretching vinyl-coated tape or 1/8-inch steel tape yields more accurate data.

Skin The skin of children differs from that of adults in several ways. The infant's epidermis is thin, poorly developed, and susceptible to irritation and infection. Sweating is scanty or may be absent. During childhood, the cohesion of epidermal cells is weak, resulting in blistering following minor trauma or staphylococcal infections. The skin is dry and susceptible to chapping due to scanty sebaceous secretions. Transition to adult skin characteristics occurs during adolescence.

Assessment of dermatologic health requires first that a history be obtained, with questions raised regarding nutrition, family allergy, occupations of family members, presence of pets, health of family members and playmates, and the patient's hygiene and habits. Although a detailed history is valuable, there is no substitute for exposure of the skin and direct examination. A pocket magnifier may be useful to the examiner. As with the adult, the child's skin is inspected for color, texture, turgor, and lesions. Scars and ecchymoses may be prevalent, although the cause of multiple bruises should be investigated thoroughly. Color provides a valuable index of some systemic disease and should be carefully evaluated. Elimination via perspiration should be assessed. Al-

Figure 15-5.
Continued.

GIRLS: BIRTH TO 36 MONTHS
PHYSICAL GROWTH
NCHS PERCENTILES*

though neonates do not perspire, month-old infants who are vigorous and cry a great deal do perspire. Inspection of the skin should be followed by palpation for nodules, deep bruises, and other lesions. Examination of the skin continues throughout the physical assessment process, as various portions of the body are exposed. In black infants, deeper pigmentation is noted in the scrotum and the nail beds.

Figure 15-5.
Continued.

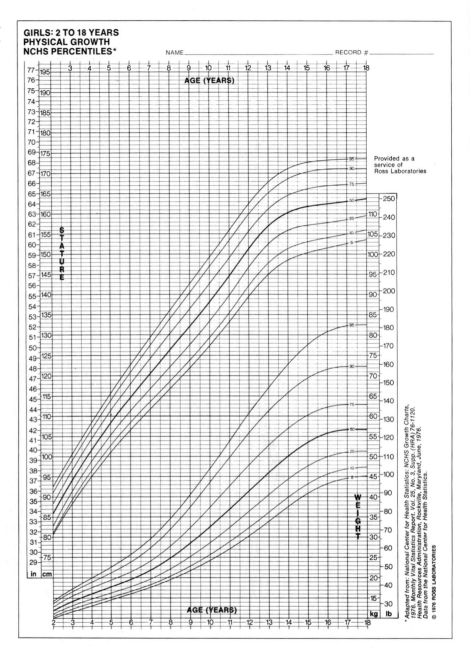

GIRLS: 2 TO 18 YEARS
PHYSICAL GROWTH
NCHS PERCENTILES*

The nails of the child should be inspected for color, evidence of trauma, nail-biting, lesions, infections of the cuticle, and clubbing. Normally hair is found only on the scalp, eyebrows, and lashes from early infancy until near puberty. Deviations from this pattern should be investigated. Evaluation should include familial characteristics and potential disease. Pubic, axillary, and facial hair develops as part of the secondary sexual characteristics. Patterns of this devel-

Figure 15-5.
Continued.

GIRLS: PREPUBESCENT PHYSICAL GROWTH NCHS PERCENTILES

opment are illustrated in the adolescent development section of this chapter. The practitioner should recall that Native Americans normally lack facial hair. The hair should be examined carefully for texture, cleanliness, and signs of infestation or disease. The scalp should be inspected for lesions and scars, then palpated for lesions and tenderness. Pubic hair should be inspected thoroughly for tinea corporis.

Figure 15-5.
Continued.

BOYS: BIRTH TO 36 MONTHS
PHYSICAL GROWTH
NCHS PERCENTILES*

Lymph node enlargement occurs readily in children with infections; therefore an attempt should be made routinely to palpate the occipital, postauricular, anteroposterior cervical, parotid, submaxillary, sublingual, axillary, epitrochlear, and inguinal lymph nodes. Frequently, discrete, shotty, nontender, cool nodes up to 3 mm in diameter are normal findings in children and usually indicate previous infections. In the inguinal and cervical regions, nodes up to

Figure 15-5.
Continued.

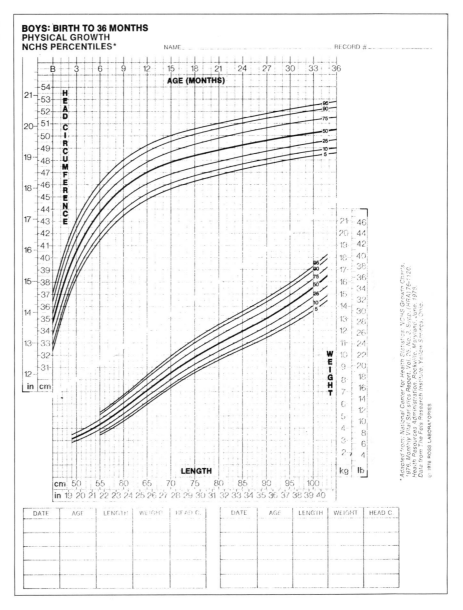

BOYS: BIRTH TO 36 MONTHS
PHYSICAL GROWTH
NCHS PERCENTILES*

1 cm in diameter are considered normal until puberty. Warm, large, tender, or isolated nodes, as well as lymphadenopathy, require medical investigation. The child should be observed for edema; fluid retention due to systemic disease is most pronounced as periorbital edema.

Good skin care includes keeping the epidermis clean, dry, and free of oils and ointments that obliterate pores. Powders are soothing and help to absorb moisture. They should be applied as a fine film so as not to become lumpy when wet. Although used extensively by parents, cornstarch tends to cake and irritate skin [1].

Figure 15-5.
Continued.

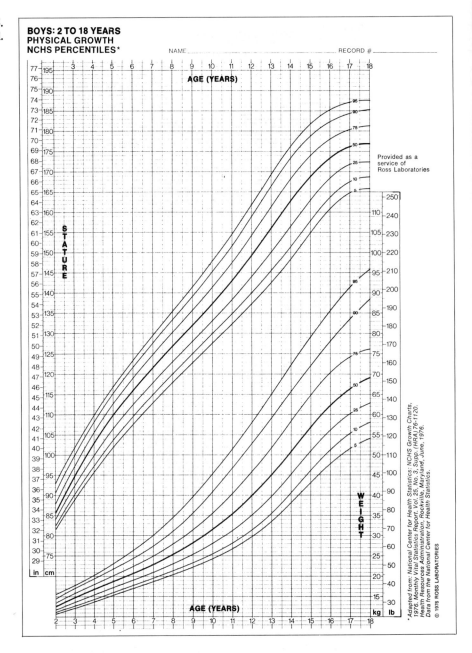

BOYS: 2 TO 18 YEARS
PHYSICAL GROWTH
NCHS PERCENTILES*

The incidence of skin problems in infants and children is second only to that of respiratory problems. Accurate examination of skin lesions includes noting distribution, configuration, topography, type of lesion (macule, papule, vesicle, pustule, nodule, wheal), nature of the lesion (hemorrhage, inflammation, tumor), and evidence of modification due to secondary infection or self-medication. The stage of lesion development is noted also, although one stage may be

Figure 15-5.
Continued.

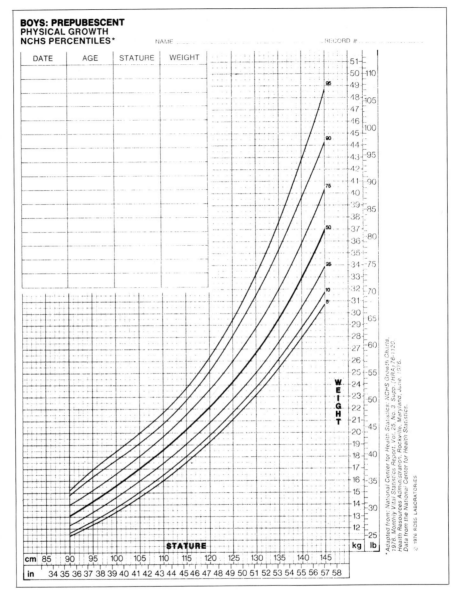

BOYS: PREPUBESCENT
PHYSICAL GROWTH
NCHS PERCENTILES*

NAME .... RECORD # ....

superimposed on another. Frequently, one skin area looks inflamed and edematous, signs of the acute stage, while other skin areas have the dry, leathery appearance of chronic dermatitis.

Transient heat rashes (miliaria rubra), caused by mechanical obstruction of excretory ducts in the epidermis, occur most commonly on the face, neck, trunk, and diaper area of infants. Treatment is directed toward keeping the infant cool by bathing, removing excessive clothing, and placing him in a cool environment. Intertrigo, characterized by raw, denuded areas resulting from rubbing of skin surfaces in moist body areas, may predispose the patient to Candida infection. The child should be kept cool with loose fitting clothing. Candidiasis (thrush) appears as white, curdlike lesions on inflamed oral mucosa or as satellite lesions with sharp margins in the diaper area. In the newborn it is caused by Candida infections of the mother, but in older infants and children it may be a complication of disease or of drug therapy. Seborrhea, relatively common in infancy and childhood, is caused by excessive secretions of the sebaceous glands. A scaling, erythematous rash covered with yellowish scales occurs over the scalp, forehead, eyebrows, eyelids, behind the ears, and on the back of the neck. This condition, known as "milk crust" or "cradle cap" in infancy, is called dandruff in older children. Contact dermatitis may be a reaction to such products as powders, soaps, or bubble bath preparations. Discontinuing their use usually results in improvement of the condition. Roseola, characterized by acute onset of high fever and a delayed erythematous macular or malculopapular rash, primarily on the neck and trunk, is common in infants and young children. Treatment is symptomatic.

In older children, skin problems include food and drug allergies, athlete's foot, and ringworm of the scalp or body. Children and adolescents are susceptible to such viral skin problems as herpes simplex, herpes zoster, viral exanthema, and warts. As children begin to explore the outdoors, contact dermatitis from insecticides, fertilizers, poison oak, and poison ivy may cause severe skin eruptions. Sunburn often results from extended periods of sun exposure during outdoor activities. Although children of any age may suffer insect bites, school-aged children are the most frequent victims of stinging insects. Children, however, rarely suffer the severe anaphylatic reactions to bites that are seen in adults.

School-age children are susceptible to contagious impetigo, a bacterial infection of the face, extremities, and exposed body surfaces, and they may infect their peers (Fig. 15-6). Anal itching, caused by poor hygiene, contact or atopic dermatitis, or pinworms, may be a childhood complaint. Atopic dermatitis (eczema), caused by allergies, irritants, and other agents, is fairly common. Characterized by erythema and a thin vesicular rash, it is usually found on the flexor surfaces of the extremities and often becomes secondarily infected from scratching.

Many communicable diseases of childhood are accompanied by skin rashes. Familiarity with rash distribution and other symptoms of common communicable diseases assists with differential diagnosis. The rashes of measles (rubeola), scarlet fever, and roseola are macular, whereas exanthema causes papular rashes. Chickenpox (varicella) in its early stages may resemble impetigo, but later develops into vesicles. Other vesicular conditions are herpes and sunburn. Impetigo and adolescent acne are pustular skin eruptions.

Relief of the itch, scratch, and secondary infection cycle is the primary treatment goal for most skin problems.

Figure 15-6. Contagious impetigo is a bacterial infection occurring usually on the face, extremities, and exposed surfaces of the skin. (Reproduced with permission from R. D. Judge, G. D. Zuidema, and F. Fitzgerald (Eds.). *Methods of Clinical Examination* (4th ed.). Boston: Little, Brown, 1982.)

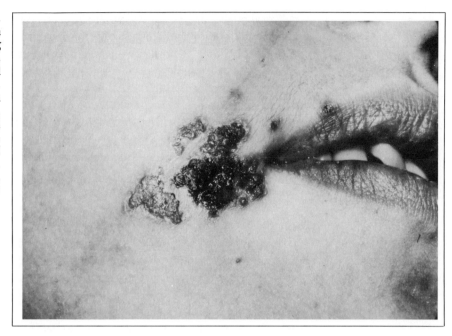

EYES, EARS, NOSE, AND THROAT

Early detection of sensory deficits is dependent on an accurate history of development and on direct observations during physical examinations.

The Eyes

Eye growth and development parallel central nervous system growth and are summarized in Table 15-7.

Table 15-7. Ocular Development from Birth to Age 4

Age	Development and Behavior
Birth	Infant resists lid opening; small pupils; soft pliable lens; doesn't cry tears, although eyes are bathed in tears; awareness of dark and light; closes eyes in bright light; blurred central vision because of incomplete macular development; peripheral vision; pseudostrabismus due to facial shape; nystagmus because of poorly developed muscle control.
1 month	Follows movement of large, conspicuous objects.
2 months	Jerky ocular movement when following moving objects.
4 months	Macula matures enough to permit fixation. Infant inspects own hands. Fixates immediately on small block brought within 12–24 inches of eye.
6 months	Pseudostrabismus disappearing; accommodation reflex present; hand-eye coordination developing; follows dropped object; fixates well in presence of competing stimuli.
1 year	Fusion developing; discriminates shapes; vision 20/180.
18 months	Convergence well established. Depth perception poor—runs into objects.
4 years	Vision 20/20. Can be screened with Snellen E Chart.

Examination of the eye varies between infants and children. Vision in the infant may be grossly ascertained by having him follow a bright light or toy. The infant is able to track an object at approximately six weeks of age. Direct and consensual pupillary reaction to light as well as blinking at a bright light are further evidence of sight.

Ocular movement is inspected. Intermittent, alternating convergent strabismus is common in the first six months of life. An ophthalmologist should be consulted for divergent, persistent, or unilateral strabismus, since vision may be sacrificed with chronic, untreated strabismus. After the age of six months, ocular movements can be inspected in all eight positions of gaze, and the cover/uncover test should be utilized in examining for strabismus. In another test, the Hirschberg test, light is directed on the pupils. Reflection should be symmetric unless strabismus is present.

Inspection of the eye begins with the lids and should follow a systematic pattern. Position and condition of the lids, including color, and retraction and closure of the upper and lower lids are noted. Position and distribution of the lashes are observed as well as the condition of the lid margins. Epicanthal folds and slant of the eyes should also be inspected. Position and condition of the brows are evaluated. The eyes are inspected for moisture without excessive tearing. The lacrimal duct is observed for redness, and the lacrimal glands and ducts are palpated.

The conjunctiva is inspected. Conjunctiva lining the lids is pink, while the bulbar portion is transparent. Lesions should be noted. Pale conjunctiva may indicate anemia, but this suspicion should be validated with laboratory data. The cornea and sclera are shiny, bright, and transparent. In black children the sclera may have a brownish tinge. The normally transparent lens may be opaque if cataracts are present. The irises are inspected for symmetry of shape and color and any markings. Brushfield spots may be indicative of Down's syndrome.

Pupils are inspected for size, shape, equality, or symmetry. Extraocular movements are noted. Inspection of the eye may best be accomplished by holding the infant upright and slowly rotating the body while holding the head midline. The infant's eyes follow the body until it ceases to rotate, at which time they look in the opposite direction.

The ophthalmoscope is used to elicit the red reflex at a distance of eight to 12 inches from the eye. Black infants normally reflect orange color; in the Caucasian child, the reflex is red. Distortion or absence of the reflex should be carefully evaluated by a skilled examiner. Although fundoscopic examination is indicated on all infants, it is best performed by an experienced examiner.

Examination of the child's eyes and vision begins with assessment of visual acuity. For the child over two years of age, the preverbal Snellen chart (illiterate E) can be used. The child indicates in which direction the "legs" of the E are pointed. Acuity assessment is followed by peripheral vision evaluation; the procedure is similar to that for the adult. Extraocular movements are inspected in the eight positions of gaze, followed by the cover/uncover test. The child looks at the examiner with both eyes open while one eye is covered with a hand or another object. After a few seconds the cover is removed and the covered eye is inspected for any movement. There should be none. The other eye is examined and the test repeated with the child focusing on a distant object. The examiner should describe the direction of deviation.

Following the cover/uncover test the eye is inspected and palpated according to the pattern already described for the infant. Since the child is more cooperative than the infant, a fundoscopic assessment can be performed by the nurse examiner.

Children complaining of eye strain require careful evaluation. Those requiring corrective lenses need help in adjusting to glasses. During the adjustment period, the child should determine the wearing time. Prior to that decision, the child should wear the glasses long enough to appreciate what corrected vision can reveal.

The Ears   Hearing at birth is similar to that of adults. Table 15-8 summarizes aural growth and auditory development.

Hearing can be measured with instrumentation that utilizes an acoustic signal. Infants react to the sound by eye blink, Moro reflex, arousal response (stirring, eye opening, limb movement), head turn, sucking activity, and cessation of movement or vocalization. By three months of age, infants begin to turn head and eye toward the source of sound and by six months fixate on the source of a soft sound. Children two to five years of age respond well to play techniques; when a sound is transmitted through earphones, they place a peg in a board or a small toy in a box. A five-year-old responds with gestures when hearing a sound through earphones if the examiner makes a game of it. Gross measurements of hearing can be made using noisemakers. A small child blinks when hearing a sharp noise made at each ear separately and out of the range of vision. An older child can hear a whispered question or simple command at eight inches. To prevent lip reading, the examiner should stand behind the

Table 15-8. Auditory Development from Birth to Age 5		
Age	Development and Behavior
Birth	Eye blinking and Moro reflex response to sounds; subcortical response to sounds because of lack of myelinization of cortical auditory pathways; anatomic maturity of auditory mechanism.
2 months	Voluntary muscle response to sound.
6 months	Infant localizes direction of sound.
5 years	Final development of auditory function; eustachian tube becoming longer and more curved; incidence of otitis media decreasing.

child. The Weber and Rinne tests, discussed in Chapter 8, are incorporated into the child's hearing assessment.

These testing procedures should be done at birth and at each visit during the first year to detect hearing deficits early. Treatment should be instituted before critical developmental periods are reached. For children who respond poorly to office testing, screening materials may be given to the parents for use in the home, where the child may be more relaxed and cooperative. Results should be reported to the nurse. Speech development can be assessed by means of the Denver Articulation Screening Examination. Speech problems or failures may be caused by lack of desire or lack of need to communicate. Muscle coordination difficulties, hearing loss, emotional disturbances, or mental retardation may also cause communication difficulties.

Because ear examinations are uncomfortable for children, especially for those who fear intrusive procedures, examination of the ear is usually postponed until the end of the physical assessment. Examination of the external ear involves inspection and palpation. Position of the pinna is assessed. It should be in line with the canthus of the eye and the occiput. Low-set ears often are indicative of congenital anomalies. Preauricular clefts, sinuses, and cysts are noted. The condition of the skin is evaluated and any discharge or lesions noted. The mastoid is inspected for redness or discharge and is palpated for tenderness or pain.

The otoscope is fitted with the largest speculum that will fit the canal. The infant is restrained in his mother's lap. The external canal is inspected using the otoscope light prior to introduction of the speculum. The canal is assessed for patency, color, and cerumen accumulation. In Oriental children cerumen may be absent. The canal is also examined for foreign bodies, lesions, edema, and discharge.

The otoscope speculum is introduced approximately 1 cm into the external canal after pulling the auricle downward. This straightens the normal upward direction of the infant's external ear. The tympanic membrane is inspected for color, luster, light reflex, bony landmarks, lesions, perforation, scars, bulging, retraction, and fluid levels. The membrane is normally pearl grey and transluscent, with the bones of the middle ear easily visible. The light reflex is diffuse in infants. Dilation of blood vessels in the middle ear of the crying infant should not be mistaken for inflammation. If infection is present, the infant requires medical therapy to prevent more serious infections.

The otoscopic examination is essentially the same for the child as for the infant. The child should be permitted to examine the otoscope. It is helpful to demonstrate ear inspection on the parent and to introduce the speculum into the child's ear without the otoscope attached. The child is restrained in the prone position on the examining table as illustrated in Figure 15-7.

Because the child's external ear canal is normally directed downward, the ear is pulled upward and backward to permit inspection of the tympanic mem-

Figure 15-7.
During the otoscopic
examination, the child
should be restrained in a
prone position on the
examining table with the
external ear canal directed
downward.

brane. In addition to the observations made in the infant, serous otitis media
may be a chronic problem and should be assessed, since it can lead to hearing
loss. Children past the age of four or five years can cooperate by sitting on the
examination table for the otoscopic assessment.

The Mouth   The oral examination begins with inspection of the lips for color, turgor, evidence of lip-biting or chewing, and specific lesions. Lip lesions are common
when infections are present. Breath odor is noted. The number, color, and
condition of the teeth are noted. Eruption of primary teeth, which is related to
genetic factors, occurs earlier in boys than in girls (Table 15-9).

However, permanent teeth erupt earlier in girls than in boys. In premature
infants eruption is generally later than in full-term infants. Sequence and site
of eruption are more important than age of eruption, gross deviations should
be evaluated carefully.

The color of the gums is noted. In black children a dark line is normally
found at the gum margin. The tongue is inspected for size, color, condition,
and movement. The condition of the tongue may indicate infection or allergy.
The buccal mucosa is inspected for color and lesions.

The hard and soft palates are examined for intactness, movement, and arch
of the hard palate. Epstein's pearls, small white epithelial nodules on the hard
palate, are normal findings in infancy.

The examination of the child's mouth is similar to that of the infant's mouth,
with the addition of tooth inspection for caries and alignment. Excessive bottle
feeding and a high carbohydrate diet increase dental caries in children. Tooth

brushing should be started about the time of the first dental visit ($2^{1}/_{2}$ to three years of age). Children continue to require assistance and supervision of oral hygiene practices until the age of six or seven years and need reinforcement again in adolescence.

The Neck   The neck is inspected for symmetry and range of motion. The thyroid and trachea are palpated. The lymph nodes are also palpated (see Chap. 6).

The Nose   Examination of the external nose of the infant is accomplished by inspection for shape, symmetry, nasal flaring, and discharge. Many infants can breathe only through the nose, and so evidence of nasal breathing should be noted. The

Table 15-9.
Dental Growth and
Development

	Primary or Deciduous Teeth					
	Calcification		Eruption*		Shedding	
	Begins at	Complete at	Maxillary	Mandibular	Maxillary	Mandibular
Central incisors	4th fetal month	18–24 months	6–10 months (2)	5–8 months (1)	7–8 years	6–7 years
Lateral incisors	5th fetal month	18–24 months	8–12 months (3)	7–10 months (2)	8–9 years	7–8 years
Cuspids	6th fetal month	30–39 months	16–20 months (6)	16–20 months (6a)	11–12 years	9–11 years
First molars	5th fetal month	24–30 months	11–18 months (5)	11–18 months (3)	9–11 years	10–12 years
Second molars	6th fetal month	36 months	20–30 months (7)	20–30 months (7a)	9–12 years	11–13 years

	Secondary or Permanent Teeth				
	Calcification			Eruption*	
		Begins at	Complete at	Maxillary	Mandibular
Central incisors		3–4 months	9–10 years	7–8 years (3)	6– 7 years (2)
Lateral incisors	Maxilla:	10–12 months	10–11 years	8–9 years (5)	7– 8 years (4)
	Mandible:	3–4 months			
Cuspids		4–5 months	12–15 years	11–12 years (11)	9–11 years (6)
First premolars		18–24 months	12–13 years	10–11 years (7)	10–12 years (8)
Second premolars		24–30 months	12–14 years	10–12 years (9)	11–13 years(10)
First molars		Birth	9–10 years	$5^{1}/_{2}$–7 years (1)	$5^{1}/_{2}$– 7 years (1a)
Second molars		30–36 months	14–16 years	12–14 years (12)	12–13 years (12a)
Third molars	Maxilla:	7–9 years	18–25 years	17–30 years (13)	17–30 years (13a)
	Mandible:	8–10 years			

(Modified from Kempe, C., et al. [6], by permission of the authors and the publisher.)
*Figures in parentheses indicate order of eruption. Many otherwise normal infants do not conform strictly to the stated schedule.

internal structures of the nose are inspected with the otoscope and a broad speculum. The septum is inspected for perforation, color of the mucosa, evidence of trauma, foreign bodies, and hemorrhage.

The examination of the child has several additional parts. Inspection of the external nose includes noting skin lesions or the allergic crease. The internal assessment includes condition of the turbinates (inferior and middle) and presence of polyps in addition to the previously mentioned observations.

In the child past the age of six years the frontal and maxillary sinuses are palpated for edema and tenderness. The technique is similar to that for the adult. The maxillary sinuses are percussed directly for evidence of air-filled cavities.

The Throat   The infant's throat is inspected for size, color, and condition of the tonsils, presence and movement of the uvula, and color of the pharyngeal mucosa. Nature of the cry indicates laryngeal status, but may reveal central nervous system problems as well. The gag reflex is elicited and its characteristics noted.

Throat examinations are sometimes difficult for young children, who resist the intrusion or gag on the tongue depressor. The examiner must develop skill in making pharyngeal observations in one quick glance, since children often do not permit a second chance. The cooperative child does not require the use of the tongue depressor, and permits more time for assessment. The older child's tonsils may have been surgically removed.

RESPIRATORY SYSTEM   Knowledge of the thoracic landmarks is essential for accurate description of respiratory findings. The landmarks are described and illustrated in the chapter on adult respiratory assessment. Inspection of the thorax of the infant includes anterior, posterior, and lateral aspects. The shape, symmetry, circumference, expansion, and scapular position are noted. The infant's thorax has an anteroposterior diameter equal to or greater than the transverse diameter, giving a round or barrel-shaped appearance. Some degree of concavity or convexity may be present normally.

Palpation of the infant's thorax yields information on masses, respiratory excursion, fremitus, crepitus, and tenderness. Because the chest wall is thinner in infants and children than in adults, it is easier to palpate respiratory findings. Fremitus is a tingling feeling over the entire thorax. Coarse fremitus indicates mucus in the upper respiratory tract; decreased fremitus is a sign of obstruction or disease.

The thorax may be percussed directly or indirectly following the technique described for respiratory appraisal of the adult (see Chap. 9). The examiner should be familiar with the various percussion sounds from tympany to flatness. Normally the breath sounds in infants are hyperresonant. The thorax should be tapped at approximately every 1/2 inch (1 cm). Posteriorly the examiner begins above the scapula and proceeds to the diaphragm, comparing the right and left sides at every level. Anteriorly the clavicle is the initiation point, with the percussion proceeding to the point of liver dullness on the right and to the tympanic stomach sounds on the left. The spleen produces left lateral dullness. Because of the small thorax size, percussion yields less helpful information in the infant than does careful inspection.

The final step in assessment of the lungs is auscultation. In the infant it is often difficult to differentiate the breath sounds because of the volume and harshness of the transmitted sounds. A pediatric stethoscope may help to localize the sounds. Breath sounds are bronchovesicular in nature and may be diminished on the side oppposite the one to which the infant's head is turned. Auscultation should proceed by comparing the same levels on both sides of the thorax. It may be necessary to restrain the infant's hands to prevent noise artifacts. A loud slapping sound may indicate a tracheal foreign body; sounds of peristalsis may be due to the proximity of the bowel or to a diaphragmatic hernia.

The technique for examination of the child's thorax is similar to that for infant and adult; the findings, however, are similar to those in the infant. After the age of six years the thorax that has a round configuration is indicative of chronic pulmonary disease. Respirations become more thoracic with advancing age. Excitement, respiratory disorders, fevers, acidosis, cardiac disease, and poisonings alter respiratory rates. The etiology of bradypnea is similar in children and adults. The child is able to cooperate for inspection and palpation of respiratory excusion, and palpation of tactile fremitus can be made a game to gain the child's cooperation.

Dyspnea. Dyspnea may be symptomatic of cardiac disease, anemia, hypothyroidism, or respiratory tract obstruction, although exercise, pain, or emotional factors also may cause difficulty in breathing. The nurse examiner should attempt to determine the cause of dyspnea. Forcing infants to cry, asking young children to run, and requesting older children to breathe deeply, forcibly exhaling a few times, gives the examiner some idea of the amount of exertion that is necessary to cause the dyspnea. Respiratory effort should be evaluated at intervals during the examination to determine whether the degree of dyspnea decreases as the child's apprehension diminishes. The position in which the child experiences the least dyspnea may be significant in determining the location of the difficulty. Young children with high airway obstruction, for example, assume a knee-chest position and cannot tolerate lying supine. Paradoxical respirations usually indicate neuromuscular disorders, necessitating more extensive diagnostic evaluation.

Cough. The frequency and characteristics of any cough are noted, and the cough reflex is tested. Infants may have a weak or poorly developed reflex, and it may be difficult to clear mucus from the airway. Because normally, infants are not mouth breathers, nasal passages must be kept clear. Mouth breathing in older children may indicate infection, allergy, or obstruction.

Respiratory Sounds. Because pitch depends on the diameter of the passageway, the small airway sizes in infants and young children cause the unique pediatric respiratory sounds. Expiratory wheezes are relatively frequent, but other sounds offer the nurse examiner clues about the location of airway obstruction. A gargling, snoring sound identifies postpharyngeal distress, such as tumor. Laryngeal stridor is usually inspiratory, high-pitched, harsh, and noisy, as is extrathoracic tracheal distress. The stridor of croup can be described as a crowing sound; intrathoracic tracheal distress and bronchial difficulties cause a prolonged expiratory phase with wheezing, like that occurring in asthma.

Infections. Infections of the respiratory tract are the most common illnesses of children, occurring with great frequency through school age. Viruses cause the majority of illnesses, and treatment is symptomatic. Children should be taught the proper use of tissues to prevent droplet spread of infection. Foreign bodies in the toddler, croup or epiglottitis in the preschooler, and allergies in children of any age may cause severe respiratory distress.

BREAST ASSESSMENT   The breasts, including the nipples, are examined in infants and children. When the pubescent female begins to develop the breast tissue that accompanies secondary sexual characteristics, she should be taught breast self-examination. This procedure is outlined and illustrated in the chapter on assessment of the female reproductive system. Adolescent girls need to be reassured about any noticeable asymmetry of the breasts. They should appreciate the fact that total symmetry is not achieved by any woman. Adolescent boys may experience some gynecomastia with the production of hormones at the onset of puberty. This usually is a transient problem, a fact that should be shared with the adolescent.

CIRCULATORY SYSTEM   Examination of the circulatory system of the infant begins with inspection and can be accomplished while the infant is quiet. The peripheral pulses are palpated for rate, rhythm, and intensity. Diminished femoral pulses are a sign of coarctation of the aorta. The point of maximum impulse is palpated, as are heaves and thrills. The size of the heart is an important indication of disease and can be ascertained with careful inspection, palpation, and percussion.

The nurse examiner must be opportunistic to auscultate the infant's heart. Ideally the infant should be quiet when this is attempted. For this reason the skilled examiner often begins the physical assessment of the infant with cardiac auscultation. The nurse should proceed deliberately and systematically to gather cardiac information. The aortic examination of the infant and child, unlike the adult examination, begins at the aortic area (second intercostal space). The examiner inches across the thorax to the pulmonic area, then to the tricuspid area and on to the apex, listening for rate, rhythm, and intensity of sounds. The examiner then repeats the process, listening for murmurs between sounds. Both of these techniques are accomplished with the diaphragm pressed against the wall of the thorax. The stethoscope is then turned to the bell, which is applied lightly, and the same areas are auscultated for low frequency murmurs. A change of the child's position may modify a murmur (Fig. 15-8).

It is often difficult to be certain of the presence of murmurs. They are classified as innocent or organic and should be described in terms of the following: (1) position in the cardiac cycle (2) location (3) point of maximum intensity (4) response to exercise and change of position and (5) radiation. Murmurs in children are graded similarly to the system used for adults. Systolic murmurs come at or after the first sound, but before the second; diastolic murmurs come at or after S_2 but before S_1. Many children have murmurs without heart disease; however, clients presenting murmurs should be referred to the pediatrician for further evaluation. Sinus arrhythmia (phase variation in the heart rate, usually associated with the respiratory cycle) is a normal finding in many children over age three and especially in young adolescents. The occasional premature beat or extrasystole has no clinical significance.

For the child, the cardiac examination steps are similar to those for the infant. The PMI is located at the fourth intercostal space until about four years of age when increased heart size moves it to the fifth intercostal space. Percussion of the border of the cardiac muscle also moves laterally with age. Auscultation should be performed with the child supine as well as in the sitting position. Third and fourth heart sounds may be heard in some children in the left lateral postion.

Figure 15-8.
Technique for auscultation of the infant's heart.
(Courtesy of Harvard Community Health Plan.)

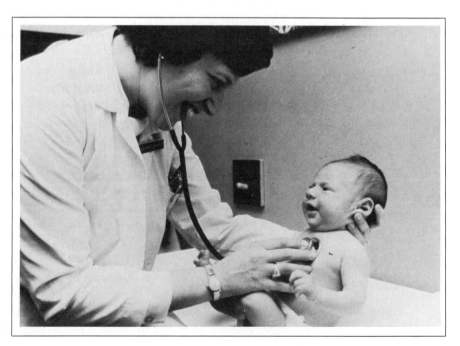

Heart sounds should be sharp and clear. During childhood, heart sounds are of a higher pitch and shorter duration than in adult life. Slurred or "mushy" heart sounds are generally characteristic of severe heart disease.

Cyanosis may be due to pulmonary disease or to cyanotic congenital heart disease. In heart disease, cyanosis may be limited to nail beds and mucous membranes or may be generalized. Cyanotic and hypoxic spells may be a frequent symptom in infants and children with specific congenital cardiac defects (e.g., tetralogy of Fallot). Characteristics of hypoxic spells include irritability, sudden increase in cyanosis, and marked dyspnea, which may progress to unconsciousness, convulsions, and coma. Clubbing of fingers and toes suggests severe cyanotic heart disease and usually is not apparent until the child is a year old.

The following signs revealed by the history may be indicative of congenital heart disease: poor weight gain; feeding problems; fainting (hypoxia) spells; difficulty in swallowing, with frequent regurgitation of curdled milk; respiratory difficulty, with increased comfort in a position of hyperextension; fatigue on exertion; and squatting (characteristic of some types of heart disease).

Signs of heart failure in young children differ from those seen in an adult. Weight gain, rapid respirations, and dyspnea in the supine position are early signs. An enlarged liver, venous engorgement, orthopnea, and gallop cardiac rhythm may or may not be present. Periorbital edema is an early sign of cardiac failure, and peripheral and pulmonary edema are late signs.

THE ABDOMEN   Since gastrointestinal functioning is not as readily observable to the examiner as functions of some other systems (cardiac, respiratory), and because gastrointestinal symptoms are frequent complaints of parents or children, a careful history is needed before the examination. Information on bowel habits and stool characteristics (consistency and color) should be obtained with the history on all infants and children. The practitioner should be familiar with the normal infant stool cycle (Ross Laboratories, 1963[5]). Diarrhea associated with systemic infections is common in children. The examiner must obtain a detailed description of frequency and characteristics of stools, since definitions of diarrhea or constipation vary widely.

Examination of the infant's abdomen can be accomplished best on a flat surface. The sequence of inspection, palpation, percussion, and auscultation varies in the abdomen. Inspection is carried out for protuberance, scars, striae, umbilical hernias, diastasis recti, hair distribution, and turgor. The contour of the umbilicus and evidence of infection or drainage are noted. The abdomen is divided into four quadrants and auscultation is performed in all four, following a systematic pattern. The diaphragm of the stethoscope is used. Medium-pitched sounds should be heard in all quadrants. Bruits and venous hums may be auscultated above the umbilicus in the midline.

Percussion also is carried out in all four quadrants. Normally the abdomen is tympanitic except for liver dullness and dullness of the bladder if it contains urine. Palpation is the final step in the examination of the abdomen. It is accomplished by flexing the infant's legs with one hand while examining with the other. All quadrants are palpated lightly and then more deeply. The examiner checks for tenderness, pain, and masses. In addition to the liver and spleen palpation, kidneys can be palpated in many infants. Fecal masses in the sigmoid colon (lower left quadrant) should not be mistaken for serious disease. Abdominal reflexes are not present during the first year of life.

The examination of the frightened young child is sometimes performed on the parent's lap, although the examination table is the preferred site. The child should be supine with his knees flexed slightly. Assessment techniques are similar to those described for the infant. Attention should be paid to hygiene of the umbilical area. Normally young children have a pot-bellied posture, which should not be confused with the protuberant abdomen of the malnourished child. Pregnancy should be considered as a possible cause of abdominal distention in adolescent girls. Palpation may be more difficult because of the child's ticklishness. Cooperation can be gained by having the child breathe deeply with his mouth open to relax the abdominal muscles, and by placing the child's hand under that of the examiner as illustrated in Figure 15-9. The examiner should attend to the child's facial expression rather than direct questioning for evidence of tenderness or pain. Palpation of the abdomen should always begin by asking the client about any painful areas and then avoiding those areas until the end of palpation. Abdominal reflexes should be elicited by stroking all four

Figure 15-9.
Technique for palpation of
the child's abdomen.

quadrants toward the umbilicus with a tongue depressor. The umbilicus should retract and move in the direction of the stroke.

Vomiting is frequently seen in children as a result of acute infections, faulty feeding techniques, fear and anxiety, and a wide range of disturbances of varying severity. Characteristics of the vomitus (color, volume, force, consistency, and time of occurrence) should be determined. It is important that the nurse ascertain whether nausea precedes or follows vomiting. In newborns, vomitus containing bile material suggests bowel obstruction. Other conditions meriting consideration when vomiting occurs at various ages are: pyloric stenosis (infancy), central nervous system disturbance, food poisoning, surgical conditions, allergies, and cardiac disease.

Episodes of abdominal pain are frequent in childhood and are often a manifestion of functional gastrointestinal illness; however, pain as a response to emotional stress should be considered. Examination during and between attacks of abdominal pain is desirable. In the young child the complaint of a "stomach ache" is used to indicate a variety of symptoms usually located in the abdominal area. Frequently, the child points directly to the umbilicus when referring to a general area of abdominal discomfort.

GENITOURINARY SYSTEM
Urinary System

Kidneys are more easily palpated in infants and young children than in adults. The lower portion of the right kidney and the upper portion of the left usually can be palpated, but in some instances they cannot be. Tumors, polycystic kidneys, congenital anomalies, infection, or renal vein thrombosis may cause enlargement of the kidney. The bladder can be percussed and palpated 1 to 4 cm above the symphysis pubis. Bladder enlargement may be due to urinary tract obstruction, voluntary retention of urine, or low spinal cord disease [9]. If urinary tract infection is suspected, a midstream specimen is required for culture or bacterial count. The finding of 100,000 or more organisms per milliliter in a clean-voided, midstream specimen indicates infection, but should be repeated [9]. Catheterization is seldom necessary and is generally avoided to prevent the possibility of trauma or introduction of infection. When a sterile urine sample is desired, suprapubic percutaneous bladder aspiration is the method of choice, but should be attempted only when the bladder is full. In all instances, urine samples are examined when fresh, since bacteria grow rapidly in vitro in a urinary culture medium, and red cells disintegrate within an hour at room temperature.

The incidence of urinary tract infections is second only to respiratory infections in childhood and may have serious consequences if untreated. Male infants are more frequently affected than females, but in childhood and adolescence, such infections are overwhelmingly more common in girls. *Escherichia coli* is the most common infecting organism, with the Klebsiella group being the next most common. Other contributing factors in females are pinworms, masturbation, the use of bubble bath preparations, and constipation. In the adolescent female, the incidence of urinary tract infections may be associated with sexual intercourse.

Urinary tract infections may be manifested by abrupt onset of fever as high as 104°F (40°C); fever may be absent in chronic infections. Infants may have vomiting, weight loss, failure to thrive, lethargy, and jaundice. Manifestations in children include urgency, frequency, dysuria, and pain or tenderness over the costovertebral angle. Toddlers are more apt to complain of abdominal pain or scream violently on urination. Fatigue and headache may occur in chronic infections. Urethral discharge indicates the presence of infection somewhere in the urinary tract.

Painless urinary tract bleeding may be evident in a number of children and can be benign. Treatment usually is not indicated, but referral to a urologist is required to rule out tumors, tuberculosis, and chronic glomerulonephritis.

Male. Examination of the male infant's genitalia includes inspection of the position and patency of the urinary meatus, force of the urinary stream (an easily obtained observation in infants), condition of the foreskin, circumcision, and shaft of the penis. The foreskin is tight and difficult to retract for several months after birth. It should not be forcibly retracted. The position of the meatal opening is normally at the tip of the glans. In hypospadias the opening is on the ventral surface of the penile shaft; in epispadias it is on the dorsal surface of the penis. Both conditions require referral to a urologist.

The scrotum is inspected for rugations, color, size, and masses. Scrotal color is darker in Blacks. Masses should be transilluminated, since hernias do not allow light to shine through and hydroceles do transilluminate. The testes are palpated in either the scrotum or in the inguinal canal. The size, consistency, and surface characteristics are noted. The epididymis can be palpated as a ridge behind the testis. Again size, consistency, and surface characteristics are noted. The spermatic cord can be palpated in the scrotum. The vas deferens is a hard cord which the examiner can trace with a finger.

The inguinal canals are inspected for bulging—evidence of direct inguinal hernias. These hernias may be auscultated for bowel sounds before palpation disturbs them. Direct and indirect inguinal hernias can be palpated in males through the scrotum and into the inguinal canal. Lymph nodes in the inguinal area are palpated for evidence of local infection.

Inspection and palpation of the male child's genitalia, until puberty are similar to these procedures for the infant. However, in suspected cases of cryptorchidism, the boy should be examined while sitting in a chair holding his knees, with his heels on the seat of the chair. This increases intra-abdominal pressure and may force the testis(es) into the scrotum. The left testis is usually lower than the right. At puberty the pattern, distribution, and condition of pubic hair is added to the observations made. The male pattern is diamond-shaped, with Native Americans having sparse pubic hair. The penile shaft, which may have appeared small in childhood, especially in obese boys, enlarges after puberty.

It should be examined carefully for lesions, and the meatus should be milked for urethral discharge, according to the procedure described for the adult. Rugations of the scrotum increase at puberty.

Female. In the female infant the urinary meatus and clitoris are inspected. The labia are inspected for size and adhesions. A large clitoris is usually a normal finding, but may indicate adrenal hyperplasia or precocious puberty. The labia minora atrophy following the neonatal period, enlarging at puberty as a result of estrogen production. The vagina is inspected for patency. Infants and children requiring vaginal examination are referred to a gynecologist. The female's labia are inspected for hernias or swellings that may have a vascular etiology. The femoral triangle is inspected and palpated for hernias. Lymph nodes are palpated in the inguinal area.

Examination of the adolescent female is essentially the same as that for adult women. Hair patterns, distribution, and conditions are noted, as well as growth of the labia. Female hair distribution is triangular. The Skene and Bartholin glands are inspected for evidence of inflammation and may be milked. Vaginal discharge is noted. A menstrual history is gathered on adolescent girls, and a sexual history should be part of the genitourinary assessment of all adolescents. Specific pubertal changes with which the examiner should be familiar are described under the section on adolescent development.

Rectal examinations are similar for both sexes and for infants and children. The perineal and anal areas are inspected for color and condition of mucosa, as well as for lesions. Sphincter tone can be checked by asking the youngster to bear down. Rectal examination should be performed using the sensitive index finger, not the small finger of the examiner's hand.

Pubertal Change

Pubertal changes vary considerably between sexes and among individuals. Growth and sexual development follow a sequential pattern, with extensive physical, psychologic, and endocrine changes. The first signs of sexual maturation appear between the ages of eight and fourteen years. The development of secondary sex characteristics in females (see Table 15-2) precedes that in males (see Table 15-3) by about two years.

Precocious Puberty. True precocious puberty refers to sexual maturation before age eight in girls and age ten in boys; that is, the hypothalamic-pituitary mechanism initiates sexual development with the potential for production of mature sperm or ova. The onset of precocious puberty may occur at any age and appears to be far more common in girls than in boys. Breast development is usually the first sign of this condition in females, but general patterns vary.

NEUROMUSCULO-SKELETAL SYSTEM

Neuromusculoskeletal examination can be a delightful part of the physical assessment for the young child who has grown restless with earlier palpation, percussion, and auscultation techniques. Many of the assessment procedures for the neuromusculoskeletal system require motor activities that can be turned into games, actively involving the child. Throughout the assessment to this point the examiner has been collecting data related to these systems. General observations should include head size and shape, level of consciousness, position of the body, especially of the head and neck, spontaneous activity, coordination of movements, muscle tone and resistance, sensation, irritability, vigor and pitch of cry, and the presence of tremors or twitching.

The infant's sucking, grasping, Moro, and Babinski reflexes, and the position of the thumb are assessed as for the newborn. Head positioning, tonic neck reflex, nuchal rigidity, hyperextension of the neck (opisthotonos), and the fullness and tenseness of fontanelles should be noted. Because the open fontanelles allow for skull expansion, intracranial bleeding or other causes of slowly increasing intracranial pressure are difficult to determine early in infants.

At birth there are six fontanelles, the anterior, posterior, two mastoid (posterolaterals), and two sphenoids (anterolaterals). Only the anterior remains palpable after several months. Normal fontanelle closures are as follows: posterior, birth to eight weeks; anterolateral, 12 weeks; posterolateral, 12 months; anterior, 18 months or earlier.

Reflexes are both superficial and deep. Examination of abdominal superficial reflexes has been discussed. The cremasteric reflex is elicited in boys by stroking the inner thigh with a pin, inspecting for the testis on the stroked side to leave the scrotum and go into the abdomen.

The deep tendon reflexes that are tested in children are the same as for adults, although they may be more difficult to elicit. Their evaluation also is similar. The illustrations of deep tendon reflexes found in the chapter on neuromuscular functioning are a helpful guide to the examiner.

Cerebellar functioning is assessed with tandem walking, with the child's finger-to-nose-to-the-examiner-finger test, and by having the child rapidly alternate supination and pronation of the hands.

Cranial nerves may be tested with the examination of the head, or with the rest of the neurologic assessment. The olfactory nerve is rarely tested in children. Cranial nerves II, III, IV, and VI are inspected during testing for visual acuity and ocular movements of the eye. The trigeminal (V) nerve's sensory branch may be tested by lightly stroking the face with cotton, asking the child, whose eyes are closed, to identify the touch. The motor portion of the fifth cranial nerve can be tested by having the child clench his teeth on a tongue depressor. The facial nerve controls expression. The child usually enjoys simulating frowns, smiles, and grimaces, especially if the examiner demonstrates the desired expression. The acoustic nerve (VIII) is tested with hearing; the vestibular branch is rarely tested unless the child complains of dizziness. Nerves IX and X are tested with the gag reflex during assessment of the pharynx; XII can be inspected by having the tongue thrust outward and to either side of the corners of the lips, looking for thrust and vesiculations. Finally the spinal accessory nerve (XI) can be assessed by having the child push his shoulders up while the examiner tries to push them down. The child is also requested to turn his head to one side. The examiner pushes the chin in the same direction with the child resisting the movement. Peripheral sensory testing is not done routinely.

Evaluation of mental development is an important part of the neurologic assessment. A careful developmental and behavioral history of the child may provide early clues about the neurologic status of the child. In the toddler and preschool child, observation of play and use of the Denver Developmental Screening Tool (see Fig. 15-2) are helpful in evaluating satisfactory mental development. Prior to the time the child begins school, his mental development must be determined to plan for appropriate educational experiences. If the child's progress appears unsatisfactory, psychologic testing should be conducted. The quality of nurturing must also be investigated. Intensive stimulation often dramatically improves the functioning of a slightly retarded child. Whenever possible, the retarded child should receive vocational training. In the past, mental retardation has been categorized by apparent degrees of severity. The current trend is to diagnose children as retarded without assigning categories.

Generally, muscle development corresponds to the state of nutrition and activity. Increase in muscle mass follows increased skeletal growth, with the weight of muscle compared with total body weight nearly doubling between infancy and adulthood. At birth muscle forms about 20 to 25 percent of the infant's total weight. Muscle examination in infants and children is the same as in adults. Pain, deformity, and limitation of function are carefully noted.

The child's posture is dependent on his age, health, and physique. As the child grows, the flexibility of the spine, the vertebral curves, and the center of gravity change. The pot-bellied appearance of the young child is less pronounced by age six, when the center of gravity becomes subumbilical.

Musculoskeletal inspection and palpation of the infant include the number of digits, full range of passive joint motion, observation for joint pain, and evaluation of the spinal column. In infants, special attention is focused on the range of motion of the hip joints. The reader is referred to Chapter 14 of this volume or to orthopedic texts for a description of the Allis and Ortalani maneuvers for identifying congenital dislocated hip. The spinal column is checked for intactness as described for the newborn. Frank defect of any joint can be differentiated from uterine position deformity by passively moving the deformed part to the neutral position or beyond. True deformities cannot be manipulated in this manner without pain or limitation of movement. Tibial torsion, apparent club feet, and flat feet are all problems of infancy that are usually self-correcting with further growth and development. Joints are inspected and palpated for tenderness and swelling. Muscles are inspected for size and atrophy, and are palpated for strength, tone, tenderness, and swelling.

Posture and tone can be observed during assessment of the infant. Symmetry should be present. After eight weeks, extension of muscles develops, adding to the repertoire of flexion postures noted in neonates; the clenched fist relaxes.

The examiner who is familiar with gross motor development in the infant can evaluate readily whether activity is progressing normally. Any deficits in muscle tone should be evaluated thoroughly.

As the child begins walking, gait is observed. The wear marks on shoes provide valuable clues to gait also. Gross and fine motor skills are noted as the child moves about the room, dresses, and plays with toys or the examination equipment.

The preadolescent growth spurt is due to androgen stimulation of bone and is usually experienced earlier by girls than by boys. Sexual maturation is related more closely to bone age than to chronologic age. As calcification of the bones continues, the incidence of fractures increases. At puberty the center of gravity is at the ilium, and the child's posture resembles the adult's.

Posture should be evaluated for genu valgum, genu varum, and club feet. The child's spine is inspected and palpated while he is bent over trying to touch his toes, but with the arms relaxed and hanging loosely. The examiner stands at the child's head. Blacks experience more lordosis than do other racial groups. Scoliosis should be a consideration when examining adolescents, especially girls. Full range of active and passive joint motion should be accomplished.

Deformities may indicate congenital anomalies or skeletal trauma and should be investigated thoroughly by radiography. Infants and toddlers often have a flat-footed appearance owing to fat pads along the longitudinal arch. These pads disappear as the muscles of the foot are exercised with walking and are no longer noticeable by the age of three years. Urging the child to stand before an interest in the upright position is displayed can strain the arch and should be discouraged. Although infants have an inward bowing of the legs from knee to ankle, usually attributable to uterine position, the bowlegged appearance is most noticeable in the two-year-old. This is a self-correcting condition and should not be confused with the deformities of rickets.

Selection of children's shoes is usually of concern to parents and opinions about the ideal shoe vary. The main purpose of shoes is foot protection. Shoes should be nonrestrictive, allowing approximately one-half inch extra in the width and three-eighths to three-fourths inch extra in the length. The shoes should be high enough to hold the heel in place and should have enough depth for the toes. The heel should not be elevated. Flexible soles provide for natural exercise of the foot muscles. If care is taken to prevent trauma, walking barefoot as much as possible on soft surfaces in the toddler and preschool years is helpful in developing a strong foot.

INFANCY, CHILDHOOD, AND ADOLESCENCE- ASSESSMENT GUIDE

INFANTS

I. HISTORY
   A. Chief Complaint
   B. Interview

*1. *Prenatal history*—X-ray exposure; medications taken; drugs, including tobacco, alcohol; diet; weight gain; BP; other symptoms
*2. *Natal history*—labor duration; delivery (vaginal, breech, c. section); cry (spontaneous, immediate); O_2 to infant; Apgar scores of infant
*3. *Neonatal history*—suck strength; feed (how taken); jaundice; age at discharge (if delayed, why)
4. *Family history*—SES; pedigree; diseases; mother's postnatal health; siblings, housing
*5. *Immunizations*
6. *Illnesses, accidents, hospitalizations*
7. *Allergies*—food, environmental factors
8. *Habits*
   a. Sleeping patterns
   b. Feeding—amount, type of food, frequency
   c. Elimination—urinary: frequency, stream, amount, characteristics; bowels: characteristics, frequency
   d. Activity—play, sleep, wake
C. Observations
   1. Parent/child interactions
   *2. Development
      a. Gross and fine motor activities—lift head, roll over, sit, etc.
      b. Vocalizations
D. Review of Systems
   1. Head, eyes, ears, nose, throat
   2. Cardiovascular
   3. Gastrointestinal
   4. Genitourinary
   5. Neuromusculoskeletal
   6. Endocrine
   7. Skin

II. PHYSICAL EXAMINATION
   *1. *Head*—fontanelles (open, closed prematurely); circumference
   2. *Eyes*—follow pupillary reflex; pupil size (glaucoma cataract); blink reflex; conjunctiva ($AgNO_3$ in newborn); sclera; lids, lashes, lacrimal apparatus (patent ducts); discharge
   3. *Ears*—position, canal, hearing (responds to sounds, not vibrations); TM (don't check in newborn usually)
   4. *Nose*—patency
   *5. *Mouth*—root, suck reflexes (present), strength; palate; teeth, present; gums; tongue; mucosa
   6. *Pharynx*—tonsils, uvula, gag reflex
   7. *Neck*—trachea, thyroid, masses, lymph nodes, ROM—check torticollis
   8. *Thorax*—symmetry, shape; check pectus; expansion;
   9. *Lungs*—respiratory rate, effort, retractions, breath sounds
   10. *Cardiovascular*—peripheral pulses, apical pulse, S_1, S_2, M, color
   *11. *Abdomen*—inguinal hernia; umbilical cord, navel (healed); masses, palpate kidney; veins
   12. *Musculoskeletal*—extremities: ROM, number of digits, position, symmetry; strength, tone, atrophy; spine (intact); hips (check congenital dislocation)
   *13. *Neurological*—Moro, Babinski, Root, suck reflexes
   14. *GU*—meatus: position, patency; foreskin; testes (present); labia (adhesions); vaginal patency; anus; sexual developmental stage/Tanner

* = different from adults

CHILDREN

I. HISTORY
  A. *Same* as infants, but less emphasis on prenatal, natal, neonatal history; more emphasis on illnesses, hospitalizations
  B. Add
    1. School performance
    2. Peer, sibling, and teacher relationships
    3. Responsibilities
    4. Restrictions, discipline

II. PHYSICAL EXAMINATION
    1. *Vital signs*, height, weight
    2. *General appearance*
    3. *Skin, hair, nails* (nail-biting, hair pulling)
    4. *Head*—shape, facial expression
    5. *Eyes*—
      a. Vision—Snellen, peripheral
     *b. EOM—cover/uncover (check strabismus)
      c. Conjunctiva, sclera, PERLA, discharge, fundoscopic
    6. *Ears*—position, canals, discharge (swimmer's ear), TM, mastoid, hearing
    7. *Nose*—flaring, turbinates, sinuses
    8. *Mouth* and *teeth*—tongue, teeth (number, condition), mucosa (color), odor, palate, tonsils (present), uvula, pharynx, larynx (voice)
    9. *Neck*—lymph nodes, trachea, thyroid, ROM
    10. *Thorax*—shape, expansion, breasts (developmental stage)
    11. *Lungs*—rate, effort, breath sounds, cough, rales, and rhonchi
    12. *Cardiovascular*—rate, rhythm; size (PMI); M; S_1, S_2; peripheral pulses; clubbing
    13. *Abdomen*—shape, scars, navel, hernia (inguinal, umbilical, femoral), peristalsis, percussion, bowel sounds, palpation (liver, kidney, spleen, masses, nodes, pulses)
    14. *GU*—discharge, adhesions, epi/hypospadius, scrotum, testes, developmental stage/Tanner, anus
    15. *Musculoskeletal*—digits, (number, condition), joint pain, ROM, strength, tone, atrophy, symmetry, gait (toe-in, ataxia), spine
    16. *Neurological*—cranial nerves (make a game); cerebral; cerebellar (make a game); LOC; DTR

ADOLESCENTS

I. HISTORY
  A. Home
    *1. Parent/sibling relationships
    2. Habits, attitudes, responsibilities, restrictions, discipline
    3. Parental occupation
  *B. Education
    1. Grade in school
    2. Curriculum, performance
    3. Favorite subjects, courses disliked
    4. Teacher/peer relationships
    5. Parental aspirations, career plans
  C. Activities—sports, hobbies, jobs
  D. Drugs—knowledge, experimentation/regular use, need, parental attitude concerning: tobacco, alcohol, drugs, chemicals, medications

* = different from adults

*E. Sex—dating, frequency, activity, sexual attitudes; knowledge of venereal disease, contraception, pregnancy
F. Diet—Basic 4; snacks
G. Accidents, hospitalizations, allergies, immunizations

II. PHYSICAL EXAMINATION

The physical examination for the adolescent is similar to that outlined for the child. For the sexually active female, cervical smears should be considered for gonorrhea and neoplasm. The examination of the male who is sexually active should include a urethral smear for gonorrhea.

REFERENCES

1. Adams, R. M. Principles and practice of topical therapy. *Pediatr. Clin. North Am.* 18:686, 1971.
2. Clark, A. L., and Affonso, D. D. *Childbearing: A Nursing Perspective* (2nd ed.). Philadelphia: Davis, 1979.
3. Drumwright, A. F. *Denver Articulation Screening Exam.* Denver: University of Colorado, 1971.
4. Frankenburg, W. K., and Dodds, J. B. Denver Developmental Screening Test. University of Colorado Medical Center, Denver, Colorado.
5. Infant Stool Cycle. Clinical Education Aid (No. 3). Columbus, Ohio: Ross Laboratories, 1963.
6. Kempe, C. H., Silver, H. K., and O'Brien, D. (Eds.). *Current Pediatric Diagnosis and Treatment* (6th ed.). Los Altos, Calif.: Lange, 1980.
7. Lowrey, G. H. *Growth and Development of Children* (6th ed.). Chicago: Year Book, 1973.
8. Malasanos, L., et al. *Health Assessment* (2nd ed.). St. Louis: Mosby, 1981.
9. McIntosh, R. M., Lum, G. M., and O'Brien, D. Kidney and Urinary Tract. In C. H. Kempe, H. K. Silver, and D. O'Brien (Eds.). *Current Pediatric Diagnosis and Treatment* (6th ed.). Los Altos, Calif.: Lange, 1980, p. 493.
10. Neuman, C. G., and Jelliffee, D. B. Symposium on nutrition in pediatrics. *Pediatr. Clin. North Am.* 24:1, 1977.
11. Report of the Committee on Infectious Diseases. Evanston, Ill: American Academy of Pediatrics, 1977.

SUGGESTED READINGS

Sachs, B. Infant and Preschool Assessment and Counseling Guide for Nurses (2nd ed.). Lansing, Mich: Bureau of Personal Health Services, Michigan Department of Public Health, 1981.
Behrman, H. T. *Practitioner's Illustrated Dermatology.* New York: Grune & Stratton, 1972.
Brazelton, T. B. Infants and Mothers. New York: Dell, 1969.
Daniel, W. A. Common problems of adolescence. *Pediatr. Ann.* 2:14, 1973.
Fraiberg, S. H. *The Magic Years.* New York: Scribner's, 1959.
Gallagher, J. R., Heald, F. P., and Garell, D. C. *Medical Care of the Adolescent* (3rd ed.). New York: Appleton-Century-Crofts, 1976.
Green, M., and Haggerty, R. J. (Eds.). *Ambulatory Pediatrics II: Personal Health Care of Children in the Office* (2nd ed.). Philadelphia: Saunders, 1977.
Kempe, C. H., and Helfer, R. *Helping the Battered Child and his Family.* Philadelphia: Lippincott, 1972.
Krugman, S., and Ward R. *Infectious Disease of Children and Adults* (7th ed.). St. Louis: Mosby, 1980.
McDonald, R. *Dentistry for the Child and Adolescent* (3rd ed.). St. Louis: Mosby, 1978.
Siffert, R. S. Orthopedic checklist for neonates and infants. *Hosp. Pract.* 5:66, 1970.
U.S. Department of Health, Education and Welfare, Office of Child Development. Infant Care. Washington, D.C.: U.S. Government Printing Office, 1976.

* = different from adults

Josephine M. Sana

16. The Elderly

GLOSSARY

aged Having lived or existed a long time; old.

aging Progressive changes produced with the passage of time.

elderly* Pertaining to people in later life; between middle age and old age.

geriatrics Branch of medicine concerned with the pathology and treatment of the aged ill.

gerontology Scientific study of the problems of aging in all their aspects—clinical, biologic, historical, sociologic, pschologic.

later maturity† Years from 65 to 74; characterized by the onset of major changes in life circumstances and patterns; physiologic changes usually occur gradually. Also called young old [10].

middle age The turning point of maturity; time of self-assessment and preparation for new and modified life patterns.

old age The final stages of the normal life span, usually 75 years or older, and a period of life with marked dependencies. Some authors divide this group into the old-old (ages 75 to 84) and very old (ages over 85 [10]).

THE clinical assessment of elderly adults necessitates consideration of multiple factors uniquely related to their age and the aging process. Knowledge of the changes characteristically associated with growing old, and of their functional implications, is essential and is the primary focus of this chapter. It is important, however, that the nurse be aware of other salient factors affecting the health and welfare of the elderly and, consequently, her practice of nursing.

POPULATION TRENDS AND IMPLICATIONS FOR NURSING

One of the most significant outcomes of the scientific advances in the health field is the extension of life expectancy. A person born in the United States at the beginning of this century had a life expectancy of less than 50 years. In 1977, the average life expectancy at birth was about 75 years for the female and somewhat lower for the male. Persons age 65 and older numbered between three and four million in 1900, constituting 4.1 percent of the total population. By 1978, this age group had increased almost eight times, to number 24.1 million, and represented 11.0 percent of the population of the United States. Population projections indicate that there may be as many as 32 million people 65 years and older in the year 2000. It is estimated that this group will constitute about 12.2 to 12.9 percent of a total population of 260 or 246 million, depending on the persistence of the current low birth rate or its continued decline [7].

Of even greater significance for the future practice of nursing is the realization that among the over-65 population, the age group of persons 75 years and older is increasing at a still faster rate. During the 30-year period from 1950 to 1980, the 65 and over group increased from 8.2% to 11.0%, whereas the group

---

*This term is used throughout the chapter in an effort to avoid ambiguity for the reader. The life periods are not absolutes and their definitions must be regarded flexibly.

†New stage in the adult life cycle defined by the noted gerontologist Clark Tibbitts, Director, Training Grant Staff, Administration on Aging, Department of Health, Education, and Welfare [11].

75 years and older increased from 2.6% to 4.1% [6]. The experienced nurse in adult care settings other than the gerontologic or geriatric, has only to pause and reflect upon the age of profile of those she serves in her daily practice to realize she encounters persons in their 80s and 90s much more frequently.

The impact of this changing population profile on nursing is already evident in the preparation for and practice of nursing. The relatively circumscribed field of geriatric nursing is growing rapidly and developing as an important specialized area of practice. Custodial and ritualistic nursing practices are being replaced by more diversified, scientifically based nursing care approaches and interventions. To assist nurses in making these practice transitions, nurse practitioner and continuing education programming has expanded.

Recognizing the special needs of the increasing number of elderly in our population, nurse educators preparing nurses at the basic level have incorporated more gerontologic content and experience in the curriculum.

The sheer magnitude and scope of the needs influencing the health and welfare of the elderly, and ultimately of the total population, mandated a priority of national attention and action. There is a concerted effort to maintain the elderly in their community and home environments as long as possible. This imposes more and more complex demands on nurses practicing in home care programs, health maintenance organizations, and community or hospital-based outpatient clinics. Intensified research into aging by other health professions, particularly in the field of gerontology, generated much new knowledge. There is, however, a growing need for parallel development of nursing research to address those clinical care and management problems of health maintenance and illness states specific to the elderly. As the numbers of nurses specializing in gerontologic nursing at the graduate level increase, the clinical translation into practice of such research generated knowledge can be expected to progress more rapidly.

COMMON MISCONCEPTIONS ABOUT THE ELDERLY

Some of the terms frequently associated with the elderly are "senile," "sick," "disabled," "dependent," and "alone." All these terms are stereotypes, and their use is often inspired by limited professional and personal experiences with the elderly. The existing data show that only about 5 percent of persons in the 65 and older age group are institutionalized for care [4]. Less than 1 percent can be appropriately described as "senile." Actually, the majority enjoy relatively good health up to the age of 70. Of those 65 years of age and older, 7 of every 10 either reside with their spouses, relatives, or friends or function as the head of the household. Generally, they are active, contributing members of society, maintaining themselves independently in their own homes or apartments and paying taxes. In many instances, they are productively employed [4].

NURSE ORIENTATIONS AND VALUES ABOUT AGING AND THE ELDERLY

It is especially important that the nurse working with older people be aware of her orientations and feelings about aging and the elderly. Close personal contacts with older people during the nurse's formative years, and the positive or negative nature of these experiences, influence the professional orientations and the attitudes she expresses in her practice. Evidence of the youth orientation of our society is overwhelming. This emphasis on youth and youthfulness is undeniably devaluative of age and aging. The demeaning effects on the elderly, and on their self-concept and functional well-being, are amply documented in the literature and will not be detailed further. It is of cardinal importance for the nurse to recognize that the elderly are particularly sensitive to expressions of these attitudes and values. However unintentional and subtle their reflection in the nurse's practice, the process and outcomes of the assessment and other care interactions with the elderly will be adversely affected.

Insight into the value systems operant in our professional endeavors as nurses is but one dimension deserving our careful consideration. As products of our culture, we need to examine our value systems in terms of their effects on society as a whole. As producers of our culture, we need to recognize our potential to impact on it, both as individuals and in our collective roles and to become responsible forces for social change. It is somewhat ironic that, as a society, we bury "trinkets" of our time in time capsules, so that those in the future will be sure to be informed about their heritage, yet attach so little value to the elderly in our midst who *are* our heritage.

HEALTH AND AGING

Some health problems are generalized as characteristic of the older population. Although knowledge of these problems is most useful to the nurse assessing the elderly, their relevance to individual patients is highly variable. Generalizations must be applied with caution, since the elderly differ as much one from another, as individuals vary in the population at large. As Fritz [8], describing one group of older people, said, "They [have] the interesting mixture of virtues and faults we find at every age."

Characteristically, the health problems of the elderly are chronic in nature and often multiple. Commonly, the functional disabilities observed in the elderly are much less incapacitating than the examining nurse would expect in view of the extent and the seriousness of the disease they have. Causes for many chronic diseases are unknown or poorly understood, limiting preventive or corrective approaches. Data obtained during assessment, however, can contribute to the early detection of these health problems and the implementation of measures to arrest or slow their progression. Disease exacerbation and complications tend to stress the old more severely than the young; recuperative abilities are reduced, and recovery is usually slower and less complete. The nurse assessing the elderly should fully appreciate the importance of her role in preventing or minimizing these crises states as well as in promoting the patient's fullest functional and coping potentials. Although serious disease may develop insidiously in older people, presenting disruptive symptoms only in late stages, many chronic problems are revealed in readily observable ways.

Generally, aging is accompanied by a decrease in the ability of an individual's body system to perform efficiently. Reserve capacities are also decreased, and there are fewer and slower reactions to stimuli from within and outside the body [1]. The onset and rate of change occurring in different body systems vary with the system as well as with the person's life experiences and heredity. Environmental, economic, and psychologic stresses often counter hereditary influences, altering the rate and nature of the aging process.

The fact that the elderly are adults warrants explicit restatement here, for it is fundamental to interacting effectively with older people in the assessment situation. The content of the chapters directly concerned with adult assessment (Section II) should be viewed as generally appropriate and applicable to the assessment of the elderly. The guides to observation, palpation, percussion, and auscultation are employed essentially as described in the preceding section. The nurse needs to adapt these assessment approaches to meet the particular needs and responses of the older person. Interpretation of clinical findings needs to be modified to take into account the changes normally occurring with increased age. Adult norms therefore have to be used flexibly and adjusted to incorporate age-related changes and individualistic aging patterns in the assessment.

INTERVIEWING THE ELDERLY

The interview with an elderly person is facilitated if the nurse examiner takes sufficient time to ensure adequate orientation and make the patient comfortable. The use of informal forms of address or given names may be distasteful to the older person, who may view it as disrespectful and demeaning. The nurse should therefore determine and respect the patient's preference.

Of prime importance is the nurse's skill in preparing the older person for the appraisal in an *unhurried* manner. Time pressures experienced by the nurse are often great, and the desire to avoid undue time entrapments is understandable. The ability of the older person to respond intelligently and cooperatively, however, can be materially impaired by being rushed. Nonverbal communications indicating that the nurse "is very busy" and "does not have much time" are quickly received by the patient. A patient's attempts to accommodate to the nurse's time frame and expectations usually conflict with his best interests and welfare. Physical findings may be inadvertently induced or intensified by unspoken demands placed on the older patient to move about and change positions quickly.

Assessment activities need advance explanation to avoid surprise and unnecessary anxiety. Instructions should be concise and uncomplicated. Questions should be clearly phrased, brief, and devoid of potentially confusing technical terminology. Sufficient time for a response must be provided; experiences accumulated over years of living may not be recalled immediately in the detail required by the nurse's questions. In other instances, the elderly may engage in extensive review, giving a great deal of information extraneous to that sought by the interviewing nurse.

Eliciting an initial history from the older individual can be unproductively and excessively time consuming for the nurse and taxing and frustrating to the client if unnecessary detailing of 50, 60, or more years of health information unrelated to his current concerns is sought. Often the older person is prompted by specific concerns to seek help and counsel, and these merit the priority attention of the nurse interviewer. There are data to support the view that an older person's perceived problems are notably congruent with those medically identified. Real or potential health problems outside the immediate verbalized concerns of the client may be evident to the nurse. If these pose a threat to the client's welfare or are emergency in nature, interview/assessment direction and action are mandated. Usually the nurse has considerable latitude in judging how selective or extensive a data base she must obtain at that first visit. In any event the nurse must deal sensitively with the informant, or important data may be lost or withheld in the communication exchange.

In one agency known to the author, clients making clinic appointments are advised that they will receive a health questionnaire by mail. They are asked to complete the questionnaire as they are able and bring it when they come for their appointed visit. This provides an unhurried opportunity for the client to give thoughtful responses to the questionnaire without the stress usually associated with an initial assessment. The questionnaire is designed to obtain specific data regarding current health practices and concerns as well as significant past health/illness experiences. The nurse and client review the data together, completing and clarifying information as necessary. The client's active participant role is thus established early and more time is available for consideration of his immediate concerns; the physical examination; problem identification; management decisions and counsel.

Understandably, not all agencies can use the approach described. Agency-specific approaches need to be designed to ensure that the necessary health history data are obtained and the assessment process is completed effectively—without undue drain of the older client's limited energies and with due consideration of staff utilization, efficient use of time, and cost containment.

Mental Performance and Aging

Early in the assessment interview, the nurse examiner should begin assessing the elderly person's ability to comprehend and respond reliably. Tentative impressions of mental functioning can be formulated while eliciting the initial social data. Specific information should be obtained routinely about the patient's family and friends, home environment, current employment or retirement status, educational background, and recreational interests and activities. During this data-gathering process, the nurse not only gains an understanding of the patient as an individual, but also evaluates his language ability, coherency, and comprehension. The patient's attention span and ability to recall and relate past and recent events are also noted. The reliability of the patient as an informant is validated by periodic rechecking of dates, times, events, and other selected data.

The following considerations should guide the nurse in assessing the mental status of elderly individuals. The older peson responds less often and more slowly than a younger person and needs more time to collect and interpret information. This slowing of reaction time with aging indicates less efficiency rather than qualitative impairment.

Learning ability and intelligence are maintained well into later years of life [2]. Generally, the learning process takes more time in the elderly because learnings amassed over years of living and experiencing must be modified or replaced by new information and ideas.

It is essential for the aging person to continue to exercise his mental abilities. Functional loss is great and rapid when the brain is not used. The consequent mental deterioration and incapacitation can be catastrophic to the total well-being of the elderly patient.

Characteristically, memory impairment with aging is for recent events, whereas past memory remains essentially intact. Frequently, the older person soon recognizes this memory change in himself even though the difficulty may be transient and mild. Some patients verbalize their concern or embarrassment freely but anxiously. When asked to recall recent occurrences, others may protect against their insecurity by dwelling on past memories.

Mental functioning declines more slowly than physical functioning. Ordinarily, marked alterations are not observed until the very advanced years. However, repetitive assaults by disease and illness are not tolerated well by the elderly and hasten the deterioration of mental functioning.

The nurse should find the methods for testing orientation, memory, and other cognitive functions described in Chapter 13 helpful in assessing the mental status of the elderly. Findings need to be carefully recorded, for functional alterations may be indicative not only of the aging process, but also of serious psychologic problems or organic disease.

Sensory Perception   Impairments of hearing or sight have direct bearing on the patient's ability to comprehend and respond appropriately during the assessment interview and examination. The nurse assessing the elderly must ascertain whether auditory or visual acuity impairments are present and, if so, obtain a gross estimate of their extent. This can be accomplished with little difficulty during the interview and assessment of mental status. A thorough assessment of the special sensory modalities includes investigation of the status of the patient's sight, touch, taste, smell, pain, temperature, and position sense (see Chaps. 7, 8, 13).

Hearing

Loss of hearing severely handicaps the overall functional ability of the elderly. The ease and safety with which the older person can move about outside his home boundaries is usually decreased markedly. Work and recreational options are more limited. Adaptive behaviors are easily misinterpreted as age-related alterations in personality and mental functioning, masking the generic problem. The social isolation associated with this sensory impairment is of significant magnitude in itself. When added to the other significant changes in the life situation generally experienced in later maturity, the effects on the individual can be overwhelming.

The incidence of hearing defects is probably much greater in the older population than available statistics indicate. Impairments of hearing are less overt than impairments of sight and less easily detected by others. Often, the older person is not immediately or acutely aware of the onset and insidious progression of hearing loss or, for reasons of embarrassment or frustration with others' response to them, will mask the problem.

Difficulties experienced in hearing may be overtly denied by some. Others may recognize the problem, but rationalize it as an aspect of aging they must accept without recourse and gradually withdraw from group activities. Too often, appropriate medical help is not sought, and the problem remains undiagnosed until other concerns bring the older person to the health care facility. The nurse testing the patient's auditory acuity may be the first to detect a hearing disorder.

The two most common hearing disorders are presbycusis and otosclerosis. *Presbycusis,* a perceptive hearing loss associated with aging, involves damage to and deterioration of the neural structures of the inner ear, the auditory nerve, or both. Initially, the ability to hear high-frequency tones is lost; hearing of low frequency tones is affected last. The patient's ability to distinguish between spoken words is diminished and further compromised by noisy environments.

The onset of *otosclerosis,* a conductive hearing loss due to changes in the structure and function of the ossicles (small bones) of the middle ear, is generally in the younger or middle years of life. Surgical correction is often possible for this hearing disorder. Neural involvements may develop over time, and the older person may demonstrate a mixed hearing loss. Audiologic testing and physician referral are arranged to determine the precise nature of the hearing deficit and the potential usefulness of a hearing aid, surgery, or other therapy. Specific examination techniques for testing hearing are described in Chapter 8.

If hearing aids are advised, the older client should be carefully counselled and given direct assistance as needed in obtaining the appropriate device. It is unfortunately true that the elderly are often victimized in the process of securing a hearing aid without adequate professional guidance. It is not an uncommon experience for the older person to have purchased, at excessive cost, aids that are inadequate, ill fitting, and essentially wastefully nonfunctional. Some older people may have a useful device, but for various reasons need help in its maintenance, i.e., battery replacement or other repairs.

Vision

Numerous changes in the eye and its function accompany the aging process, with great impact on the quality of life of the elderly. Visual acuity, as does hearing acuity, decreases with age, and the psychosocial effects of this sensory deprivation are as wide-ranging and complex. Depending on the severity of visual impairment, new constraints may be experienced by the older person. Independence and safety in ambulation and driving is often lessened. Diversional and occupational activities are more restricted, and self-care demands new and difficult adjustments. It must be remembered that many older people have excellent vision. However, those who have severe visual field defects and severe defects in macular vision may be eligible for special financial and tax benefits. The nurse needs to be aware of the nature of these benefits and of the criteria for eligibility, so that she can counsel patients appropriately (see Chap. 7).

In addition to the problem of impaired macular vision, the two other eye conditions most frequently seen with aging are glaucoma and visual field defects. The potential for blindness associated with untreated glaucoma mandates routine examination for increased intraocular pressure in adults over 40 years of age. Particular attention to the patient's family history and symptomatology is warranted, since glaucoma has a familial tendency and presents alerting symptoms.

Lens opacities (cataracts) develop with aging and eventually interfere with vision. Well-developed cataracts may be observed by the nurse without added illumination. The patient needs to be referred for precise diagnosis and evaluation for surgery.

The ophthalmoscopic examination has particular significance for the elderly. The high incidence of diabetes and vascular disease in later years is well recognized. Consequently, fundoscopic examination should be done routinely to detect changes indicative of vascular changes and retinal damage. (See Chap. 7.)

Other Senses

Perception of taste, smell, touch, temperature, and pain and proprioception (movement and position) alter with aging. In general, the nature of change is one of blunting and loss.

After age 45 the number of taste cells gradually decreases, and sensitivity to tastes is correspondingly less. This loss, combined with the decreasing ability to sense and differentiate odors, often affects the older person's eating habits and nutrition. Previous desires for and satisfaction with various foods are lost, and appetite is diminished.

The highly interrelated sensory mechanisms of touch, temperature, and pain are dulled. Consequently the older person's alerting system to environmental danger and tissue injury is impaired. The value of pain as a signal of disease and damage is great, and the seriousness of reduced pain perception and response to pain should not be underestimated. It is not uncommon for the elderly to frequently sustain cuts, burns, and bruises; these should be noted carefully and the circumstances of their occurrence clarified.

Adaptation to external temperature changes is diminished, and extremes of heat and cold are poorly perceived and tolerated. Body temperature adjusts more slowly in illness, and fever may appear later than normally expected. For this reason, fever in the elderly patient has added significance as a finding and should be evaluated medically for its underlying cause. Metabolism is slowed in the elderly, and temperature-regulating mechanisms function less efficiently.

The person with altered proprioception is less secure about his body positioning in space. This impairment of position-sensing ability is compensated for by slower, more cautious body movement. The slowing of movement allows the patient added time for sensory input, so that more information about the environment can be gathered and processed by the nervous system. The nurse examiner may be cued to this problem by the patient's notable tendency to use visual input as a substitute for the impaired position sense. This is demonstrated by the older person who looks down to watch the placement of his feet when walking. Specific testing methods to be used are detailed in Chapter 13.

Skin Changes   As with other biologic aspects of aging, changes in the skin vary greatly from one older person to another. However, alterations in the skin are among the most readily discernible changes in the aging process.

In the aging skin, subcutaneous fat and water are lost, and there is decreased turgor. As a result, the skin becomes lined and wrinkled. Skin folds hang loosely, giving the appearance of flabbiness. Diminished glandular function and dehydration result in skin dryness. Elasticity is reduced; the skin is more friable, subject to excoriation, and easily traumatized. The skin becomes less vascular, and healing time is prolonged. Alterations in skin pigmentation are noticeable in the blotchy, spotty patterning. Both skin and hair thin, the latter losing pigment and becoming gray. Some skin areas become thickened, and keratotic lesions may be observed on the face and body.

Elderly persons may be distressed by generalized itching, commonly caused by excessive dryness of the skin. However, if the itching is localized, there is greater likelihood of other causes. Dermatitis and fungal infections are among the more common skin problems in aging and should be considered in the assessment. Skin cancer is a major problem, and the lesions are generally found on skin areas exposed to the sun and weathering.

Assessment of the skin of the elderly must include careful examination of the feet. The examining nurse should make a special point of inquiring about any foot problems the elderly person is experiencing and should be attentive to any complaints. Ability "to get around" is crucial to independence in self-care activities. Ambulation may be compromised by the discomfort of foot conditions amenable to improvement, if not to actual prevention or correction. The older person may have special problems in caring for the skin and nails of the feet. These problems are to be identified and appropriate instruction and assistance provided. At times assistive equipment is indicated, and consultation with a physical or occupational therapist should be arranged. Excessive sweating and foot odor may pose an embarrassing and troublesome problem, necessitating special foot care and treatment. Cuts, blisters, and fissures are easily infected, and treatment should not be delayed. The presence of calluses and corns should be noted and an attempt made to determine and remedy their cause. Because these conditions may become painful and incapacitating, referral to a dermatologist or podiatrist may be indicated.

Motor Performance and Musculoskeletal Considerations

Loss of muscle mass and strength is a major change with aging. Energies are depleted more quickly, and tolerance for physical activity is lowered. The complaint of not being able to do as much as before is commonly heard from the elderly. Muscles move with less smooth coordination, and speed of muscle movement is decreased, resulting in poorer performance of motor activities. The change is generally noticed first in loss of motor skills for more complex tasks and for activities demanding precise, coordinated movement.

Osteoarthritic changes in the joints with associated pain on movement is particularly debilitating. Joint stiffening and impaired range of motion may be severely incapacitating and distressful. The nurse has to examine the patient's joint function with special care and gentleness to minimize discomfort and anxiety. Decreased range of motion should be quantitated whenever possible and measurements recorded for making comparisons and noting changes.

Intervertebral disc changes occur with the "wear" of years, and normal spinal curvatures are exaggerated. The stooping posture is apparent in many older people.

Hormonal changes with aging are important in assessing older women. Postmenopausal females, particularly Caucasians, are predisposed to osteoporosis. This loss of minerals from bone increases the elderly person's vulnerability to fractures, and a careful history of recent trauma, no matter how slight, should be elicited.

Cardiovascular and Respiratory Function

Heart disease is a health problem common to the elderly and is the major cause of death in people over 65. Changes in cardiovascular functioning in the older person are usually the result of a combination of factors, the aging process being only one [5].

The ability of the heart to function efficiently decreases with advancing years. Usually, there is some degree of fibrosis of the myocardium, with a decrease in its contractility. Cardiac output is less at rest, and the heart's ability to respond to increased work demands by increasing its output is decreased. The decrease in cardiac reserve in the elderly person has significant implications for their ability to adapt to sudden stresses, either physical, mental, or emotional [5]. The nurse's understanding of what these stresses might be for the patient she is examining should guide her in providing care and counsel. Elderly patients frequently need help in identifying what modifications in their life-style could be made to minimize or prevent stress. Available community services are often unused because the older person is unaware of them or does not know how to arrange for them. The nurse can be extremely helpful in facilitating the patient's use of these resources.

When examining the older patient for peripheral vascular function, several facts should be kept in mind. Vessel lumens may become narrowed and partially occluded by the deposit of fatty substances. Symptoms of circulatory insufficiency may be experienced by the older patient, but may not be considered sufficiently important to mention unless he is asked about them. Fibrotic changes also occur in the vessel walls, making them hard and pipelike. These can be seen and palpated easily. With the loss of elasticity in arteries, there is an increased peripheral resistance to blood flow and the systolic blood pressure usually becomes elevated.

Care must be exercised by the nurse in having the elderly patient change position during the assessment. Usually, older people do not compensate well for the effects of gravity on the circulatory system and may readily experience orthostatic hypotension, sustaining preventable injury.

Two of the most common cardiac symptoms found in the elderly are chest pain (angina) and dyspnea. The nature and circumstances surrounding either of these symptoms must be explored thoroughly with the patient. He should be asked specifically whether the dyspnea occurs at night, has an acute onset, is accompanied by chest pain, is precipitated by exertion, and if so, with what kind and how much exertion. If exertional dyspnea is the complaint, it is important to clarify whether this has been previously experienced with the activities described.

Cardiovascular changes affecting pulmonary circulation influence the respiratory status of the older patient. Much of the comprehensive descriptions of the respiratory and cardiovascular examinations given in Chapters 9 and 10 has relevance for the nurse assessing the elderly. It may be helpful to the nurse assessor to examine these two areas of patient function in sequence.

Ordinarily, respiratory function is adequate in the elderly unless disease is present. However, it should be recalled that the loss of elasticity in the body musculature of the elderly also pertains to the respiratory muscles and chest wall, and some impairment of respiratory excursion may be present. The patient's history of smoking and exposure to occupational and other dangerous pollutants should be documented by the nurse. The elderly are more susceptible to respiratory infections than are younger patients and often suffer more serious consequences from them [3]. Any indication of a recent need to curtail activities should be probed for respiratory function implications.

Throughout the assessment process the nurse working with older adults can find rich guidance in this principle [9]:

". . .there are distinctions to be made between the state of being old, the process of becoming old and changing potentials for the future old."

Mindful of these distinctions, the nurse in her assessment role can contribute in some knowledgeable and planned way to the quality of each for her patient. . . and for herself.

THE ELDERLY- ASSESSMENT GUIDE

I. Interview
  A. Determine client's preferred way of being addressed
  B. Avoid "hurrying" older people
  C. Start with client's immediate concerns
  D. Be alert to nonverbal communication behaviors
  E. Provide clear explanations before "handling" the client
  F. State questions simply in nontechnical language
  G. Allow enough time for client to recollect and answer
  H. Monitor client closely for energy depletion to prevent undue client fatigue.
II. Mental Performance
  A. Comprehension and response reliability
  B. Language ability, coherence
  C. Attention span
  D. Recent or remote memory
  E. Orientation

Note: Much assessment of mental status can be done while eliciting data about client's social history, educational/occupational background, activities and interest, etc.

III. Sensory Perception
  A. Hearing
    1. Acuity tests
    2. Impact on life activities and functional abilities
    3. Disorders
      a. Presbycusis: nerve/perceptive deficit
      b. Otosclerosis: conductive deficit
    4. Hearing aid: procurement and maintenance concerns
  B. Vision
    1. Acuity tests
    2. Impact on life activities and functional abilities
    3. Disorders
      a. Visual field defects
      b. Glaucoma
      c. Cataracts
      d. Retinal changes
    4. Legal Definition of blindness and benefits to blind
  C. Other Senses
    1. Taste and smell
      a. Blunting of sensitivity
      b. Effects on nutrition and eating habits

2. Touch and Pain
    a.   Decreased sensitivity and discrimination
    b.   Impaired alerting system to tissue injury and environmental danger
3. Temperature
    a.   Diminished adaptation to temperature changes—susceptible to extremes of cold and heat
    b.   Slowed metabolism and body temperature regulation so fever cue is slowed in illness
4. Proprioception
    a.   Position sense altered so movements are slow and cautious; i.e.: tends to watch foot placement when walking
    b.   Safety concerns

IV. Skin
   A. Loss of subcutaneous fat and H_2O; decreased turgor, skin lined, wrinkles
   B. Loss of elasticity, more friable, easily excoriated
   C. Decreased vascularity–delayed healing
   D. Decreased glandular function–skin dry and less protective
   E. Decreased hair pigment; graying, and thinning
   F. Pigmented skin–liver spots
   G. Skin lesions: kerotosis, purpura; other benign, premalignant, cancerous lesions
   H. Itching, dermatitis and fungal infections
   I. Finger and toenail changes
   J. Importance of foot care (podiatrist referral)

V. Motor Performance
   A. Loss of muscle mass, strength
   B. Diminished energy level and activity tolorance
   C. Coordination and balance less
   D. Diminished motor skills for complex, precision tasks
   E. Joint changes: osteoarthritis, decreased ROM
   F. Bone loss and changes in disc with loss of height, stooped posture, vulnerability to fracture

VI. Cardiovascular and Respiratory
   A. Cardiac output is less at rest; response to cardiac demand is less
   B. Cardiac reserve is less–less ability for adaptation to sudden stress
   C. Vessels may become fibrotic appearing pipelike and hard
   D. Systolic blood pressure elevation is common. Prone to orthostatic hypotension
   E. Angina and dyspnea are common symptoms. Detail circumstances of these symptoms thoroughly
   F. Decreased respiratory excursion
   G. Susceptibile to respiratory infections
   H. Smoking history

REFERENCES

1. Botwinick, J. *Aging and Behavior* (2nd ed.). New York: Springer, 1978. Chap. 12, P. 185.
2. Burnside, I. M. *Nursing and the Aged.* New York: McGraw-Hill, 1976. Pp. 49-50.
3. Busse, E. W., and Pfeiffer, E. (Eds.). *Behavior and Adaptation in Late Life* (2nd ed.). Boston: Little, Brown, 1977. P. 99.
4. Butler, R. N., and Lewis, M. I. *Aging and Mental Health* (2nd ed.). St. Louis: Mosby, 1977. P. 8.
5. Chinn, A. B. (Ed.). *Working with Older People: A Guide to Practice.* Vol. IV. Clinical Aspects of Aging. Washington, D.C.: Department of Health, Education, and Welfare, Public Health Service, Publication No. 1459, June, 1971.
6. Current Population Reports, Special Studies Series P-25, Nos. 311, 519, 614, and

601. *Demographic Aspects of Aging and the Older Population in the U.S.* U.S. Department of Commerce, Bureau of Census.

7. *Facts About Older Americans.* U.S. Department of Health and Human Services, Administration on Aging, Publication No. (80-20006), 1979. Pp. 2–12.
8. Fritz, D. B. *Growing Old is a Family Affair.* Richmond, Va.: John Knox Press, 1972.
9. Riley, M. W., Riley, J. W., and Johnson, M. E. (Eds.). *Aging in Society.* New York: Russell Sage Foundation, 1969.
10. Schrock, M. M. *Holistic Assessment of the Healthy Aged.* New York: Wiley, 1980. Pp. 6–7.
11. Tibbitts, C. *Middle-Aged and Older People in American Society.* In F. G. Scott and R. M. Brewer (Eds.), *Perspectives in Aging II: An Operational Focus.* A Continuing Education Book, Corvallis, Ore., 1971. Chap. 3, pp. 13–21.

SUGGESTED READINGS

Atchley, R. C. *The Social Forces in Later Life* (2nd ed.). Belmont, Calif.: Wadsworth, 1977.

Brown, M. *Readings in Gerontology* (2nd ed.). St. Louis: Mosby, 1978.

Burnside, I. M. (Ed.). *Nursing and the Aged* (2nd ed.). New York: McGraw-Hill, 1981.

Burnside, I. M., Ebersole, P., and Monea, H. E. (Eds.). *Psychosocial Caring Throughout the Life Span.* New York: McGraw-Hill, 1979.

Carotenuto, R., and Bullock, J. *Physical Assessment of the Gerontologic Patient.* Philadelphia: Davis, 1980.

Ebersole, P., and Hess, P. *Toward Healthy Aging.* St. Louis: Mosby, 1981.

Gerontological Nursing. *The Nursing Clinics of North America.* Philadelphia: Saunders, 1979. Vol. 14, No. 4.

Hess, B. B., and Markson, E. W. *Aging and Old Age.* New York: Macmillan, 1980.

Hogstel, M. (Ed.). *Nursing Care of the Older Adult.* New York: Wiley, 1981.

Kart, C. S., Metress, E. S., and Metress, J. G. *Aging and Health.* Reading, Mass.: Addison-Wesley, 1978.

Neugarten, B. L. *Middle Age and Aging.* Chicago: University of Chicago Press, 1973.

Weber, H. *Nursing Care of the Elderly.* Reston, Va.: Reston, 1980.

Index

Index